Affective and Non-Psychotic Disorders

Recent topics from
Advances in Psychiatric Treatment Volume 2

Edited by Alan Lee

Gaskell

British Library Cataloguing-in-Publication Data
A catalogue record for this book is available from the British Library.

ISBN 1 901242 17 X

Gaskell is an imprint of the Royal College of Psychiatrists, 17 Belgrave Square, London SW1X 8PG
•
The Royal College of Psychiatrists is a registered charity (no. 228636).

The views presented in this book do not necessarily reflect those of the Royal College of Psychiatrists, and the publishers are not responsible for any errors of omission or fact. This volume is produced by the Publications Department of the College; it should in no way be construed as providing a syllabus or other material for any College examination.

Printed by Henry Ling Limited, Dorchester, Dorset.

Contents

Contributors

Gwen Adshead Honorary Senior Lecturer and Consultant in Forensic Psychotherapy Broadmoor Hospital, Crowthorne, Berkshire RG45 7EG.

Ian Anderson Senior Lecturer in Psychiatry, Department of Psychiatry, University of Manchester, Rawnsley Building, Manchester Royal Infirmary, Oxford Road, Manchester M13 9WL.

A. J. Bell Consultant Psychiatrist, Whitecliff Centre, East Cleveland Hospital, Alford Road, Brotton, Cleveland TS12 2XT.

P. J. Cowen Honoray Consultant Psychiatrist and MRC Clinical Psychiatrist, Psychopharmacolology Research Unit, University of Oxford, Warneford Hospital Headington, Oxford OX3 7JX.

C. Duggan Professor of Psychiatry and Honorary Consultant, East Midlands Centre For Forensic Mental Health, Arnold Lodge, Cordelia Close, Leicester LE5 0LE.

Guy Edwards Honorary Senior Lecturer in Psychiatry and Member of the Mental Health Group, Faculty of Medicine, Health and Biological Sciences, University of Southampton, Royal South Hants Hospital, Brintons Terrace, Southampton SO14 0YG.

Christopher Fairburn Wellcome Principal Research Fellow, University of Oxford, Department of Psychiatry, Warneford Hospital, Headington, Oxford OX3 7JX.

I. Nicol Ferrier Head of Department of the Department of Psychiatry, School of Neurosciences and Psychiatry, University of Newcastle, The Royal Victoria Infirmary, Queen Victoria Road, Newcastle upon Tyne NE1 4LP and Honarary Consultant Psychiatrist, Newcastle City Mental Health NHS Trust.

John Henry Professor of Accident and Emergency Medicine at Imperial College, South Wharf Road, London W2 1NY.

Jeremy Holmes Consultant Psychiatrist/Psychotherapist, North Devon District Hospital, Raleigh Park, Barnstaple, Devon EX31 4JB.

Allan House Senior Lecturer in Liaison Psychiatry, University of Leeds and Consultant Liaison Psychiatrist, Leeds General Infirmary, Great George Street, Leeds LS1 3EX.

Rachel Jenkins Director, WHO Collaborating Centre and Honorary Senior Lecturer, Institute of Psychiatry, De Crespigny Park, Denmark Hill, London SE5 8AF.

Navneet Kapur Research Registrar, Department of Liaison Psychiatry, Leeds General Infirmary, Great George Street, Leeds LS1 3EX.

Cornelius Katona Deputy Head of Department, Department of Psychiatry and Behavioural Sciences, University College London Medical School, 2nd Floor Wolfson Building, 48 Riding House Street, London W1N 8AA and Dean of the Royal College of Psychiatrists, 17 Belgrave Square, London SW1X 8PG.

Alan Lee Consultant Psychiatrist and Special Senior Lecturer, University Hospital, Nottingham NG7 2UH.

Keith Llyod Senior Lecturer in Mental Health, University of Exeter, Department of Mental Health, Wonford House Hospital, Dryden Road, Exeter, Devon EX2 5AF.

Toni Lock Consultant in General Adult Psychiatry, Crosshouse Hospital, Kilmarnock, KA2 0BE

Stirling Moorey Consultant, Psychotherapy Department, City & Hackney Community Services, 50–52 Clifden Road, Hackney, London E5 0LJ.

Gethin Morgan Emeritus Professor of Mental Health, Division of Psychiatry, University of Bristol, 41 St Michael's Hill, Bristol BS2 8DZ.

Kingsley Norton Consultant Psychotherapist, Henderson Hospital, 2 Homeland Drive, Brighton Road, Sutton, Surrey SM2 5LT.

David Owens Senior Lecturer in Psychiatry, Division of Psychiatry and Behavioural Sciences in Relation to Medicine, School of Medicine, University of Leeds, 15 Hyde Terrace, Leeds LS2 9LT.

Bob L. Palmer Senior Lecturer at the Department of Psychiatry, University of Leicetser, Brandon Mental Health Unit, Leicester General Hospital, Gwendolen Road, Leicester LE5 4PW.

Richard Porter Lecturer, John Elliott Unit, Birch Hill Hospital, Rochdale OL12 9QB

Duncan Raistrick Clinical Director, Addiction Unit, 19 Springfield Mount, Leeds LS2 9NG.

Jan Scott Head of Department at the Department of Psychiatry, Academic Centre, Gartnavel Royal Hospital, 1055 Great Western Road, Glasgow G20 6DW.

Graeme Smith Professor of Psychological Medicine, Monash University, Department of Psychological Medicine, 246 Clayton Road, Clayton Melbourne, VIC 3168, Australia.

S. P. Tyrer Consultant Psychiatrist, Department of Psychiatry, Royal Victoria Infirmary, Queen Victoria Road, Newcastle upon Tyne NE1 4LP.

Preface

Alan Lee

This is the second volume of a series which brings together selected topics from the popular journal *Advances in Psychiatric Treatment*. Readers will again find expert advice from leading clinicians on key elements of general adult psychiatric practice. The advice is backed by up to date and balanced reviews of the relevant literature, presented in a clear, concise and well organised format.

The first volume, with a focus on the challenges of engaging and treating those with severe psychotic disorders and schizophrenia, provides a cogent reply to those who have feared that general adult psychiatry occupies a no-mans land, and is heading for imminent demise. This companion volume should act as a counterbalance, addressing the equal concern that general psychiatry might be seen as no more than a psychosis or schizophrenia service, overly concerned with the administrative problems of risk management.

It is sometimes assumed that the term 'non-psychotic', like its unfashionable predecessor neurotic, must imply a lesser degree of morbidity. This can lead to sufferers being marginalised as 'merely' the 'worried well'. However, there is now good evidence that those most severely affected with depressive and non-psychotic disorders have levels of disability and enduring suffering comparable to those with schizophrenia. In addition, the less severe variants of these disorders are so widespread that their cumulative morbidity has a massive impact on the public health.

This book will address some of the most problematic areas in treating individuals with affective and non-psychotic disorders. The crucial elements of a contemporary approach are emphasised throughout; primary and secondary prevention, balanced integration of diverse models, and a combination of biomedical and psychosocial treatments. There is also a focus on carefully managing the interface between psychiatrists and those in primary care, general medicine and other professions. Taken together, the ensuing chapters leave little doubt that general psychiatry can now offer a great deal of sensitive, effective and evidence-based treatment across a very broad range of disorders.

Thanks are due to all the expert contributors, many of whom have generously updated their original articles so as to enhance the value and relevance of this volume. Thanks also to Professor Andrew Sims the founding Editor of *Advances in Psychiatric Treatment*. The members of the Editorial Board of the Journal have been responsible for maintaining the high standard of articles throughout. Professor Gethin Morgan, previously Chief Examiner for the Royal College of Psychiatrists, and now retiring as Director of Continuing Professional Development, has kindly written very helpful introductions to both this volume and its predecessor.

Finally, it is important to acknowledge the excellent Publications Team at the Royal College of Psychiatrists. Whilst their praises are often unsung, they continue to provide quality support and expertise of the highest order. Thanks are especially due to Zoë Stagg, Andrew Morris, Louise Whalley and Gillian Blease who has now taken over as Editorial Assistant for *Advances in Psychiatric Treatment*.

Alan Lee
August 1999

Foreword

Gethin Morgan

This second volume of selected papers from *Advances in Psychiatric Treatment* is concerned first with many practical aspects of affective disorders, and later proceeds to consider a number of important clinical topics that feature prominently in the day to day practice of general psychiatry. As in the first volume, the emphasis throughout is on systematic consideration of the delivery of clinical care, against a background of succinct and up to date reviews of the relevant literature.

No comprehensive discussion of affective disorders would be complete without consideration of self-harm and it is appropriate to find here a paper on this topic. Based on the 1994 College *Consensus Statement on Standards of Service Provision* it is indeed salutary to match our own clinical practice with recommended standards of care as set out in this document. The inter-play of psychological and social factors relevant to primary and secondary prevention of depression is then considered in a brief overview, following which the problems involved in trying to provide effective care and prevention of affective disorders in general practice are set out vividly: practical guidelines are provided on how we might best focus our scarce expertise in liaising with primary care. Consideration is also given to depression in the elderly, including important practical topics such as the negative effects of ageism on the proportion of patients with depression who remain untreated, the need to be assertive in clinical approach given the proven positive value of psychotherapy and antidepressive drugs, and problems related to obtaining valid consent for electroconvulsive therapy (ECT) in elderly patients. It is particularly helpful to see a concise and clear consideration of treatments useful in emergency treatments of depression.

The many issues concerning efficacy and potential toxicity of antidepressant drugs are set out clearly. The relative values of new and old antidepressants, as based on research findings from both individual studies as well as meta-analysis of the literature are discussed from the perspective of the clinician who has to take in so many considerations such as efficacy, adherence, toxicity and cost. It is useful to find a chapter on treatment-resistant depression, especially one which sets out a plan of action based on a wide range of pharmacological agents, enabling us to consider all options thoroughly and systematically. The comprehensive evaluation of antidepressant medication is rounded off by a chapter on relapse prevention, including issues such as long-term medication, drug interactions and other adverse effects as well as cognitive–behavioural benefits. Those who have seen the way in which ECT has developed over the years will understand how grateful we should all be for the initiative of the College, from the early audits to the more recent work of its Special Committee on ECT: the lucid review of research and audit findings to be found in this volume deserve careful reading. The chapter on lithium therapy is also a very important contribution, one which helps us to keep up to date in prescribing this drug: clinicians need to be more aware that the potential medico-legal hazards resulting from its toxic effect. A consideration of brief dynamic psychotherapy encourages us to acknowledge the potential of a psychotherapeutic approach under even the busiest conditions of clinical practice. The principles of cognitive–behavioural therapy are also set out, with emphasis on how to select patients who may benefit from this approach as well as the value of self-help manuals.

The management of obsessive–compulsive disorders is the first of several other important topics considered in this volume. Behaviour therapy, so often seen as too specialised and time-consuming to be included in a generalist's day to day clinical practice, is demystified and rendered feasible for us all to consider using. Likewise we are encouraged to approach anew and think again about the problem of somatisation, which has long been seen as an unrewarding interface between physicians and psychiatrists. We are also enabled to tackle the problem of personality disorder with vigour. So often this label can mean disqualification from active therapy: we are helped here to realise that provided we observe basic clinical guidelines and remain aware of the pitfalls which may occur, particularly by not attempting the impossible, then even when difficulties loom large much therapeutic gain can still be achieved in patients who have acquired this diagnostic label. The closely related theme of alcohol misuse is discussed in the context of substance dependence which is presented as a purely psychological concept, distinct from tolerance and withdrawal phenomena. All psychiatrists are encouraged to adopt a positive therapeutic stance to alcohol misuse which will surely convey to the patient that help is available and can be effective. A chapter on the management of anorexia nervosa avoids a rigid theoretical approach which makes many texts seem hidebound. It discusses with sensitivity the many issues which can arise in face to face contact with the sufferer. The result is both refreshing and encouraging. Generalists will surely feel more certain about what needs to be done, the limit and the extent of their skills and the indications to seek more specialist advice in this perplexing condition which can raise anxieties even in the most expert. The general psychiatrist is only too aware of the frequency with which bulimia nervosa and other binge eating problems present in

day to day practice, and there may not be easy access to a specialist service. The latest research findings are described here briefly and clearly, and we are given valuable practical advice on how we might begin a stepped care approach in the first instance, again with welcome referral to the role of self help manuals. The many dilemmas which we face in assessing and managing post-traumatic states are also discussed briefly yet critically in a way which is very helpful to the generalist.

This second volume, like the first, should have an immediate appeal to those who have the responsibility of providing effective clinical care for patients with psychiatric disorders. Good clinical practice must certainly be based on up to date evidence derived from systematic scientific study. we need to ensure that this includes thorough evaluation of day to day clinical practice and the actual delivery of care if it is to be fully effective. The great strength of this volume, like its partner, is that in a relatively few pages it describes systematically the day to day, face to face aspects of clinical psychiatric practice in the light of up to date theory and evidence. Such an approach is surely the underlying reason why *Advances in Psychiatric Treatment* has itself so quickly become highly valued as a clinical journal. The selected papers presented here are testament to that well-deserved success.

Assessment of deliberate self-harm in adults

David Owens, Allan House & Navneet Kapur

Deliberate self-harm remains a common problem in the UK, with rates in the order of 250–300 per 100 000 per year (Hawton & Fagg, 1992). Since the suicide rate in the 12 months after hospital attendance for deliberate self-harm is around 1% (Hawton & Fagg, 1988), each year approximately 2–3 per 100 000 of the population die by suicide within a year of attending hospital with a non-fatal episode of deliberate self-harm. This is about a quarter of the overall suicide rate of 11 per 100 000. There is, therefore, an easily definable group at risk of suicide who should be the focus of a suicide prevention strategy.

Conscious of a need to improve services for self-harm patients, the Royal College of Psychiatrists has examined standards of care. The then Audit Working Group of the College and its Liaison Psychiatry Special Interest Group arranged a consensus conference of mental health and public health professionals to consider and set standards for the hospital management of adult deliberate self-harm patients. Many of the steps towards better care and the standards suggested below are drawn from the agreed statement which resulted from that meeting (Royal College of Psychiatrists, 1994). All those who are involved with services for deliberate self-harm should examine the recommendations of the College closely.

Organisation of services

Despite the scale of the problem, services for deliberate self-harm have not been coherently planned or well delivered. Blake & Mitchell (1978) audited the management of self-poisoning by 10 psychiatric teams in Nottingham hospitals and found wide variations in the decisions made by each team. For example, further follow-up was arranged for almost all patients by one team but for less than half by another. Twenty years later, figures from our own study suggest that service provision around the country remains in disarray (Kapur et al, 1998). We examined the hospital management of deliberate self-poisoning in four large hospitals in the Midlands and the north of England and found a four-fold difference in the proportion of patients discharged directly from the accident and emergency department (18–76%), and a two-fold difference in the proportion of patients leaving hospital without a psychosocial assessment (32–64%). This striking variability in management was not accounted for by differences in patient characteristics.

Variations in the actions of clinicians are paralleled by inconsistencies in the organisation of services. A survey around the Yorkshire region revealed that less than half of the districts had written guidelines on management of deliberate self-harm, or had a named consultant psychiatrist with responsibility for the service. Hawton & James (1995) found that only one of the nine hospitals in the Oxford region had a local group for planning and overseeing the service for self-harm patients.

A national survey of practice in the late 1980s suggested that there had been little movement towards the use of specific self-harm teams and only a quarter of health districts reported the use of multi-disciplinary assessment as suggested in the 1984 Department of Health and Social Security guidelines (Butterworth & O'Grady, 1989)

This is unfortunate because there is evidence that staff other than psychiatrists can make satisfactory psychosocial assessments of self-harm patients. These staff are most commonly social workers (Newson-Smith & Hirsch, 1979) and psychiatric nurses (Catalan et al, 1980). Non-psychiatric medical staff have been shown to be competent in assessing in-patients (Gardner et al, 1977) and attenders in accident and emergency departments (Gardner et al, 1982; Waterhouse & Platt, 1990; Owens et al, 1991).

Whatever the style of assessment and after-care, self-harm services need to be planned, and responsibilities defined. Because of the scale and importance of deliberate self-harm, those who commission and purchase hospital services are increasingly likely to want specifications for minimum quality. Each hospital or trust should take a number of steps.

Self-harm services planning group

A deliberate self-harm services planning group should be set up. A consultant and a nurse from the accident and emergency department, general medicine and psychiatry are the obvious clinical members of the planning group, together with a social worker. Also essential are a senior manager and a representative of purchasers. The involvement of several distinct parts of the hospital or trust points to inclusion of an information officer to help with service monitoring.

A designated clinical team

Two aspects of the work have led some hospitals to set up a designated, multi-disciplinary deliberate self-harm clinical team – staffed by a variety of psychiatrists, nurses, social workers and others. First, such teams can coordinate and deliver prompt services for the hundreds of patients to be assessed across the different settings in the hospital. Second, interventions following self-harm differ from those used in general psychiatric practice. Although identifying and instituting treatment for severe mental illness is among the most important tasks in the assessment of deliberate self-harm patients, in a majority of patients the precipitating events are psychosocial problems which are not amenable to routine treatments for mental illness. Self-harm clinical teams must offer psychosocial interventions, often based around helping patients to learn new ways to solve problems, through a mixture of cognitive–behavioural and counselling techniques.

Specialist multi-disciplinary teams can improve the quality of care for deliberate self-harm patients and each planning group should consider setting one up. A specialist team may not be feasible in small districts, particularly in rural areas. In those circumstances sectorised multi-disciplinary mental health teams may more appropriately offer the assessment and after-care. In larger hospitals it is difficult for multiple sector mental health teams to offer the full range of interventions swiftly and to communicate adequately with the relevant departments. In either case – special teams or regular mental health services – the planning group must

ensure the support of psychiatric colleagues so that the general adult psychiatric service provides necessary backup in accident and emergency and on in-patient wards (for example, out-of-hours and holiday cover) for the assessment of self-harm patients.

Policy on direct discharge

Reports from around the country indicate that between a quarter and three-quarters of all self-harm patients are discharged directly from the accident and emergency department (Owens, 1990; Kapur *et al*, 1998). A high proportion of these patients are not assessed by specialist mental health staff before their discharge. Often this practice is not openly acknowledged; discharge without specialist referral will occur from some accident and emergency departments, but there should always be a written policy, and cases should be documented so that rates of discharge and referral can be monitored and audited.

Recovery time

Some patients will need time to recover their equanimity before a decision can be made about what to do next. Sometimes a relative or other informant is awaited, or there may be social needs which must be organised. It is therefore important that there are facilities to allow some patients time either in the casualty department or a medical ward for a degree of recovery. Short-stay wards may be a useful setting for brief admissions; patients should not spend many hours in an accident and emergency department.

Training and supervision

Opinions vary on how best to carry out psychosocial assessment of patients who attend hospital as a result of deliberate self-harm (usually self-poisoning, less often self-injury). Although there has been a good deal of argument about who should carry out such assessments, these issues were largely resolved before the latest set of official guidelines were issued 10 years ago (Department of Health and Social Security, 1984). In particular, evidence was accepted that in some circumstances adequate assessment could be carried out by non-psychiatrists (Black & Pond, 1980). As the current guidance stands, "the consultant who has charge of the patient whether in the accident and emergency department or in a ward will be responsible for ensuring that a full physical assessment is made and that before patients are discharged from hospital, a psychosocial assessment is carried out by staff *specifically trained for this task"* (Department of Health and Social Security, 1984).

In reality, patients are often not assessed by staff with adequate training and supervision in psychosocial assessment before their discharge. Even when patients are referred for specialist psychiatric assessment, whether in an accident and emergency department or on an in-patient ward, they are frequently seen by junior psychiatrists with indifferent supervision.

Non-specialist staff

Where accident and emergency staff and other non-psychiatric medical staff undertake psychosocial assessment of self-harm patients they should undergo post-qualification training. The planning group in each hospital should arrange for newly appointed accident and emergency and general medical staff to receive training before they are expected to carry out this task, probably within days of taking up a post.

As well as training, accident and emergency medical staff who carry out assessments need supervision by senior staff who have themselves had designated training in psychiatry. It is now commonplace for those appointed as consultants in accident and emergency to have spent a period of post-qualification training in psychiatry, but where they have not, appropriate supervision needs to be identified. If physicians opt to undertake psychosocial assessment of in-patients without calling in the specialist self-harm team or a psychiatrist, that assessment then becomes a major part of the patient's management and must be dealt with by the medical team as a whole (involving nurses, senior doctors and other staff), and not by an unsupervised house officer.

Specialist staff

In many cases, however, a specialist mental health worker will be called to the accident and emergency department or an in-patient ward in order to assess deliberate self-harm patients. This person should be suitably trained and supervised, but need not be a psychiatrist. There are numerous services in which nurses and social workers act as specialist assessors. Whatever the professional background of the specialist assessor, there are minimum standards for their training. Someone new to the task should undertake observed assessments, that is, under

direct supervision, until they are judged as being competent. New specialist staff should be provided with or directed to relevant literature.

During the first six months of carrying out specialist assessments, every case should be supervised, and the management should be discussed in detail with a designated supervisor. Out of hours, when cases can be particularly complex, self-harm assessments by new staff should routinely be discussed with the on-duty consultant or specialist registrar. Rotational senior house officers who have previously undertaken work of this kind do not need to discuss every case in detail but they should routinely discuss, over the telephone or face-to-face, the management with a designated supervisor.

The planning group should set a policy for supervision of non-medical staff once they are adequately trained for self-harm assessments. These arrangements will vary according to the experience of the specialist nurse or social worker, and the views of senior psychiatrists – both in the planning group and within adult psychiatry in the district.

Tricky areas of clinical responsibility arise when specialist staff are asked to make an assessment. First, is the specialist providing advice to the accident and emergency or medical team, or acting autonomously and making management decisions? Second, is a training-grade doctor or a non-medical specialist acting independently or on behalf of a consultant psychiatrist? Local views on these issues will vary. Written guidance is essential – preferably agreed across the service; another job for the deliberate self-harm services planning group.

Assessment of patients

The purpose of psychosocial assessment is to identify among self-harm patients those who have a psychiatric illness, are a high suicide risk or have coexisting problems (for example alcohol or drug problems), and those in social crisis. Those with mental illness or a substance use problem may need prompt and effective psychiatric treatment, and, where other psychosocial problems are identified, patients should have access to various forms of social and psychological help.

The first task in an accident and emergency department and on a medical or short-stay ward will usually be to provide prompt assessment and effective treatment of the patient's physical condition in order to minimise risk of death and disability. However, not far behind in importance and urgency are detection of suicide risk and of severe mental illness. Patients in accident and emergency departments include some who may leave the hospital precipitately due to an abnormal mental state. Therefore, when the presenting complaint is deliberate self-harm, prior to any consultation a member of the accident and emergency staff (probably a nurse) should answer three questions immediately after the patient's arrival:

(a) Is the person physically fit to wait?
(b) Is there obvious distress?
(c) Is the person likely to wait until seen by the accident and emergency doctor?

This process should lead to rapid medical assessment for some patients and for some a request for psychosocial assessment while in the accident and emergency department. Nurses on general medical and short-stay wards should be trained in the nursing of suicidal patients and be able to produce a nursing care-plan which assesses immediate risk and recognises that risk fluctuates.

When a psychosocial assessment is undertaken in an accident and emergency department or on a ward, the physical environment needs to be adequate. Each patient should be interviewed in a setting which accords with privacy, confidentiality and respect. There should be a designated room to which patients can be directed for the necessary interview. In an accident and emergency department the room should be close to, or part of, the main receiving area and should have a suitable security system. Psychosocial assessment should be carried out in such a room unless it is inappropriate (for example, when a patient is threatening and/or abusive and it is necessary for other staff to be present or immediately available).

Information to be documented

Whether psychosocial assessment is carried out by accident and emergency medical staff, psychiatrists or specialist non-medical staff, it should be systematic. The information highlighted in Box 1 should always be collected and documented in either accident and emergency or standard hospital case notes. A pre-printed check-list prepared by the planning group may assist with this task.

The most important information is level of consciousness. If the drugs or alcohol taken have impaired the patient's consciousness then much of the assessment may be rendered unreliable or be impossible to carry out. Where an intoxicated deliberate self-poisoning patient wants to leave the accident and emergency department or a ward without assessment, staff nevertheless have an obligation to carry out as much assessment as is possible – and to take appropriate action, especially

if the patient continues to express suicidal intent.

It is particularly important for accident and emergency and medical staff to recognise that deliberate self-harm patients with impaired consciousness must be able to stay in hospital until they are fully assessed, even if assessment needs to be delayed for physical, psychiatric or social reasons. If monitoring reveals that discharge of in-patients who have not undergone specialist assessment is commonplace, regular meetings between general medical staff and the specialist self-harm team should be held.

Risk assessment

Assessing the degree of risk for an individual patient remains an important part of the overall psychosocial assessment. Risk is not easily quantified but attention needs to be paid to three key areas: (a) suicidal intent at the time of the self-harm; (b) present psychiatric state; and (c) social support.

Suicidal intent has been studied closely by Beck *et al* (1974) and their intent scale is widely used in clinical practice; it is reproduced in the excellent book on self-harm by Hawton & Catalan (1987). Assessing the present psychiatric state requires a full history and mental state examination. Particular attention needs to be paid to depressive features, especially hopelessness. Adverse social circumstances add to despair and it is essential to enquire into the extent of the patient's social support. Useful guides to interviewing self-harm patients, with specific questions about intent, present state and social support, are included in one of the Health of the Nation publications – a review on the theme of suicide prevention, carried out by the Health Advisory Service (Williams & Morgan, 1994). Table 1 sets out some examples of important questions about intent, psychiatric state and social support.

Risk factor check-lists predicting repetition of self-

Box 1. Information to be collected and documented during assessment

Consciousness level
Psychiatric history and mental state examination
Social situation and events
Risk
Alcohol and drug use
Decisions taken
Specific arrangements for any follow-up

Table 1. Estimating risk of further suicidal behaviour: examples of enquiry[1]	
Risk factors	Past psychiatric contact or admission, previous self-harm, advancing age, living alone
Suicidal intent of self-harm episode	Premeditation, risk of discovery, calls for assistance, patient's stated intent, actual lethality of method and patient's perception
Present psychiatric state	Recent history of depressive features, guilt, hopelessness, desperation, suicidal thoughts or plans
Social support	Housing, employment, support from family or partner, isolation or solitude, professional helper (e.g. social worker)

1. These are only examples – see text for references to more complete lists.

harm or subsequent suicide (Buglass & Horton, 1974; Kreitman & Foster, 1991) may sometimes be a useful adjunct to assessment. However, although factors such as psychiatric history, past episodes of self-harm, or advancing age may indicate increased risk among groups of patients, the predictive value of risk factors is poor and consequently they are of limited clinical value (Owens *et al*, 1994).

High-risk approach to assessment

Our current approach to deliberate self-harm assessment is a good example of a 'high risk' strategy. We aim to identify demographic and clinical variables thought to be predictive of future suicidal behaviour (Owens *et al*, 1994) and target our interventions at this so called 'high risk' group. Since only 20% of individuals are identified as being at high risk by the best available screening instruments (Kreitman & Foster, 1991), a large proportion of hospital attendees are now neither admitted to hospital nor offered psychosocial follow-up (Kapur *et al*, 1998). Restricting intervention in this way has advantages. It reduces the immediate burden on psychiatric services and might represent an efficient use of resources; it also avoids unnecessary treatment, and is well suited to current models of service provision in psychiatry.

However, there are serious problems with an exclusively high risk strategy for deliberate self-harm patients. Targeting high-risk groups, such as those with enduring affective disorder or those with other specific risk factors, results in large numbers of people at supposedly low risk being defined out of care, reducing the impact of psychosocial intervention. For example, those identified as being at high risk using the Kreitman & Foster (1991) risk assessment scale account for only 26% of cases of future suicidal behaviour, the much larger 'low risk' group accounting for the remainder. With intervention restricted to the high-risk group, even assuming that it is totally

effective (which is improbable), we will reduce the overall rate of suicidal behaviour by at most one quarter. The high risk strategy is also dangerous because it assumes an artificial distinction between high- and low-risk groups, and fails to take into account degrees of risk.

An alternative would be to adopt a more inclusive approach to assessment. In preventive medicine, population based strategies target whole populations rather than just vulnerable (high risk) individuals (Rose, 1992). This is potentially powerful because of the numbers of subjects involved; even very small population shifts can have large effects. Such a strategy for deliberate self-harm would mean offering effective psychosocial interventions to everyone following an episode of deliberate self-harm and not just those perceived to be at high risk.

Other considerations in assessment

Certain groups of patients can be particularly difficult to assess. For patients aged over 65 years, and those with a learning disability, referral to the specialist service as a matter of routine is recommended. Some would advocate routine referral to specialists of all deliberate self-harm patients aged under 18 years.

In many hospitals a large proportion of self-harm patients are discharged directly from the accident and emergency department. The evidence is that those who return home are, in general, a group whose risk of further suicidal behaviour is lower than those who are admitted to medical or short-stay wards; they are younger and have less history of self-harm or of psychiatric care (Owens *et al*, 1991). Where the patients discharged from an accident and emergency department are being selected appropriately, there must be a corresponding concentration of morbidity and risk within the remainder who are admitted to medical or short-stay beds. This in turn will make the task of assessing these patients more difficult.

Accident and emergency staff must have immediate access to telephone advice, either from a psychiatrist whose designated duties include attendance in the accident and emergency department, or from another designated self-harm health specialist (a nurse or social worker) who is equipped to undertake psychosocial assessment and management. A request for emergency attendance should result in the prompt arrival of a member of the self-harm specialist team or a duty psychiatrist. There should also be available social services assistance for those self-harm patients who have significant social difficulties (for example, homelessness).

If all in-patients are referred for specialist assessment, there will be no need for the general medical staff to do more than make the initial assessment of immediate risk and disturbance of mental state. The system for referring patients should be efficient and clearly understood by physicians, nurses and others on medical wards, psychiatric clerical staff, and those who undertake the assessment.

Patients should be seen for assessment on the same working day provided that the referral is made from the ward during the first part of the morning. At weekends and public holidays in small hospitals it may not be possible to arrange for a daily round of routine assessment. However, when a psychiatric emergency arises with a deliberate self-harm patient – as it does from time to time – it should be agreed policy that a member of the self-harm specialist team or a duty psychiatrist will attend any hospital ward within one hour of an urgent request for consultation from the medical team in charge of the patient's care.

Where there is no designated self-harm team, the rota for routine assessments of self-harm patients should name the consultant team responsible for the assessment rather than the names of trainee psychiatrists. This step helps to emphasise that assessment of those patients should be a scheduled team activity with adequate time and supervision set aside.

Intervention

It is unfortunate that neither official guidelines nor research findings have led to uniformly high standards of service, because the research evidence strongly suggests that psychiatric intervention can improve psychiatric and social function after deliberate self-harm; whether it can reduce repetition rates or suicide rates is not yet clear. Five randomised controlled trials of psychosocial after-care have been undertaken in the UK. Although they used widely differing interventions, each showed significant improvements among those receiving the psychosocial intervention, compared with the patients receiving routine care. The studies, their interventions, and findings are summarised in Table 2.

In the two earliest studies (Chowdhury *et al*, 1973; Gibbons *et al*, 1978) repetition rates were similar in those receiving new and established interventions. Three more recent studies found markedly less repetition among those receiving the new intervention. All five studies were, however, far too small to ensure a definite answer on lowering repetition (House *et al*, 1992); and intervention to reduce suicide following non-fatal self-harm cannot be demonstrated without a study of many thousands of patients. In the likelihood of a continued lack of such a study, demonstrable improvements in outcomes such as repetition might be taken as a reasonable proxy measure of reduction in suicides. The world literature of clinical trials involving every kind of intervention aimed at reducing repetition of deliberate self-harm was recently systematically reviewed by a Cochrane Review Group (Hawton *et al*, 1998*a,b*). The methodological quality of the trials reviewed was poor: highly selected patient groups were used, sample size was low, few incorporated standardised measures of outcome, and analysis was not by 'intention-to-treat'. The main message of the Cochrane review and the recent Effective Health Care Bulletin (1998), which systematically reviewed non-trial literature, was the need for considerably more clinical research about management of patients who commit deliberate self-harm. Three interventions emerge from the systematic review process showing some promise: problem-solving therapy, dialectic behaviour therapy, and providing patients with written guidance on how to gain access to psychiatric help at times of crisis. In the case of problem-solving and dialectic behaviour therapies small studies have suggested benefit, but confirmation from better designed and larger studies is required before implementation in clinical practice. Written guidance (in the form of a brief card given out to patients) has been found in successive studies from Bristol to be potentially beneficial and potentially harmful (Morgan *et al*, 1993; Evans *et al*, 1999); plainly, routine implementation would be inadvisable at present. Other research priorities might include the effect of discharge from accident and emergency, and attention to the widely disregarded clinical problems of self-injury.

In the meantime, what should be done? In a practical way Hawton & Catalan's (1987) book indicates how the specialist deliberate self-harm

Table 2. Five randomised treatment trials in deliberate self-harm: details of methods and outcome

Study	n	Nature of intervention	Repetition rate (%) Treatment	Control	Other outcomes (benefits seen in treatment group)
Chowdhury *et al* (1973)	197	General psychiatry	24	23	More improvement in social circumstances
Gibbons *et al* (1978)	400	Task-centred social work	14	15	Less psychiatric contact More satisfaction with services More improvement in social problems
Hawton *et al* (1981)	96	Brief problem-oriented counselling (domiciliary *v.* out-patient care)	10	15	More improvement in social adjustment
Hawton *et al* (1987)	80	Brief problem-oriented counselling (out-patient *v.* general practitioner care)	7	15	More improvement in target problems (in women) More improvement in symptoms (GHQ) and mood (BDI) scores More improvement in social adjustment
Salkovskis *et al* (1990)	20	Problem-solving therapy	0	38	More improvement in mood (BDI) scores Greater reduction in hopelessness

GHQ, General Health Questionaire (Goldberg, 1972); BDI, Beck Depression Inventory (Beck *et al*, 1961).

counsellors in Oxford approach the real problems encountered by their patients. The authors describe how to formulate problems and tackle them with brief psychotherapeutic and social interventions. Further description of problem-solving after self-harm is provided by Salkovskis *et al* (1990) in a report of a small but successful intervention study using cognitive–behavioural techniques.

After-care

One of the established findings about after-care for self-harm patients is the tendency of many to default from follow-up appointments. In a recent study in our hospital of almost 200 self-harm patients who repeated within one year of an index episode, their median time to repetition was 12 weeks; a quarter had repeated by only three weeks from the index episode (Gilbody *et al*, 1997). This means that where any kind of follow-up appointment is arranged, it must be very prompt to be effective, probably within seven working days of discharge from hospital.

On leaving hospital, the patient should be given written information about how to seek further help, together with written details of the treatment plan and who to contact if in doubt about the arrangements. Whoever makes the decision to discharge the patient should ensure that the patient's general practitioner (GP) is contacted promptly, often telephoning during the next 24

hours. A discharge letter (including all the information mentioned previously in Box 1) should be sent out within a few days. To assist both GP and patient, the letter should record whether the GP agreed to see the patient, and what action the patient was told to take in order to see the GP.

It should be standard practice for a relative or other informant to be contacted, in order to obtain details about the circumstances of the self-harm event, and to discuss any after-care or discharge. Where medical or accident and emergency staff undertake psychosocial assessments, they need to be able to produce a practical management plan which shows awareness of local facilities (such as psychiatric clinics, social work services, and voluntary services).

References

Beck, A. T., Ward, C. H. & Mendelson, M., *et al* (1961) An inventory for measuring depression. *Archives of General Psychiatry*, **4**, 561–571.
—, Schuyler, D. & Herman, J. (1974) Development of suicidal intent scales. In *The Prediction of Suicide* (eds A. T. Beck, H. L. P. Resnick & D. J. Lettierite). Bowie, MD: Charles Press.
Black, D. & Pond, D. (1980) Management of patients after self-poisoning. *British Medical Journal*, **281**, 1141.
Blake, D. R. & Mitchell, J. R. A. (1978) Self-poisoning: management of patients in Nottingham, 1976. *British Medical Journal*, **i**, 1032–1035.
Buglass, D. & Horton, J. (1974) A scale for predicting

subsequent suicidal behaviour. *British Journal of Psychiatry*, **124**, 573–578.

Butterworth, E. & O'Grady, T. J. (1989) Trends in the assessment of cases of deliberate self-harm. *Health Trends*, **21**, 61.

Catalan, J., Marsack, P., Hawton, K., *et al* (1980) Comparison of doctors and nurses in assessment of deliberate self-poisoning patients. *Psychological Medicine,* **10**, 483–491.

Chowdhury, N., Hicks, R. C. & Kreitman, N. (1973) Evaluation of an after-care service for parasuicide (attempted suicide) patients. *Social Psychiatry*, **8**, 67–81.

Department of Health and Social Security (1984) *The Management of Deliberate Self-Harm* (HN(84)25). London: Department of Health and Social Security.

Effective Health Care Bulletin (1998) *Deliberate Self-Harm*. Volume 4, number 6. York: NHS Centre for Reviews and Dissemination, University of York.

Evans, M. O., Morgan, H. G., Hayward, A., *et al* (1999) Crisis telephone consultation for deliberate self-harm patients: effects on repetition. *British Journal of Psychiatry,* **175**, 23–27.

Gardner, R., Hanka, R., O'Brien, V. C., *et al* (1977) Psychological and social evaluation in cases of deliberate self-poisoning admitted to a general hospital. *British Medical Journal*, ii, 1567–1570.

—, —, Roberts, S. J., *et al* (1982) Psychological and social evaluation in cases of deliberate self-poisoning seen in an accident department. *British Medical Journal*, **284**, 491–493.

Gibbons, J. S., Butler, P., Urwin, P., *et al* (1978) Evaluation of a social work service for self-poisoning patients. *British Journal of Psychiatry*, **133**, 111–118.

Gilbody, S., House, A. & Owens, D. (1997) The early repetition of deliberate self-harm. *Journal of the Royal College of Physicians*, **31**, 171–172.

Goldberg, D. P. (1972) *The Detection of Psychiatric Illness by Questionnaire (GHQ)*. Maudsley Monograph 21. Oxford: Oxford University Press.

Hawton, K., Bancroft, J., Catalan, J., *et al* (1981) Domiciliary and out-patient treatment of self-poisoning patients by medical and non-medical staff. *Psychological Medicine,* **11**, 169–177.

—— & Catalan, J. (1987) *Attempted Suicide: a Practical Guide to its Nature and Management* (2nd edn). Oxford: Oxford University Press.

——, McKeown, S., Day, A., *et al* (1987) Evaluation of out-patient counselling compared with general practitioner care following overdoses. *Psychological Medicine*, **17**, 751–761.

—— & Fagg, J. (1988) Suicide, and other causes of death, following attempted suicide. *British Journal of Psychiatry*, **152**, 359–366.

—— & —— (1992) Trends in deliberate self poisoning and self

injury in Oxford, 1976–90. *British Medical Journal*, **304**, 1409–1411.

––– & James, R. (1995) General hospital services for attempted suicide patients: a survey in one region. *Health Trends*, **27**, 18–21.

——, Arensman, E., Townsend, E., *et al* (1998*a*) Deliberate self-harm: systematic review of the efficacy of psychosocial and pharmacological treatments in preventing repetition. *British Medical Journal*, **317**, 441–417.

—, —, —, *et al* (1998*b*) Deliberate self-harm: the efficacy of psychosocial and pharmacological treatments. In *The Cochrane Library. Cochrane Database of Systematic Reviews*, Issue 3. Oxford: Update Software.

House, A., Owens, D. & Storer, D. (1992) Psychosocial intervention following attempted suicide: is there a case for better services? *International Review of Psychiatry*, **4**, 15–22.

Kapur, N., House, A., Creed, F., *et al* (1998) Management of deliberate self-poisoning in adults for teaching hospitals: a descriptive study. *British Medical Journal*, **316**, 831–832.

Kreitman, N. & Foster, J. (1991) The construction and selection of predictive scales, with special reference to parasuicide. *British Journal of Psychiatry*, **159**, 185–192.

Morgan, H. G., Jones, E. M. & Owen, J. H. (1993) Secondary prevention of non-fatal deliberate self-harm. The green card study. *British Journal of Psychiatry*, **163**, 111–112.

Newson-Smith, J. G. B. & Hirsch, S. R. (1979) A comparison of social workers and psychiatrists in evaluating parasuicide. *British Journal of Psychiatry*, **134**, 335–342.

Owens, D. (1990) Self-harm patients not admitted to hospital. *Journal of the Royal College of Physicians of London*, **24**, 281–283.

——, Dennis, M., Jones, S., *et al* (1991) Self-poisoning patients discharged from accident and emergency: risk factors and outcome. *Journal of the Royal College of Physicians of London*, **25**, 218–222.

——, ——, Read, S., *et al* (1994) Outcome of deliberate self-poisoning. An examination of risk factors for repetition. *British Journal of Psychiatry* , **165**, 797–801.

Rose, G. (1992) *The Strategy of Preventive Medicine*. Oxford: Oxford University Press.

Royal College of Psychiatrists (1994) *The General Hospital Management of Adult Deliberate Self-Harm. A Consensus Statement on Standards for Service Provision*. Council Report Number 32. London: Royal College of Psychiatrists.

Salkovskis, P. M., Atha, C. & Storer, D. (1990) Cognitive–behavioural problem solving in the treatment of patients who repeatedly attempt suicide. A controlled trial. *British Journal of Psychiatry*, **157**, 871–876.

Waterhouse, J. & Platt, S. (1990) General hospital admission in the management of parasuicide. A randomised controlled trial. *British Journal of Psychiatry*, **156**, 236–242.

Williams, R. & Morgan, H. G. (1994) *Suicide Prevention: the Challenge Confronted. A Manual of Guidance for Purchasers and Providers of Mental Health Care*. London: HMSO.

Prevention of depression: psychological and social measures

Jan Scott

The role of pharmacotherapy in the management of depressive disorders is well-established and frequently reviewed. This paper focuses on the prospects for reducing the incidence, prevalence and morbidity of depression through psychosocial interventions. A central requirement in prevention is a knowledge of the epidemiology of the disorder being investigated. This data can be used to identify high-risk groups. By comparing the number of known cases with population levels of morbidity, it allows comment on help-seeking behaviour and accessibility of services. Also, differences in incidence and prevalence rates give some indication of the chronicity of the disorder.

Risk of depression

Epidemiology

About 3% of general practitioner (GP) attendees have a recognised, depressive disorder, while an equal number of sufferers go unrecognised. The median age of onset of affective disorders is early adulthood (about 23 years). Unipolar disorders are twice as common in women as men. Marital history has a powerful influence on depression rates, with continuously married subjects, cohabitees and never married subjects demonstrating the lowest morbidity. There is an inverse relationship between depression and social disadvantage. When the latter is controlled for, there is minimal evidence of racial or ethnic differences in the prevalence of depression. Eighty per cent of individuals who experience a minor episode later suffer a major depression.

Associated psychobiosocial factors

Bipolar disorder and severe unipolar disorders are the most familial forms of affective disorder.

However, even where genetic influences are strong environmental factors are still important in determining whether a depressive disorder occurs and the form it takes. Psychosocial factors influencing vulnerability to depression include life events, social support networks, early environment and premorbid personality. Key risk and protective factors are summarised in Box 1.

Life events

In comparison with the general population, depression sufferers experience a significant excess of independent undesirable life events in the six months prior to episode onset, or they report chronic difficulties (Paykel & Cooper, 1992). An increase in such events may also be implicated in recurrence or maintenance of depression (Scott & Paykel, 1994). However, in the community, only about 10% of individuals who experience an 'exit' event develop a clinical depression. Hence, mediating factors need to be explored (Scott & Paykel, 1995).

Box 1.   Risk factors and protective factors

Risk factors
**Close biological relative with depression
    (due to genetic or environmental effect)
Severe stressors
Low self-esteem
Female gender
Social disadvantage**

Protective factors include
**Presence of a confidante
Coping skills – problem-solving ability and
    personal resilience**

Social support

Many people with depression demonstrate pre-morbid deficits in interpersonal relationships. However, research suggests that lack of support does not directly predispose to depression. Social support reduces depression risk by buffering individuals against the impact of adversity (Alloway & Bebbington, 1987). A specific form of support, namely the presence of a confidante, is known to reduce vulnerability to onset and may also protect against recurrence of depression. Other characteristics of effective support are that it has to be perceived by the individual as adequate, and it has to be available to them at times of crisis.

Level of expressed emotion in a key relative at the time of a depressive episode is a significant predictor of outcome in patients with unipolar and bipolar illnesses.

Early adversity

Brown (1989) suggested that loss of the mother before an individual is 11 years old is associated with increased risk of adult depression because of the adverse effect on the individual self-esteem. There is no evidence from recent reviews (Parker, 1992) that childhood bereavement or parent–child separations specifically predispose to adult depression. While such events may be associated with a number of disorders, any negative effects are probably a consequence of inadequate post-loss parenting. Childhood exposure to a parental style of 'affectionless overcontrol' is associated with an increased risk of neurotic disorders, particularly non-melancholic depression, in adult life. Physical or sexual abuse in childhood also increases the risk of adult depressive and other mental disorders.

Premorbid personality and coping strategies

While personality factors may affect the course of an affective disorder, no personality characteristics have been found to be specifically associated with onset of depression. Individuals who develop a first depressive episode differ from 'never ill' controls in showing higher levels of neuroticism, lower levels of emotional stability, less resilience and higher levels of interpersonal dependency (Hirschfeld & Shea, 1992). Cognitive theory highlights that high levels of neuroticism are associated with chronic low self-esteem, global negative affect and enhanced recall of negative self-related material. This may partly explain the role of this trait in the development of depression.

Alternative models of vulnerability to depression focus on perceived self-efficacy, coping and problem-solving strategies. Coping consists not only of what an individual does but also of what psychological and social resources are available. Individuals differ in the extent and efficacy of their coping responses. For example, those who generate fewer and less effective alternative solutions to problems may be at increased risk of depression and deliberate self-harm (Scott & Paykel, 1995).

Key concepts in prevention

Epidemiological data are used initially to identify those people at greatest risk of affective disorder (the target population). Historically, three forms of prevention have been defined:

(a) Primary: aimed at reducing the incidence of the disorder;
(b) Secondary: aimed at reducing prevalence;
(c) Tertiary: aimed at reducing associated disabilities.

The strategies used in secondary and tertiary prevention are essentially those employed in good clinical practice. Primary preventive interventions are less well defined, but may be categorised as 'pro-active' or 'reactive' (Jenkins, 1994).

For example, improving parenting skills, which may in turn enhance a child's self-esteem and reduce the risk of depression in adulthood, is a pro-active intervention. Counselling recently bereaved individuals to reduce the risk of abnormal grief reactions is a reactive intervention. Selecting

---

Box 2. Issues for clinicians

A sound knowledge of epidemiology helps clinicians understand which psychosocial factors may predispose to, or protect against, the onset of depressive disorder

The introduction of self-rating question-naires is an inexpensive way of improving the detection of depressive disorders in community settings. To be truly effective this strategy probably needs to be linked to training that improves treatment

Even where genetic or biological influences are strong, taking a psychosocial (dis-tressed person) as well as a biomedical (diseased organ) approach improves patient outcome

candidates for such approaches is a critical consideration. Three targeting strategies are recognised:

(a) Universal – measures regarded as desirable for all members of the community (e.g. health promotion, improved housing);
(b) Selective – measures appropriate to high-risk groups within the community (e.g. young female single parents);
(c) Indicated– measures targeting an individual at very high risk (e.g. someone with a strong genetic predisposition).

These preventive interventions operate at different levels within the social order. Macro-level interventions are aimed at changing the society and culture. Psychiatrists may seek to operate at a macro-level by trying to influence government policies to reduce poverty, unemployment and poor housing. Micro-level interventions are aimed at individuals, primary groups or social networks. It is easier to show the efficacy of micro-level interventions with individuals in their immediate environment, particularly if the strategy is highly targeted as in selective or indicated measures (Jenkins, 1994; Scott & Leff, 1994).

Specific psychosocial preventive strategies may comprise individual or family therapy or may focus on general behavioural change in the individual (e.g. social skills training) or significant others. The social environment may also be modified either by enhancing existing support systems or creating a new more protective environment (e.g. through changes in lifestyle).

Systematic research on psychosocial aspects of prevention is limited. In the biological field, there is a small literature on primary prevention (regarding the role of genetic counselling) while secondary and tertiary preventive strategies are described in the detailed research on the benefits of different drugs in the acute, continuation and maintenance phases of depression treatment. The increasing awareness of psychosocial factors associated with onset and maintenance of depression means that the development of prevention programmes is likely to expand in the next decade. Potential strategies are reviewed below (Effective Health Care, 1997).

Preventive strategies in depressive disorder

Primary prevention

Primary prevention strategies may target early aspects of the lifespan (genetic or constitutional vulnerability or childhood adversity), or may focus on individuals experiencing specific life events (see Table 1).

Interventions in parent–child relationships

The impact of poor parenting may not specifically predispose a child to depression in adulthood. However, if parental care could be improved, or self-esteem of the child at risk enhanced, it might have a long-term primary preventive effect. Rutter (1985) highlights how problems experienced by one individual may adversely affect another individual in the immediate environment, which may further worsen the interaction and problems of both people. Strayhom & Weidman (1991) attempted to intervene in this vicious cycle by targeting distressed mothers who were having difficulty managing children who had identified behaviour problems. Support for the mothers was associated with reduced levels of behavioural disturbance in the offspring.

School programmes with 'at risk' children and adolescents

In the USA, Shure & Spivack (1982) described improved problem-solving skills with a programme targeted at over 200 young children with behaviour problems who came from disadvantaged backgrounds. Others describe small projects which

Table 1. Primary prevention strategies

Strategy	Example
Reduce individual vulnerability	School programmes to improve coping skills in adolescents
Improve parent–child interactions	Supporting mothers of children with behaviour
Offer event centred interventions	Counselling for individuals:
	(a) at risk of abnormal grief;
	(b) facing severe trauma, e.g. cancer surgery;
	(c) with risk factors for depression, e.g. divorce.

reduced neurotic traits in adolescents through the use of rational emotive therapy. School programmes that educate children and adolescents in how to cope with conflict and crises and improve life skills may benefit women more than men (Mrazek & Haggerty, 1994). School-based suicide prevention programmes are not deemed effective.

Event-centred interventions

Most life events implicated in studies of depression are inevitable consequences of the life-cycle. However, the occurrence may signal a period of increased risk of onset of depression and preventive interventions may be feasible. This approach lies on the border between primary and secondary prevention (Effective Health Care, 1997).

Support and counselling reduces depression and other psychiatric morbidity in those at high risk of abnormal grief reactions (Raphael, 1977; Parkes, 1981). Futhermore, research showed that treated individuals at high risk were less symptomatic than controls who were not treated up to 20 months post-intervention. Morbidity rates in the counselled group were reduced to the same levels as found in individuals at low risk of an abnormal grief reaction.

In the USA, Bloom *et al* (1985) describe a programme of pre-divorce counselling targeted at adults demonstrating other risk factors for depression. A four-year follow-up study of 150 individuals demonstrated fewer symptoms of anxiety and depression and better vocational outcomes in the intervention group.

Maguire *et al* (1980) randomly assigned women having surgery for breast cancer to counselling or to practical advice. The prevalence of anxiety and depression was similar in both groups, but episodes were of shorter duration in the counselled women and they showed better social and psychological adjustment at post-operative follow-up after 18 months. However, the reduced morbidity during episodes

might have been a function of early recognition and prompt referral (i.e. secondary prevention), rather than representing primary prevention.

Secondary prevention

The secondary prevention of affective disorders encompasses early case detection and early initiation of treatment (see Table 2).

Early detection

Early detection of affective disorders depends in part on the attitude of the individual towards any symptoms which develop, and the behaviour of the professional they present to. As few as 50% of those developing depressive disorders seek help (Scott & Paykel, 1994). Individuals with endogenous symptoms, limitations in ability to work, impaired functioning and lower levels of social support are more likely to consult. Between 25 and 50% of individuals with depressive disorder will remain undetected by their GP. Depression is more frequently missed in young men, people presenting with somatic symptoms and those 00who mention emotional disturbance late in the interview.

The use of self-report or simple observer-rated questionnaires such as the General Health Questionnaire (GHQ; Goldberg, 1978), the Beck Depression Inventory (BDI; Beck *et al*, 1961), or the Hospital Anxiety and Depression Scale (HADS; Zigmond & Snaith, 1983) offer a cost-effective method (a GHQ costs about two pence to complete) of helping primary care staff detect depression. Importantly, research has shown that notifying a GP that a patient meets the criteria for psychiatric caseness produces a better outcome than non-notification.

An alternative approach is to use educational programmes to improve case recognition. In Sweden,

Table 2. Secondary prevention strategies	
Strategy	Example
Improve early case detection	Screening questionnaires, e.g. Beck Depression Inventory Education and interview skills training for GPs Increase awareness of depression and enhance help-seeking, e.g. Defeat Depression campaign
Offer early intervention	Support and monitoring of at-risk mothers or pregnant women e.g. NEWPIN project Improve access to professional help e.g. self-referral, liaison attachment to primary care

Rutz *et al* (1989) described a programme that improved detection and management of depression and suicide risk. Evidence from England (Scott & Paykel, 1994) suggests that a package aimed at improving the interviewing skills of primary care physicians produces similar results. At a national level, professional colleges (American Psychiatric Association; Royal College of Psychiatrists) initiated the 'DART' (Depression Awareness, Recognition and Treatment) and the 'Defeat Depression' campaigns. These aimed to improve knowledge and treatment skills of professionals, and to raise awareness, reduce stigma and encourage help-seeking by sufferers.

Early intervention

Early intervention offers possibilities both of interrupting distress before it reaches the level of clinical depression (at the border of primary/secondary prevention) and of markedly shortening clinical depressive episodes.

Newton (1988) describes befriending projects where parents who are at risk are supported in the community in an attempt to enhance child development and improve parental functioning. The NEWPIN project in London relates most closely to those at risk of depression. Mothers who were vulnerable to depression according to the Brown & Harris model (Brown, 1989) formed a contract with a volunteer supporter from a similar social background who offered input over an extended period. Self-evaluation by the women suggested that self-esteem, self-confidence and interpersonal relationships had improved and that the mothers related better to their children (Newton, 1988; Scott & Paykel, 1995).

In New South Wales, Barnett & Parker (1985) undertook a project with primiparous women who had been shown to be at greater risk of neurotic and depressive disorders. The women were assigned postnatally to either professional support, lay support or a control group with no additional help offered. Overall, those who received professional help showed a significant reduction in postnatal anxiety levels compared to the other groups; those receiving lay support showed a non-significant improvement.

Access to services

Increasing direct access to mental health services (e.g. offering self-referral or providing liaison sessions in primary care) is another way of increasing detection and early intervention. More information is needed about the accessibility or acceptability of the services to certain high-risk groups. For example, young Asian women have higher suicide rates than young Asian men, but attend GPs less often than any other subgroup in the general population.

Tertiary prevention

Although the measures described in this section lie more in the realm of treatment, they have preventive implications since the interventions reduce prevalence rates of symptomatic disorder. Recent studies confirm that at least 50% of those with first episodes of depression have a further episode, while the median prevalence of chronicity is 12% (Scott, 1992). About 15% of deaths are due to suicide, and mortality rates from other causes are also increased in people with affective disorders (Jenkins, 1994).

Prevention of recurrence and relapse

The role of pharmacotherapy in preventing further episodes has been well studied and clear guidelines exist. Psychosocial approaches are less clearly evaluated, but the literature is expanding rapidly (see Table 3). Interpersonal psychotherapy was of significant value in reducing recurrence in one study, but did not reduce early relapse in a controlled study of continuation medication (Scott & Paykel, 1994). There is accumulating evidence that cognitive therapy may reduce relapse rates in mild to moderately severe unipolar depressions (US Department of Health and Human Services, 1993). Evans *et al* (1992) demonstrated that the relapse rate with cognitive therapy was no different from that of patients receiving continuous drug treatment and was only half that of the patients who stopped their drug treatment immediately after their depression remitted. If cognitive therapy alone reduces risk of relapse this will be the first time any form of antidepressant treatment has been shown to have an effect beyond the point of termination of the intervention. Whether the combined use of cognitive therapy and pharmacotherapy bestows any additional benefit over either treatment alone is inconclusive. However, a cognitive approach may significantly enhance coping skills, lithium adherence and outcome in bipolar and unipolar cases (Scott, 1992, 1995).

The research on expressed emotion demonstrated that (in contrast to schizophrenia) people with unipolar or bipolar disorders with relatives who have a high level of expressed emotion were not protected by drug treatment or by reduced contact. However, Jacobson *et al* (1993) reported that marital therapy alone or in combination with individual cognitive therapy offers effective treatment of the acute depressive episode and may prevent relapse.

Table 3. Tertiary prevention strategies	
Strategy	Example

Reduce relapse and recurrence	Psychotherapies alone or as an adjunct to pharmacotherapy:
	     Cognitive therapy
	     Couples therapy/interpersonal therapy
	     Family therapy

Provide vocational rehabilitation	Establish meaningful daytime activities
Develop support programmes	Psychoeducation programmes Network therapy Social skills training Befriending schemes Assertive outreach Lifestyle counselling

Rehabilitation

There has been a failure to investigate the residual disabilities of individuals with affective disorders (Scott, 1992, 1995). Vocational rehabilitation of these patients focuses less on the role of work performance and more on its potential for restoring confidence, improving self-esteem and enhancing feelings of mastery. Only broad guidelines are available, but meaningful daytime activity seems important. Re-employment may reduce depression in socially isolated men who have been made redundant, and women working outside of the home show less impairment following depression than housewives.

Educational and support programmes

Psychoeducational programmes for hospital-treated patients and their families may be associated with better resolution of the index affective episode and better global outcome (Glick *et al*, 1994). Also, individuals with chronic neurotic disorders and their families benefit more from home-based support of a community psychiatric nurse rather than intermittent symptom-oriented out-patient appointments. Improving individual coping repertoires, network therapy (where each member of the sufferer's primary group takes responsibility for initiating specific social changes), befriending projects and social skills training have been advocated but not fully evaluated. Finally, in some individuals, reducing stress can only be achieved through significant changes in lifestyle (e.g. taking a less demanding job). However, care is required. Change should not be made until the individual's mental state is stable, and it must not condemn the individual to an unfulfilling existence.

Conclusions

Analysis of epidemiological data identifies high-risk groups and potentially allows the development of primary, secondary and tertiary preventive strategies

---

Box 3. Controversial issues

No model of depression onset is robust enough to allow mental health services to introduce cost-effective primary preventive programmes

Many unrecognised cases of depression are mild and self-limiting. To be perceived as clinically relevant preventive strategies must ensure that either:

(a) early detection of mild cases is matched by early detection of severe cases

(b) the long-term outcome of the mild cases detected is significantly improved

Few bipolar patients receive psychosocial interventions in day to day clinical practice, yet the limited research data available shows that outcome is improved if such approaches are provided (Scott, 1995). The effect may be due to the indirect improvement in treatment adherence, but even so, shouldn't we employ such approaches more often?

across the lifespan. Evidence of the prevention of first episodes of depression is not available.

Promising lines of primary prevention research relate to trying to improve coping skills, and enhancing 'protective' factors during times of increased vulnerability to depression onset. Individuals with a wide range of coping strategies and resources available to them are less likely to reach the pathological end-state of depression in response to stress (Scott, 1992; Scott & Paykel, 1994).

Event-centred interventions, which fall on the boundary between primary and secondary prevention, are the most relevant approaches for clinical psychiatrists. There is a possibility that major affective disorders may be prevented by interventions at the subclinical level. Psychosocial input to individuals at high risk for depression who have experienced, or are about to experience, a significant life event seems to reduce morbidity rates to the same level as low-risk individuals.

Prospects for secondary prevention vary. Accessibility of services can be modified. Primary care professionals can be encouraged to improve detection rates of affective disorders, and help-seeking behaviour may be promoted through public education. However, improving case recognition must be linked to training that improves the management of depression. Only 30% of recognised cases of depression in primary care currently receive adequate treatment.

While the mechanisms of action of putative risk factors in the onset of depression are unresolved, the role of psychosocial variables in the presentation and maintenance of the disorder is less contentious. Clinically, the prompt introduction of multimodal treatment during the acute depressive phase and rigorous attention to after-care of the individual and their family are the most effective preventive strategies currently available. As such, there is no substitute for following 'good practice' guidelines in an attempt to reduce the morbidity and mortality associated with affective disorders.

Acknowledgements

I thank Professor E. S. Paykel for his input. Many of the ideas expressed in this paper draw on our previous joint writings on this topic.

References

Alloway, R. & Bebbington, P. E. (1987) The buffer theory of social support: A review of the literature. *Psychological Medicine*, **17**, 91–108.

Barnett, B. & Parker, G. (1985) Professional and non-professional intervention for highly anxious primiparous mothers. *British Journal of Psychiatry*, **146**, 287–293.

Beck, A. T., Ward, C. H., Mendelson, M., *et al* (1961) an inventory for measuring depression. *Archives of General Psychiatry*, **4**, 561–571.

Bloom, B. L., Hodges, W. F., Kern, M. B., *et al* (1985) A preventive intervention program for the newly separated. *American Journal of Orthopsychiatry*, **55**, 9–26.

Brown, G. W. (1989) Depression: A radical social perspective. In *Depression: An Integrative Approach* (eds K. R. Herbst & E. S. Paykel), pp. 21–44. Oxford: Heinemann Medical Books.

Effective Health Care (1997) *Mental Health Promotion in High Risk Groups*, pp. 1–12. Plymouth: Latimer Trend & Co.

Evans, M., Hollon, S., Derubeis, R., *et al* (1992) Differential relaps following cognitive therapy and pharmacotherapy for depression. *Archives of General Psychiatry*, **49**, 802–808.

Glick, I. D., Burti, L., Okonogi, K., *et al* (1994) Effectiveness in psychiatric care III. Psychoeducation and outcome for patients with major affective disorder and their families. *British Journal of Psychiatry*, **164**, 104–106.

Goldberg, D. (1978) *Manual of the GHQ*. Slough: NFER–Nelson.

Hirschfeld, R. & Shea, M. (1992) Personality. In *Handbook of Affective Disorders*, 2nd edn (ed. E. S. Paykel), pp. 185–194. Edinburgh: Churchill Livingstone.

Jacobson, N. S., Fruzetfi, A. E., Dobson, K., *et al* (1993) Couple therapy as a treatment for depression II: The effects of relationship quality and therapy on depressive relapse. *Journal of Consulting and Clinical Psychology*, **3**, 516–519.

Jenkins, R. (1994) Principles of prevention. In *Prevention in Psychiatry* (eds E. S. Paykel & R. Jenkins), pp. 11–24. London: Gaskell.

Maguire, P., Tait, A., Brooke, M., *et al* (1980) The effect of counselling on the psychiatric morbidity associated with mastectomy. *British Medical Journal*, **281**, 1454–1456.

Mrazek, P. J. & Haggerty, R. J. (1994) *Reducing Risks for Mental Disorders: Frontiers for Preventive Intervention Research*. Washington, DC: National Academy Press.

Newton, J. (1988) *Preventing Mental Illness*, pp. 134–196. London: Routledge.

Parker, G. (1992) Early environment. In *Handbook of Affective Disorders*, 2nd edn (ed. E. S. Paykel), pp. 171–84. Edinburgh: Churchill Livingstone.

Parkes, C. M. (1981) Evaluation of a bereavement service. *Journal of Preventative Psychiatry*, **1**, 179–188.

Paykel, E. S. & Cooper, Z. (1992) Life events and social stress. In *Handbook of Affective Disorders*, 2nd edn (ed. E. S. Paykel), pp. 149–170. Edinburgh: Churchill Livingstone.

Raphael, B. (1977) Preventative intervention with the recently bereaved. *Archives of General Psychiatry*, **34**, 1450–1454.

Rutter, M. (1985) Resilience in the face of adversity: Protective factors and resistance to psychiatric disorder. *British Journal of Psychiatry*, **147**, 598–611.

Rutz, W., Van Knorring, L. & Walinder, J. (1989) Frequency of suicide on Gotland after systematic postgraduate education of general practitioners. *Acta Psychiatrica Scandinavica*, **80**, 151–154.

Scott, J. (1992) Social and community approaches. In *Handbook of Affective Disorders*, 2nd edn (ed. E. S. Paykel), pp. 525–538. Edinburgh: Churchill Livingstone.

—— (1995) Psychotherapy for bipolar disorder. *British Journal of Psychiatry*, **167**, 581–588.

—— & Leff, J. (1994) Social factors, social interventions and prevention. In *Prevention in Psychiatry* (eds E. S. Paykel & R. Jenkins), pp. 25–31. London: Gaskell.

—— & Paykel, E. S. (1994) Affective disorders. In *Prevention in Psychiatry* (eds E. S. Paykel & R. Jenkins), pp. 53–66. London: Gaskell.

—— & —— (1995) Depression: risks and possibilities for prevention. In *Handbook of Studies on Preventative Psychiatry* (eds B. Raphael & G. Burrows), pp. 514–530. Oxford: Elsevier.

Shure, M. B. & Spivack, G. (1982) Interpersonal problem-solving in young children: A cognitive approach to prevention. *American Journal of Community Psychology*, **10**, 341–356.

Strayhom, J. M. & Weidman, C. S. (1991) Follow-up one year after parent–child interaction training: Effects on behaviour of preschool children. *Journal of the American Academy of Child and Adolescent Psychiatry*, **30**, 138–143.

US Department of Health and Human Services (1993) *Depression in Primary Care: Treatment of Major Depression*, pp. 71–123. Rockville, MD: Agency for Health Care Policy and Research Publications.

Zigmond, A. & Snaith, R. (1983) The hospital anxiety and Depression Scale. *Acta Psychiatrica Scandinavica*, **67**, 361–370.

Chronic depression in primary care: approaches to liaison

K. Lloyd & R. Jenkins

Much attention has focused on prompt, accurate identification and treatment of depression and anxiety in primary care settings. Less is known about what to do when treatment is unsuccessful or the initial opportunity to intervene is missed. The long-term prognosis of depression and anxiety in primary care settings is not good: half of sufferers experience a relapsing remitting course and a quarter become chronic. There is also a relationship between chronicity and high service utilisation. The label 'heartsink' has sometimes been applied to these patients, often pejoratively.

Initiatives such as the Defeat Depression Campaign (Paykel & Priest, 1992) and Health of the Nation (Department of Health, 1994) have raised expectations and concerns about the morbidity to be addressed. It is important that strategies be developed within primary care to detect and manage these conditions so as not to divert secondary care resources from so-called severe mental illness. This chapter looks at available practical strategies.

What problems do these patients have?

Between a third and a quarter of the workload of the average general practitioner (GP) concerns mental health problems (Sharp & Morrell, 1989). Depression and anxiety are the most common mental illnesses seen in primary care while patients with psychosis constitute less than 10% of general practice psychiatry. A GP with a list size of 2500 identifies approximately 300 patients with a non-psychotic mental illness per year. This is termed 'conspicuous psychiatric morbidity'. Almost as many attendees again have an undiagnosed mental illness, most commonly depression or anxiety. This is the 'hidden psychiatric morbidity'. Only a small proportion of people with mental disorders who consult GPs reach the specialist psychiatric services. The majority are managed in primary care (see Fig. 1) (Goldberg & Huxley, 1992).

Setting	Period prevalence (n/1000 at risk/year)
Level 1: The community	260–315
1st filter . . . . The decision to consult	
Level 2: Total primary care morbidity	230
2nd filter . . . . GP recognition	
Level 3: Conspicuous psychiatric morbidity	101.5
3rd filter . . . . The decision to refer	
Level 4: Mental illness services	20.8
4th filter . . . . Admission to psychiatric beds	
Level 5: Psychiatric in-patients	3.8–6.7

Fig. 1. Goldberg & Huxley's (1992) five levels and four filters on the pathways to psychiatric care

When chronicity is defined as persistence of the index episode for more than two years, the greatest number of patients with chronic illnesses are encountered in primary care settings, as are the greatest opportunities for prevention and treatment (Lloyd & Jenkins, 1994). Depression and anxiety are among the most common chronic conditions seen in primary care (Lyons et al, 1992; Scott et al, 1992). However, many primary care patients do not fit easily into a diagnosis of major depression or generalised anxiety disorder but have some symptoms of both. For practical purposes it is probably most helpful to think of depression and anxiety as dimensions rather than categories, although some disagree (Goldberg & Huxley, 1992). Such patients may not reach the threshold for either disorder but show considerable morbidity and persistent symptoms (Johnstone & Goldberg, 1976). Many experience symptoms of other physical and psychiatric disorders during their lifetimes.

Poorer short-term outcome is associated with initial severity of symptomatology, significant concomitant physical illness, severe social problems and material circumstances, genetic risk score and personality factors (Mann et al, 1981; Goldberg & Huxley, 1992). Mortality is also increased among patients with conspicuous psychiatric morbidity referred on to psychiatric out-patients (Sims, 1973). According to US figures minor depression results in more days lost from work than major depression because of the former's greater prevalence. Only chronic heart disease produces more disability (Eisenberg, 1992). These patients are clearly not the 'worried well'.

The importance of intervention

There is a clear health gain for the patient from improved detection and management because detection improves prognosis and effective management improves the prognosis still further (Paykel & Priest, 1992; Freemantle et al, 1993; Drummond, 1994). It is important to improve management in order to avoid the consequences of chronicity, such as considerable stress and a low quality of life. Additionally there are considerable occupational problems such as absence due to sickness, labour turnover, problems with colleagues, poor performance and accidents. There can be problems for children with chronically ill parents; they are more vulnerable to emotional and cognitive impairment, which in turn can predispose to adult mental illness on maturity, as well as having an adverse effect on the children's ultimate intellectual attainment

(Jenkins, 1992; Lloyd & Jenkins, 1994). Besides persistent morbidity, a small proportion commit suicide. It has been argued that 90% of people who complete suicides have some form of mental disorder, most frequently depression; 66% had consulted their GP in the previous month; 40% had consulted their GP in the last week; and 33% expressed clear suicidal ideation (Department of Health, 1994). This remains a controversial area.

Chronic depression, persistent unresolved grief states, chronic phobias and tranquilliser dependency may also place an excessive burden on health services. A survey of women aged 20–45 years registered with two south London general practices found that high attendance (defined as more than 10 consultations per year) was significantly associated with psychiatric morbidity, young age, lower socioeconomic group, concomitant physical symptoms, and receipt of a prescription for psychotropic medication within the last 12 months (Corney & Murray, 1988). High attendees were more likely to have sought help from other agencies in addition to their GP. Patients with predominantly somatic presentations of depression are more likely than non-somatisers to use both medical and mental health services (Bass, 1994).

Resources available to GPs and primary care teams

Having emphasised the scale of the problem, the particular advantages of the GP's position, and the scope for preventive activity in general practice, how can busy GPs possibly deliver, in the midst of all the other competing obligations? They clearly need help and support, and plenty of it. How can this best be achieved?

Several developments in the past have arisen from this need, and some have been thoroughly evaluated. They have generally built on the practice of attaching secondary care personnel to the primary care team. So, for example, schemes of attached social workers have proven valuable in the treatment of people with chronic depression related to chronic social difficulties (Corney, 1984). Schemes of attached psychologists have been evaluated in the treatment of anxiety disorders, and in cognitive therapy of depression (Robson, 1992). Community psychiatric nurse (CPN) attachments are now probably the most common form of attachment. A recent thorough evaluation by Gournay & Brooking (1994) demonstrated the enormous opportunity cost entailed in withdrawing CPNs from the long-term severely mentally ill to treat depression and anxiety

A problem of numbers

There is a problem with the attachment of secondary care personnel to the primary care because of the sheer numbers involved. There are approximately 30 000 GPs in the country, each of whom will have 300–600 patients with depression and anxiety in any one year, and there are 2000 consultant general psychiatrists. Therefore each psychiatrist would need to have close links with 15 GPs, and could realistically only help each GP with a tiny proportion of all their patients with depression. Similarly, there is one CPN to 5–10 GPs (the precise ratio varying across the country). If we take the best case of one CPN to every five GPs, we know that on average each GP has seven patients with chronic severe mental illness (mostly chronic schizophrenia) who require supervision, support and family interventions and so on from a CPN (Kendrick *et al*, 1991). He or she then already has a caseload of 35. It is easy to see that if each GP also refers three or four patients with depression, the CPN's working week has been overloaded (unless care is withdrawn from those with severe mental illness). Meanwhile, only a tiny dent is made on the GPs load of several hundred patients with depression. The severely mentally ill now, more than ever, need concentrated efforts in continuing care during and after they leave hospital. CPNs will often be their case managers and/or key workers, and there are substantial concerns that this important work is being jeopardised by the shift of CPNs' caseloads from being primarily focused on the severely mentally ill to being focused on those with minor psychiatric morbidity (Gournay & Brooking, 1994).

The role for the psychiatrist

Out-patient referral is the traditional route for obtaining a psychiatric opinion on a patient with chronic anxiety or depression. Strathdee (1994) surveyed 154 GPs in Camberwell to ask them what they wanted from out-patient services (see Box 1). Many of the GPs concerns related to communication. At a simple level, the referral letter and reply can help improve communication (King & Pullen, 1994). One approach is to use a standardised letter one A4-side in length giving details of problems, management (physical, psychological and social) and a care programme.

The main limitation of the out-patient referral route is the small numbers of patients who can

---

> **Box 1. General practitioner (GP) requirements from out-patient services (after Strathdee, 1994)**
>
> **Rapid assessment**
> **Shorter referral–appointment interval**
> **Better communication**
> **Clear management guidelines**
> **Statement of objectives of treatment**
> **Predicted response, complications and side-effects**
> **Six monthly review plans for patients with chronic illnesses**
> **Clearly stated role in the treatment for GPs and specialists**
> **Clarification of prescribing responsibilities**
> **Information booklets of therapies available**

be managed in this way. As outlined above, a significant increase in the numbers of referrals dealt with via this route would seriously impair the secondary care team's ability to manage patients with psychotic mental illness. The alternative is to move into primary care.

Over the last 25 years more and more psychiatrists have established attachments to primary care settings and a variety of liaison models have emerged (see Box 2). The 'shifted out-patients' model, the most simple and common arrangement, was first described by Tyrer (1984). The psychiatrist conducts a usual out-patient clinic except that it takes place in a surgery. He or she can offer assessment, crisis intervention and 'hands on' management in the surgery. Patients often prefer being seen in a primary care setting and supervision of trainees is relatively easy. However, no research has been conducted to see if this method helps the primary heath care team improve their own management skills. A major problem is providing this kind of service to all the practices in a sector. According to the 'consultation model' the psychiatrist advises the GP about management at regular intervals and also sees patients in primary care if required.

> **Box 2. Models of primary care liaison**
>
> **Informal meetings**
> **Shifted out-patients consultation model**
> **Consultation–liaison model**

In the 'consultation–liaison' model the psychiatrist attends practice meetings to discuss management problems with the primary health care team. He or she may then see the patient accompanied by the GP or another member of the primary health care team or the CPN associated with the practice (Creed & Marks, 1989). More patients can be discussed in this way and there is better GP–psychiatrist contact (Goldberg & Huxley, 1992).

A framework for liaison

Having decided upon one of these approaches, the specific needs of the liaison setting need to be considered. A suggested framework for assessing referrals is given in Box 3 and explained in more detail below.

The referral

The psychiatrist may wish to think about: why the person is being brought to attention now? What are the major concerns about this person? What is the relevant history? Is there a history of challenging behaviour or self-harm? How does this person respond to new professionals or changes in their management?

Diagnoses and personality

What is the likely psychiatric diagnosis? Does this person have comorbid disorders such as alcohol or substance misuse or tranquilliser dependency? What is the role of personality factors and coping style? It is important to emphasise that a diagnosis of personality disorder does not mean that the individual is 'untreatable', nor does it exclude other psychiatric

diagnoses or physical and social problems. Tyrer (1994) proposed a simple classification of personality disorders seen in general practice (antisocial, withdrawn, dependent or inhibited and outlined simple management strategies).

Physical factors

Does the person have comorbid physical illnesses? If so, how are they being treated and has the management of psychiatric problems been given an equal priority?

Somatisation

Does this person have medically unexplained physical symptoms? Is the practice agreed on how far they should investigate those symptoms? Is it appropriate to educate the patient to re-attribute their symptoms?

Psychological factors

What is the role of life events and developmental factors? What are the coping strategies and cognitive style? Are there relevant family and partner issues which should be addressed? What do the family/partner/carer understand about the person's condition? What psychological interventions has the person received from health social services or voluntary sector providers? What does the person stand to gain and lose by recovery?

Social factors

What are the sources of stress and support in this person's life? Consider particularly occupation relationships, marital/cohabitation, family, social life, money and housing. What is the relevance of gender, ethnic and social class factors?

Level of functioning

How well does this person function in their activities of daily living? Do they need further support or might recovery mean losing some of their existing support?

Medication

Has the patient had an appropriate course of an appropriate drug at adequate doses for long enough? How does the patient view the role of medication, what is adherence like and what

---

Box 3. A framework for consultation–liaison

The referral
Diagnoses and personality
Physical factors
Somatisation
Psychological factors
Social factors
Level of functioning
Medication
Organisation of care

side-effects are they experiencing? Are they receiving treatments that will exacerbate their psychiatric condition?

Organisation of care

Who currently sees this person, how often and what for? How often do they consult and what happens in the consultation? Would regular booked appointments with a member of the primary health care team help structure interaction? Is there a role for interview skills training? What patient literature does the practice have available? Does the practice have a directory of available health, social and voluntary sector agencies and what is locally available? How could communication about this patient be best improved?

Identifying patients

In addition to the patient-specific help suggested above, it might also be helpful to think about the practice's strategy for identifying patients with chronic anxiety and depression. A number of simple screening instruments exist which can facilitate this process (Lloyd & Jenkins, 1994). Computerised screening may have an increasing role to play in the future. Patients who consult very frequently can be identified from the practice computer and may merit screening for undiagnosed chronic depression and anxiety. Frequent consulters known to the GPs may have under-treated depression and anxiety.

Above all, the main aim is to support the primary health care team in their management of difficult cases by reviewing what the issues are, what has been tried so far and what other possibilities there are. The intention is to offer assessment advice and support rather than active intervention in the majority of cases. This approach can be supplemented with teaching and educational materials for the primary health care team.

Educational materials for the primary health care team and patient

An alternative strategy to shifting secondary care personnel into the primary care setting is for secondary care personnel to teach the primary care teams to handle these patients themselves, that is,

to have a supportive and educational role rather than a direct 'hands on' role in relation to these patients with minor psychiatric morbidity.

A number of initiatives have been developed that can be adapted for local use or approached for advice. For example, the Royal College of Psychiatrists has produced educational material for patients and professionals on depression and anxiety. Much self-help literature is available for the management of anxiety disorders (Drummond, 1994). A special primary care version of the 10th revision of the International Classification of Diseases (ICD–10 PHC) has been developed which presents simple diagnostic and management guidelines for common mental disorders such as depression and anxiety (Goldberg, 1994).

There is a national network of regional GP mental health fellows coordinated by Dr Andree Tylee. They are available as a resource for practices to develop their care of mental illness. Facilitators have been assisting primary care teams in developing their management of common chronic physical illnesses. A study has been undertaken to see if they can take on the same task of helping practices manage mental health (Lloyd & Jenkins, 1995).

Gask (1992) in Manchester developed a method to train GP-trainers to teach communication skills using video and audio feedback techniques. Teaching packages have been developed to improve the detection and management of common mental disorders. These techniques are also available for experienced practitioners.

Psychological treatments developed in hospital settings are not always appropriate or available in primary care. Problem-solving therapy has been developed in Oxford as a simple, brief effective treatment that can be carried out by the primary health care team. It has been shown to be an effective treatment for anxiety disorders of otherwise poor prognosis (Mynors-Wallis & Gath, 1992).

Making more help available

The GP needs more 'helping hands', and these can be obtained by strengthening the primary care team by the employment of practice nurses and counsellors and strategic deployment of health visitors and district nurses. The growth of counsellors in general practice is now well established, although we still need more careful evaluative studies of the effectiveness of brief psychotherapies used by counsellors, and the indications for such treatment (Freemantle *et al*, 1993). Most GPs already employ practice nurses, health visitors and district nurses, but these have traditionally only been used for physical and not psychological problems. There are a number of studies under way which can be brought to the GP's attention as practical strategies for improving the care of chronic mental illnesses in primary care.

A study at the Institute of Psychiatry examined whether practice nurses can identify those patients at risk of chronicity. The University of Exeter has developed and evaluated a general package to audit the quality of mental health care for depression. Oldfield Park Surgery, Bath, was funded to create a 'model' general practice for the purposes of optimal care of patients with psychological illness and related emotional problems consulting in that practice. The Royal College of Psychiatrists' and the Royal College of General Practitioners' five-year Defeat Depression campaign comprised both professional and public education initiatives. The aims were to increase knowledge among health care professionals about recognition and treatment of depressive illness and to enhance public awareness of depressive disorders.

Sometimes it is not possible to sort the problem out locally. The Maudsley Hospital has a specialist tertiary referral service led by Professor Anthony Mann for general practice patients with chronic depression and anxiety. The key to the service is that it is extremely flexible and tailored to the individual patient. For some patients an afternoon spent at the GP's surgery with staff from the centre might be sufficient to enable them to continue being treated at primary care level. Others might require a longer assessment during which the aim is to listen, measure, watch and gain trust, not to reassure or treat.

Conclusions

The best treatment of chronic anxiety and depression is prevention (Lloyd & Jenkins, 1994). Simple strategies exist to improve the detection and management of depression and anxiety which are among the most common chronic disorders encountered in primary care settings. Yet they are less likely to be practice priorities than other common disorders such as asthma, diabetes, coronary heart disease and cancer. Much ignorance and stigma are attached to depression and anxiety. Sufferers are sometimes unwilling to seek help. People may feel embarrassed to mention their problems. They may feel there is not enough time or that the doctor will be unsympathetic. Doctors are only too aware of the importance of not missing physical illnesses, but

depression and anxiety are often overlooked, leading to chronicity and increased morbidity. This may be due to time constraints, the belief that nothing can be done, or the notion that they are understandable and therefore do not require treatment. The psychiatrist has a key role to play in getting the balance right.

References

Bass, C. (1994) Somatisation. In *Prevention in Psychiatry* (eds E. Paykel & R. Jenkins), pp. 188–197. London: Gaskell.

Corney, R. (1984) The effectiveness of attached social workers in the management of depressed female patients in general practice. *Psychological Medicine*, **14** (Monograph Suppl. 6.), 1–47.

—— & Murray, J. (1988) The characteristics of high and low attendees at two general practices. *Social Psychiatry & Psychiatric Epidemiology*, **23**, 39–49.

Creed, F. & Marks, B. (1989) Liaison psychiatry in general practice: a comparison of the liaison attachment scheme and the shifted out-patient clinic models. *Journal of the Royal College of General Practitioners*, **39**, 514–517.

Department of Health (1994) *Health of the Nation Key Area Handbook of Mental Illness* (2nd edn), pp. 19–24. London: HMSO.

Drummond, L. M. (1994) Anxiety. In *Psychiatry and General Practice Today* (eds I. Pullen, G. Wilkinson, A. Wright, *et al*), pp. 112–134. London: Gaskell.

Eisenberg, L. (1992) Treating depression and anxiety in primary care: closing the gap between knowledge and practice. *New England Journal of Medicine*, **326**, 1080–1084.

Freemantle, N., Long, N., Mason, J., *et al* (1993) The treatment of depression in primary care. *Effectiveness Health Care Bulletin*, **5**, 2–12.

Gask, L. (1992) Teaching psychiatric interview skills to general practitioners. In *Prevention of Depression and Anxiety – the Role of the Primary Care Team* (eds R. Jenkins, J. Newton & J. Young), pp. 39–45. London: HMSO.

Goldberg, D. (1994) Epidemiology of mental disorder in general practice. In *Psychiatry and General Practice Today* (eds I. Pullen, G. Wilkinson, A. Wright, *et al*), pp. 36–44. London: Gaskell.

—— & Huxley, P. (1992) *Common Mental Disorders*. London: Routledge.

Gournay, K. & Brooking, J. (1994) Community psychiatric nurses in primary health care. *British Journal of Psychiatry*, **165**, 231–238.

Jenkins, R. (1992) Depression and anxiety: an overview of preventive strategies. In *Prevention of Depression and Anxiety – the Role of the Primary Care Team* (eds R. Jenkins, J. Newton, & R. Young), pp. 11–21. London: HMSO.

Johnstone, A. & Goldberg, D. (1976) Psychiatric screening in general practice: a controlled trial. *Lancet*, *i*, 605–608.

Kendrick, T., Sibbald, P., Burns, T., *et al* (1991) Role of general practitioners in care of long-term mentally ill. *British Medical Journal*, **302**, 508–510.

King, M. & Pullen, I. (1994) Communication between general practitioners and psychiatrists. In *Psychiatry and General Practice Today* (eds I. Pullen, G. Wilkinson, A. Wright, *et al*), pp. 251–264. London: Gaskell.

Lloyd, K. & Jenkins, R. (1994) Primary Care. In *Prevention in Psychiatry* (eds E. Paykel & R. Jenkins), pp. 198–209. London: Gaskell.

—— & —— (1995) The economics of depression in primary care: Department of Health Initiatives. *British Journal of Psychiatry*, **166** (suppl. 27), 60–62.

Lyons, R. A., Caroll, D., Doherty, K., *et al* (1992) General practice estimates of the prevalence of common chronic conditions. *Irish Medical Journal*, **85**, 22–24.

Mann, A. H., Jenkins, R. & Belsey, E. (1981) The 12 month outcome of patients with neurotic disorder in general practice. *Psychological Medicine*, **11**, 535–550.

Mynors-Wallis, L. M. & Gath, D. H. (1992) Brief psychological treatments. *International Review of Psychiatry*, **4**, 301–306.

Paykel, E. S. & Priest, R. G. (1992) Recognition and management of depression and general practice: consensus statement. *British Medical Journal*, **305**, 1198–1202.

Robson, M. (1992) Counselling in general practice: options for action. A clinical psychology. In *Prevention of Depression and Anxiety – the Role of the Primary Care Team* (eds R. Jenkins, J. Newton & R. Young), pp. 77–81. London: HMSO.

Scott, J., Eccleston, D., & Boys, R. (1992) Can we predict the persistence of depression? *British Journal of Psychiatry*, **161**, 633–637.

Sharp, D., & Morrell, D. (1989) The psychiatry of general practice. In *Scientific Approaches in Epidemiological Psychiatry. Essays in Honour of Michael Shepherd* (eds P. Williams, G. Wilkinson & K. Rawnsley), pp. 404–419. London: Routledge.

Sims, A. (1973) Mortality and neurosis. *Lancet*, *ii*, 1072–1075.

Strathdee, G. (1994) Psychiatry and general practice – a psychiatric perspective. In *Psychiatry and General Practice Today* (eds I. Pullen, G. Wilkinson, A. Wright, *et al*), pp. 22–35. London: Gaskell.

Tyrer, P. (1984) Psychiatric clinics in general practice: an extension of community care. *British Journal of Psychiatry*, **145**, 9–14.

—— (1994) Personality problems. In *Psychiatry and General Practice Today* (eds I. Pullen, G. Wilkinson, A. Wright, *et al*), pp. 180–193. London: Gaskell.

Managing depression in older people

Cornelius Katona

Although common and disabling, depression in old age remains both underdetected and under-treated. This is particularly regrettable in view of its high risk of chronicity, recurrence and suicide, as well as the considerable burden of associated health care costs. Despite the availability of a variety of physical and psychological treatment options of well-established efficacy, there is little recent evidence of improvement in either clinical practice or patient outcome. An understanding of the principles of management of depression in elderly patients requires some knowledge of the differences between such patients and their younger counterparts. The clinical presentation and diagnosis of depression in old age, its epidemiology and prognosis are reviewed briefly below, before focusing on the practicalities of treatment.

The importance of improving detection and management of depression in old age (particularly in the primary care setting) has been highlighted by the publication, under the auspices of the 'Defeat Depression' campaign, of a consensus statement on recognition and management of depression in late life in general practice (Katona *et al*, 1995). The key points of the statement are summarised in Box 1.

Assessing depression

Depression may present in less obvious ways in older people, probably reflecting a combination of cultural factors, pathoplastic effects of ageing and differences between birth cohorts. This provides some explanation for its underdetection, although failure by patients to acknowledge their own depression (or to be aware of its potential for treatment) may also be important. Presentations with prominent lethargy or hypochondriacal complaints are common. Both phobic and generalised anxiety disorders (but not panic disorder) frequently coexist with depression in older people (Katona *et al*, 1997). 'Neurotic' complaints such as subjective nervousness and irritability may also reflect

underlying depression. The distraught, 'importuning' elderly patient with depression may present a particularly difficult challenge to the tolerance as well as the diagnostic skills of the clinician. Formal comparisons of symptom pattern between older and younger patients with established diagnoses of depression show the former to have greater initial insomnia, agitation and hypochondriasis but less depersonalisation, suicidal intent and loss of libido. Crucially, depressed mood is frequently not reported by elderly people who otherwise have all the clinical features of depression. This may be as a result of alexithymia (the inability of patients to verbalise or fantasise affective experience) or of rigid defense mechanisms. A further diagnostic trap is presented by the pattern of 'affective flattening', characterised by unchanging facial expressions, reduced motility, lack of eye contact or expressive gestures, loss of emotional reactivity, and monotonal voice. This presentation is particularly characteristic of depression in older people in residential care and in those with severe coexistent physical illness –

Box 1. Consensus statement on recognition and management of depression in late life in general practice

Depression is harder to diagnose in old age

Its prevalence is higher in general practice surgery attenders than in community samples

Risk is increased by poor health and life events

Ageist attitudes may impede appropriate management

Physical and psychological treatments are as effective as earlier in life

Depression in old age is a relapsing condition and must be monitored closely

---

both representing circumstances associated with increased risk of developing depression. The most important differences in presentation between older and younger depressed patients are summarised in Box 2.

An issue of particular importance in assessment is the question of suicide risk. Although the absolute numbers of elderly suicides in the UK are relatively low and the suicide rates in young men have recently risen dramatically, the highest suicide rates are still in men aged over 65. The relationship between depression and both suicide and attempted suicide is also closest in old age. Factors known to be associated with suicide in older people are bereavement, increasing social isolation, deteriorating physical health and pain. Any deliberate act of self-harm in an older person should be taken seriously, with particular attention to the exclusion or treatment of underlying depressive illness.

Is depression in old age amenable to screening?

Since depression in old age is both common and (see below) eminently treatable it is an ideal target for screening and, in particular, for attention within the mandatory over-75 health check that now forms part of the GP contract. Screening instruments designed for use in younger subjects, like the Montgomery–Åsberg Depression Rating Scale (MADRS; Montgomery & Åsberg, 1979) or the Zung Depression Scale (Zung, 1965) may be used, although these have received relatively little formal validation in older subjects. A number of

screening questionnaires for depression have been designed for and validated in elderly subjects. One of these, the Geriatric Depression Scale (GDS; Yesavage *et al*, 1983), has not only been extensively validated but appears to retain its validity in the physically ill elderly. It is quick to administer and highly acceptable to patients and has been recommended for hospital use by the Royal College of Physicians and the British Geriatrics Society and in primary care by the Royal College of General Practitioners. It exists in 30- and 15-item versions. The original 30-item version (with the 15-item version in bold) is shown in the Appendix.

Screening instruments like the GDS are undoubtedly of potential use in avoiding underdetection and undertreatment of depression in old age. It must however be borne in mind that screening alone probably has little or no effect in improving subsequent GP behaviour or patient outcome. Iliffe *et al* (1994) have shown that depression screening in older primary care patients did not have a significant impact either on GP behaviour or on individual patient outcome. The utility of screening would be enhanced enormously by increased public awareness of its potential for treatment and the more widespread adoption of accepted principles for its management. A summary of such principles is provided in the recent consensus statement on depression in old age (Katona *et al*, 1995).

Subtypes of depression in old age

Conventional diagnostic subtypings of depression, such as 'endogenous/non-endogenous' or 'severe/mild' appear less appropriate in elderly depressed patients. A much higher proportion of older patients are classified as 'endogenous' than would be the case for depression earlier in adult life and agreement between diagnostic systems over the endogenous/non-endogenous distinction is poor in older depressed subjects. The severe/mild distinction may also be less informative in old age. In a large community survey, subjects fulfilling criteria for dysthymia (chronic mild depression) according to DSM–III (American Psychiatric Association, 1980) had HDRS scores very similar to those with major depression. A classification of depression in old age based on age at first onset may be more informative (Alexopoulos, 1989). Subjects becoming depressed for the first time in late life are less likely to have first-degree relatives with depression. In addition, late first onset has been reported to be associated with more frequent cognitive impairment, lower treatment response, magnetic resonance imaging (MRI) signal intensities and 'silent' cerebral infarction (Fujikawa *et al*, 1996;

Box 2. **Differences in clinical features of depression between older and younger people**

More common in old age:
  Anxiety
  Insomnia
  Agitation
  Hypochondriasis
  Lethargy
  Irritability

Less common in old age:
  Depressed mood
  Depersonalisation
  Overt suicidal ideation

Krishnan *et al*, 1997). This has lead to the suggestion that some older patients should be considered to suffer from 'vascular depression'.

Prevalence

Estimates of the prevalence of depression in elderly people have varied widely, reflecting differences in sample selection, screening instruments and caseness criteria. In particular, studies using criteria designed for and field-tested in younger subjects usually report high levels of depressive symptomatology in old age, but very low prevalence rates for major depression. These anomalous results have encouraged the development of diagnostic interviews and diagnostic algorithms specifically for the elderly, of which the most widely used is the Geriatric Mental Status Schedule (GMS; Copeland *et al*, 1986). Studies using the GMS are much more consistent and suggest a community prevalence (for depression sufficiently severe not to be out of place in a psychiatric out-patient clinic) of about 15% (Katona, 1994*a*). As in younger subjects, the prevalence of depression is higher (by a factor of 1.5) in women than in men. Some studies suggest increasing prevalence with increasing age, but this probably reflects concomitant physical illness (discussed below) rather than a direct age effect.

Prevalence rates drawn from community samples are likely to underestimate the scale of the problem since there is consistent evidence for much higher rates in institutional care. Depression is particularly likely to be missed in an institutional setting in which apathy, agitation and irritability are liable to be misinterpreted as part of a dementing illness.

Elderly primary care attenders also appear to have higher prevalence rates for depression (Macdonald, 1986), suggesting that frequent surgery visits (usually with predominantly physical symptomatology) are a characteristic behaviour pattern in elderly people with depression.

Depression and physical illness

Studies in community, primary care and general hospital samples all suggest that depression is about twice as common in physically ill than in healthy elderly subjects. The main predictors of depression in the physically ill elderly appear to be positive psychiatric history and severity of the physical illness itself.

Depression in elderly medical patients may have an adverse effect on physical prognosis. Associations have been reported with increased length of admission, poor rehabilitation, increased risk of transfer to residential care and increased mortality. Coexistent depression may also distort elderly patients' attitudes to life-sustaining medical therapy, and its presence should always be excluded in patients refusing such treatment.

Depression in elderly medical patients is frequently missed. Rapp *et al* (1988) found that fewer than 10% of a series of depressed medical in-patients were correctly recognised by house physicians. Screening questionnaires such as the GDS may be particularly useful in medical settings.

The management of depression in physically ill elderly patients is particularly difficult. Tricyclic antidepressants (TCAs) are frequently contra-indicated and, where used, are associated with particularly high side-effect rates. Clinical trials have been few and small.

Depression in people with dementia

Wragg & Jeste (1989) have reviewed several studies examining depressive symptoms and signs in people with established Alzheimer's disease; they reported a median prevalence for depressed mood of 41% and for depressive disorder of 19%. Most studies suggested a higher prevalence of depression than in control subjects without dementia. Depression may present prodromally as well as in established dementia. Severe depression may also present with a dementia-like picture (depressive pseudo-dementia) initially responsive to treatment but with a high subsequent risk of true dementia. Depression may be difficult to assess in patients with severe dementia because of their loss of verbal skills. A number of rating scales, such as the Cornell Scale (Alexopoulos *et al*, 1988) have been devised, utilising informant history to supplement patient interview and clinical observation. Depression is clinically important in established dementia since it may result in increased behavioural disturbance and loss of daily living skills. Antidepressant treatment in such patients may improve cognitive function as well as depressive symptoms.

Prognosis

Depression in old age is associated with high chronicity and a considerable risk of relapse even after recovery. Cole (1990) systematically reviewed 10 follow-up studies, the combined results showing that although 60% of subjects remained well or had relapses with recovery, about 25% developed chronic depression. Elderly patients with depression have a mortality rate approximately double that found in age- and gender-matched community subjects. At least some of the excess appears to be related directly to the depression since it remains apparent after allowance is made for concurrent physical illness (Murphy *et al*, 1988).

Several factors have been identified as being of prognostic significance within depression in old age. Notable among these are the negative effects of poor physical health and the positive ones of appropriate treatment.

General principles of management

Depression as identified in community surveys is hardly ever treated. Community studies have reported that as few as 4% of patients with depression receive appropriate treatment (Copeland *et al*, 1992). Treatment is almost as unlikely to occur in general practice attenders with depression, with rates as low as 10% reported (Macdonald, 1986) even though the GPs are almost invariably able to recognise their patients' depression on direct questioning.

The first challenge is therefore to break down attitudes in patient and doctor alike which mitigate against treatment being instituted. These include lack of public awareness that depression, even in old age, is a distinct and treatable illness. 'Ageist' medical beliefs to be addressed include the notions that misery is a legitimate response to becoming old, that older people are mentally too rigid to benefit from psychological intervention and that drugs are too hazardous for 'frail' elderly people.

All the treatment options relevant to depression earlier in life remain effective in old age and, as in younger people, may be more effective combined than in isolation. Drug treatments are most widely available and are most frequently used as 'first-line' management, particularly in primary care. Their use should not, however, preclude consideration of psychological treatments, particularly cognitive behavioural therapy (CBT) and electroconvulsive therapy (ECT).

Drug treatment

Although the same principles of antidepressant drug treatment apply as for younger patients, several particular problems (relating mainly to age-related changes in drug handling and in cognitive function) need to be considered when planning the treatment of individual older patients.

Antidepressant drugs currently in use include: 'older' drugs such as TCAs, related heterocyclic antidepressants (mianserin, maprotiline) and monoamine oxidase inhibitors (MAOIs); a relatively newly introduced TCA (lofepramine); the selective serotonin reuptake inhibitors (SSRIs); and a novel MAOI, moclobemide. The evidence regarding the efficacy and tolerability of these groups will be discussed, with particular emphasis on the question of whether the advantages of the newer drugs in elderly patients might be sufficient to outweigh their higher cost.

Efficacy

Controlled antidepressant trials in the elderly published up to 1986 have been reviewed by Gerson *et al* (1988) and those between 1987 and 1992 by Anstey & Brodaty (1995). TCAs such as amitriptyline and clomipramine and the heterocyclic antidepressants such as mianserin and trazodone have established efficacy in older patients as does the MAOI phenelzine. Similar efficacy is also evident for SSRIs and for moclobemide. Placebo-controlled evidence is relatively scant, although some evidence is available for a number of TCAs (nortriptyline, imipramine, amitriptyline), for the MAOI iproniazid and for the SSRIs citalopram, fluvoxamine and fluoxetine. Overall, all antidepressant drugs formally evaluated in the elderly seem effective in 50–60% of patients with, in particular, no clear difference in efficacy between 'older' and 'newer' drugs (Mittman *et al*, 1997).

Caution must be used in extrapolating the results of such trials to routine practice, since trials only include patients with relatively severe depression (sufficient to warrant a diagnosis of major depression) who are also physically fit enough to be free of contraindications. Virtually no antidepressant trials have examined very old (aged 80+) samples since such patients, while remaining an important treatment target in clinical practice, almost invariably fulfil one or more of the exclusion criteria for drug trials. Clinical experience suggests however that antidepressant efficacy is similar to that in clinical trial populations.

Tolerability

Elderly patients are particularly likely to suffer side-effects when taking TCAs or MAOIs and are more vulnerable to serious adverse consequences as a result. The most important of these side-effects are shown in Box 3. Perhaps most crucial is the fact that elderly patients are more vulnerable to accidents, particularly to falls, which in turn carry an increased risk of osteoporosis-related long bone fracture. This relates mainly to the drugs' potency

---

Box 3. Side-effects of tricyclic antidepressants of particular relevance in older patients

Anticholinergic
Confusion
Urinary retention
Precipitation/worsening of glaucoma
Blurring of vision

Antihistamine
Sedation

Antiadrenergic
Postural hypotension
Dizziness
Falls

---

in blocking α_1-adrenergic receptors, thereby exacerbating postural hypotension, which is often present anyway in old age. The antihistaminic effect of most TCAs renders them sedating, which may be helpful in agitated depression, but may also worsen cognitive function and further increase vulnerability to falls and accidents.

Age-related decreases in protein synthesis can increase free plasma TCA levels, as may reduced creatinine clearance and hepatic blood flow. Inter-individual variability in blood levels is, however, considerable in elderly as well as younger subjects and (with the exception of nortriptyline which has a well-established optimal therapeutic range) titration to maximum tolerated dose may be as necessary in elderly as in younger subjects, though the average dose required will be smaller.

It should, however, be remembered that while the above considerations are broadly applicable to TCAs (and also to heterocyclic antidepressants and MAOIs), not all of these drugs have identical side-effect profiles. Lofepramine, for example, has a conventional tricyclic structure but appears in both in-vitro studies and trials in non-elderly subjects to be relatively free of anticholinergic side-effects and to cause significantly less impairment in cognitive functioning. However, the cost of treatment with lofepramine is much higher than that of most other TCAs and approaches the cost of SSRIs.

Age-associated pharmacokinetic and pharmaco-dynamic changes are, in general, less clinically important for newer antidepressants, most of which can be administered in the same dose to elderly as to younger patients. SSRIs and moclobemide are also relatively free of anticholinergic effects and cardiotoxicity, and cause much less postural hypotension than TCAs and MAOIs. The main

side-effects of the SSRIs, as in younger patients, are headache and nausea. The reviews by Anstey & Brodaty (1995) and Mittman *et al* (1997) examine the overall and adverse effect-related withdrawal data from several trials comparing newer antidepressants (mainly SSRIs, but also moclobemide) with TCAs and/or heterocyclic antidepressants in elderly patients with depression. Several of these trials report lower withdrawal rates in the SSRI (or moclobemide) groups, although in most of the studies the differences are quite modest. Anstey & Brodaty and Mittman *et al* emphasise the methodological limitations of the data as reported in the published trials. 'Fitness to treat' on the basis of datasheet indications is another measure of tolerability which can be applied in more representative populations. A study by Mullan *et al* (1994) suggested that a higher proportion of elderly patients are fit to take SSRIs than TCAs, reflecting their relatively few contraindications.

Practical aspects of treating older patients with antidepressants

Adherence to treatment with antidepressants is often problematic in old age. This reflects higher vulnerability to troublesome side-effects, particularly in the context of comorbid physical illness and coadministration of other drugs with potential adverse interactions. The onset of therapeutic action may take even longer in the elderly, with useful effects sometimes only emerging in the 7th and 8th week of treatment. Patients unaware of such response delay can hardly be blamed for stopping taking tablets which make them feel worse.

The new generation of antidepressant drugs represent a modest step forward in the treatment of depression in elderly patients. This relates mainly to a reduction in practical problems associated with their use in relatively frail patients which may enable a higher proportion of such patients to be treated effectively (Mullan *et al*, 1994). The question of whether such superiority is sufficient in cost–benefit terms to justify their use as first-line drugs for depression in old age remains open.

Psychological treatments

It is widely thought that elderly people are not amenable to psychological treatments because their 'mental set' is too rigid to be amenable to therapeutic change. Controlled trials of cognitive, psycho-dynamic and behavioural treatments, however, reveal them to have similar magnitudes of effect to those found in younger depressed patients. The psychotherapeutic focus may be different to that in younger patients, often concentrating on the losses to which older people are particularly vulnerable (bereavement, physical health, financial security etc.) and on fears of impending death.

The best efficacy evidence (Koder *et al*, 1996) is for CBT, which has been shown to be an effective treatment for depression in older subjects in a group setting as well as individually, and may thus be economically viable as well as effective in older people. CBT in old age has also been found superior to less specific therapies such as craft or music groups. Depression in old age is associated with the same pattern of negative cognitions (about self, the world and the future) as earlier in life, and a similar cognitive shift with CBT has also been demonstrated.

Electroconvulsive therapy

Although widely used in old age, ECT remains a particularly controversial treatment option in this age group because of concerns about its safety and about the validity of consent procedures. There is no denying that ECT is less safe in old age than in younger people, but this comparison is irrelevant: the crucial issue is the safety of ECT compared with other treatments or to leaving depression in old age untreated. The safety profile of ECT in the elderly is in fact surprisingly good. It should, however, be borne in mind that such safety relies on good liaison with the anaesthetist. For example, it may be appropriate to delay the procedure until the patient's physical condition is optimised.

The efficacy of ECT in old age is beyond doubt. Mulsant *et al* (1991) carried out a meta-analysis of 1025 elderly patients receiving ECT in 14 separate studies and reported a favourable outcome in 83%, with full recovery in 62%. This is at least as good an acute response as can be expected in younger patients. ECT may be effective in a broader range of older than younger patients with depression. In contrast with what would be expected earlier in life, prominent comorbid anxiety is associated with a good response to ECT.

ECT is a particularly important treatment option in elderly patients unresponsive to antidepressants and in those with very severe illnesses. It may be lifesaving in patients who are acutely suicidal and those who, in the context of depressive retardation or stupor, have stopped eating and drinking. Particular care must be taken to ensure that the consent obtained is properly informed and that patient and relatives' anxieties about the procedure are fully addressed.

Elderly patients treated with ECT appear to have a surprisingly favourable long-term prognosis; one study (Godber *et al*, 1987) reported 59% of subjects entirely well at three-year follow-up; most of the remainder (29%) had only mild residual symptoms and only 3% had either died or developed a dementia. ECT does not in itself provide any protection against depressive relapse except if given monthly as 'maintenance', a procedure seldom used in the elderly because of increased risk of cumulative memory side-effects. The question of prophylactic treatment (reviewed below) should not be forgotten in patients with a good acute response to ECT.

There is less evidence in old age for bilateral electrode placement being more effective (though this may simply reflect a lack of studies) but unilateral electrode placement is, in the elderly, clearly associated with a reduction in the cognitive side-effects (acute confusion and loss of recent memory) to which older people receiving ECT are particularly vulnerable.

Refractory depression

In patients failing to respond to first-line treatment, a full review of the appropriateness and adequacy (in terms of dosage, duration and adherence) of such a treatment trial should be undertaken. Where appropriate, psychological treatments and/or ECT should be considered. Depression is particularly likely to become refractory in the context of coexistent organic brain disease, particularly cerebral infarction (Fujikawa *et al*, 1996; Baldwin & Simpson, 1997).

The many drug combination treatments used in younger patients have received little evaluation in elderly subjects in whom they are also more likely to be hazardous. Lithium augmentation and, to a lesser extent, MAOIs have, however, shown promise in open studies of resistant depression in old age. It must however be borne in mind that older people (particularly those with comorbid dementia and/or Parkinson's disease) are particularly vulnerable to lithium neurotoxicity. Where lithium is used, the initial dose should be low (100–200 mg/day) with gradual dosage titration to achieve blood levels within a downward-adjusted therapeutic range (0.4–0.8 mmol/l). A wide variety of pharmacological augmentation strategies have been subjected to limited clinical evaluation in older subjects; these are reviewed by Flint & Rifat (1995).

Continuation treatment

As discussed above, depression in old age is a relapsing condition and recovered patients should be monitored closely. In a placebo-controlled study of dothiepin (Old Age Depression Interest Group, 1993) the relapse rate over two years was reduced by a factor of 2.5 in the dothiepin group. Most other antidepressants so far evaluated appear to have similar prophylactic efficacy; these are reviewed by Katona (1994*b*) and include a placebo-controlled trial of phenelzine and open studies of fluoxetine, doxepin and lithium.

Other treatments may also result in low relapse rates. These include CBT in several of the studies reviewed by Morris & Morris (1991) and supportive psychotherapy. A recent four-arm randomised comparison of nortriptyline and interpersonal psychotherapy (both separately and in combination) against placebo over three years attests to the effectiveness both of the combination and of nortryptiline alone (Reynolds *et al*, 1999). Ong *et al* (1987) randomly allocated 20 elderly in-patients with depression at the point of recovery and discharge to attend a psychotherapy support group or to act as controls. In the subsequent nine months, none of those in the psychotherapy group had to be readmitted, compared with six out of the 10 in the control group.

It should be emphasised that the case for continued antidepressants is based on evidence from relatively severe, hospital treated patients and it must also be borne in mind that long-term use of antidepressants can pose problems as physical health deteriorates with increasing age. As far as milder depression responsive to antidepressants is concerned, the conclusion of the consensus statement on recognition and management of depression in late life in general practice (Katona *et al*, 1995) is that they should continue on the same dose of antidepressant to which they responded for at least six months. Following this, antidepressant treatment may be tapered slowly. In view of the high risk of depressive recurrence in older people, opportunistic monitoring of mood and questioning about symptoms associated with depression should form part of any subsequent clinical contact with a patient who has recovered from a depressive ilness in old age.

Conclusions

Despite being both common and life-threatening, depression in old age is hardly ever treated. A variety of treatments (particularly antidepressants, CBT and ECT) have, however, been shown to be effective, despite the particular challenges to be met in treating such a relatively vulnerable group. Specific treatments should be considered within an overall treatment plan rather than used in isolation. Even in apparently treatment-resistant cases, the response to more aggressive treatment approaches can be

gratifying and not necessarily associated with excessive hazard. The high risk of recurrence of depression in old age can be significantly reduced by close monitoring and the judicious use of prophylactic treatments.

Appendix

The Geriatric Depression Scale

30-item version score 1 for answers in capitals.
0–10: not depressed; 11–20: mild depression; 21–30: severe depression.
15-item version in bold. 0–5: not depressed; 6–15: depressed.

Are you basically satisfied with your life?	**yes/NO**
Have you dropped many of your activities and interests?	**YES/no**
Do you feel that your life is empty?	**YES/no**
Do you often get bored?	**YES/no**
Are you hopeful about the future?	yes/NO
Are you bothered by thoughts you can't get out of your head?	YES/no
Are you in good spirits most of the time?	**yes/NO**
Are you afraid that something bad is going to happen to you?	**YES/no**
Do you feel happy most of the time?	**yes/NO**
Do you often feel helpless?	**YES/no**
Do you often get restless and fidgety?	YES/no
Do you prefer to stay at home, rather than going out and doing new things?	**YES/no**
Do you frequently worry about the future?	YES/no
Do you feel you have more problems with memory than most?	**YES/no**
Do you think it is wonderful to be alive now?	**yes/NO**
Do you often feel downhearted and blue?	YES/no
Do you feel pretty worthless the way you are now?	**YES/no**
Do you worry a lot about the past?	YES/no
Do you find life very exciting?	yes/NO
Is it hard for you to get started on new projects?	YES/no

Do you feel full of energy?	**yes/NO**
Do you feel that your situation is hopeless?	**YES/no**
Do you think that most people are better off than you are?	**YES/no**
Do you frequently get upset over little things?	YES/no
Do you frequently feel like crying?	YES/no
Do you have trouble concentrating?	YES/no
Do you enjoy getting up in the morning?	yes/NO
Do you prefer to avoid social gatherings?	YES/no
Is it easy for you to make decisions?	yes/NO
Is your mind as clear as it used to be?	yes/NO

GDS, reprinted with permission from *Journal of Psychiatric Research*, Vol. 17, Yesavage *et al*, 1983 'The Geriatric Depression Scale'. Oxford: Elsevier Science Ltd.

References

Alexopoulos, G. S. (1989). Biological abnormalities in late life depression. *Journal of Geriatric Psychiatry*, **22**, 25–34.

——, Abrams, R. C., Young, R. C., *et al* (1988) Cornell Scale for depression in dementia. *Biological Psychiatry*, **23**, 271–284.

American Psychiatric Association (1980) *Diagnostic and Statistical Manual of Mental Disorders* (3rd edn) (DSM–III). Washington, DC: APA.

Anstey, K. & Brodaty, H. (1995) Antidepressants and the elderly: double-blind trials 1987–1992. *International Journal of Geriatric Psychiatry*, **10**, 265–279.

Baldwin, R. C. & Simpson, S. (1997) Treatment-resistant depression in the elderly. A review of its conceptualisation, management and relationship to organic brain disease. *Journal of Affective Disorders*, **46**, 163–173.

Cole, M. G. (1990) The prognosis of depression in the elderly. *Canadian Medical Association Journal*, **142**, 633–639.

Copeland, J. R. M., Dewey, M. E. & Griffith-Jones, H. M. (1986) A computerised psychiatric diagnostic system and case nomenclature for elderly subjects: GMS and AGECAT. *Psychological Medicine*, **16**, 89–99.

——, Davidson, I. A., Dewey, M. E., *et al* (1992) Alzheimer's disease, other dementias, depression and pseudo dementia: prevalence, incidence and three-year outcome in Liverpool. *British Journal of Psychiatry*, **161**, 230–239.

Flint, A. & Rifat, S. (1995) Augmentation strategies in refractory depression. *International Journal of Geriatric Psychiatry*, **10**, 137–146.

Fujikawa, T., Yokota, N., Muraoka, M., *et al* (1996) Response of patients with major depression and silent cerebral infarction to antidepressant drug therapy, with emphasis on central nervous system adverse reactions. *Stroke*, **27**, 2040–2042.

Gerson, S. C., Plotkin, D. A. & Jarvik, L. F. (1988) Antidepressant drug studies 1946 to 1986: empirical evidence for aging patients. *Journal of Clinical Psychopharmacology*, **8**, 311–322.

Godber, C., Rosenvinge, H., Wilkinson, D., *et al* (1987) Depression in old age: prognosis after ECT. *International Journal of Geriatric Psychiatry*, **2**, 19–24.

Iliffe, S., Mitchley, S., Gould, M., *et al* (1994) Evaluation of the use of brief screening instruments for dementia, depression and problem drinking among elderly people in general practice. *British Journal of General Practice*, **388**, 503–508.

Katona, C. L. E. (1994a) The epidemiology of depression in old age. In *Depression in Old Age* (ed. C. L. E. Katona), pp. 30–41. Chichester: Wiley.

——— (1994b) The prognosis of depression in old age. In *Depression in Old Age* (ed. C. L. E. Katona), pp. 123–140. Chichester: Wiley.

——, Freeling, P., Hinchliffe, K., *et al* (1995) Recognition and management of depression in late life in general practice: consensus statement. *Primary Care Psychiatry*, **1**, 107–113.

——, Manela, M. & Livingston, G. (1997) Comorbidity with depression in older people: the Islington Study. *Aging and Mental Health*, **1**, 57–61.

Koder, D.-A., Brodaty, H. & Anstey, K. J. (1996) Cognitive therapy for depression in the elderly. *International Journal of Geriatric Psychiatry*, **11**, 97–107.

Krishnan, K. R. R., Hays, J. C. & Blazer, D. G. (1997) MRI-defined vascular depression. *American Journal of Psychiatry*, **154**, 497–501.

Macdonald, A. J. D. (1986) Do general practitioners "miss" depression in elderly patients? *British Medical Journal*, **292**, 1365–1367.

Mittman, N., Hermann, N., Einarson, T. R., *et al* (1997) The efficacy, safety and tolerability of antidepressants in late-life depression: a meta-analysis. *Journal of Affective Disorders*, **46**, 191–217.

Montgomery, S. A. & Åsberg, M. (1979) A new depression scale designed to be sensitive to change. *British Journal of Psychiatry*, **134**, 382–389.

Morris, R. G. & Morris, L. W. (1991) Cognitive and behavioural approaches with the depressed elderly. *International Journal of Geriatric Psychiatry*, **6**, 407–413.

Mullan, E., Katona, P., D'Ath, P., *et al* (1994) Screening, detection and management of depression in elderly primary care attenders. 2. Detection and fitness for treatment: a case record study. *Family Practice*, **11**, 267–270.

Mulsant, B. H., Rosen, J., Thornton, J. E., *et al* (1991) A prospective naturalistic study of electroconvulsive therapy in late-life depression. *Journal of Geriatric Psychiatry and Neurology*, **4**, 3–13.

Murphy, E., Smith, R., Lindesay, J., *et al* (1988) Increased mortality rates in late-life depression. *British Journal of Psychiatry*, **152**, 347–353.

Old Age Depression Interest Group (1993) How long should the elderly take antidepressants? A double-blind placebo-controlled study of continuation/prophylaxis therapy with dothiepin. *British Journal of Psychiatry*, **162**, 175–182.

Ong, Y. K., Martineau, F., Lloyd, C., *et al* (1987) A support group for the depressed elderly. *International Journal of Geriatric Psychiatry*, **2**, 119–123.

Rapp, S. R., Walsh, D. A., Parisi, S. A., *et al* (1988) Detecting depression in elderly medical in-patients. *Journal of Consulting and Clinical Psychology*, **56**, 509–513.

Reynolds, C. F., Frank, E., Perel, J. M., *et al* (1999) Nortriptyline and interpersonal psychotherapy as maintenance therapies for recurrent major depression: a randomised controlled trial in patients older than 59 years. *Journal of the American Medical Association*, **281**, 39–45.

Wragg, R. E. & Jeste, D. V. (1989) Overview of depression and psychosis in Alzheimer's disease. *American Journal of Psychiatry*, **146**, 577–586.

Yesavage, J. A., Brink, T. L., Rose, T. L., *et al* (1983) Development and validation of a Geriatric Depression Screening Scale: a preliminary report. *Journal of Psychiatric Research*, **17**, 37–49.

Zung, W. W. K. (1965) A self-rating depression scale. *Archives of General Psychiatry*, **12**, 63–70.

Emergency treatment of depression

Richard Porter & Nicol Ferrier

Psychiatric emergencies are common and each case presents particular problems and difficulties. This chapter focuses on one subset of psychiatric emergencies, that of severe depression, and on the role of and use of antidepressant treatments in these conditions. The clinical situations to be discussed in this chapter include active suicidality, severe psychomotor retardation (with associated problems of hydration and nutrition), affective psychosis, bipolar depression and behavioural disturbance.

All these situations require careful assessment, frequent monitoring and involvement of carers and the multi-disciplinary team. The setting in which treatment should take place and the role of admission, the Mental Health Act, observation and the medical needs of patients with depression in these situations are important, but are beyond the scope of this chapter. All patients in emergency situations need careful, sympathetic and empathic handling and, on occasions, firm guidance. Supportive psychotherapy is useful, but the role of specific psychotherapeutic techniques in these situations is not clear. It seems likely that such patients require both the instillation of hope and the skilled challenging of negative thoughts or guilty ruminations. There is a clear need for nursing research on the benefits and utility of such approaches.

Treatments

There is a long-standing view that there is a lag period of 2–3 weeks to a significant benefit of antidepressant treatment compared with placebo. This has been challenged by Parker (1996) who argued that early responses to antidepressants may be obscured by a number of factors inherent in clinical trials. For instance, in clinical trials, a positive treatment effect in some individuals may be obscured by a number of non-responding patients. Parker further argues that in cases where there is no early response: "the dose may be insufficient or that particular drug may be ineffective". We would argue that the treatments for which there is evidence of an 'earlier' onset of antidepressant action have in common either early high doses or a broad spectrum of pharmacological activity. Such regimes may induce a more rapid response in a significant proportion of patients if used more commonly.

Electroconvulsive therapy

Although double-blind comparisons with placebo or other antidepressants have not directly addressed the issue of early response, there is evidence to support the widely held clinical impression that electroconvulsive therapy (ECT) often results in a relatively rapid antidepressant effect. How rapid this effect is varies considerably between patients, but a substantial and sustained improvement has been demonstrated after 1–3 treatments (Rodger et al, 1994) with nearly maximum improvement in some patients after two weeks of ECT three times a week (Post et al, 1987). This makes ECT useful in emergency situations and it seems to work particularly well in situations which are likely to be emergencies, such as psychomotor retardation and psychosis. It has been suggested that it is only effective in these situations (Buchan et al, 1992), but more recent evidence has challenged this (Sobin et al, 1996), suggesting an early improvement in all subtypes of major depression. It should, therefore, be considered as a possible first-line treatment in all emergency situations (see Box 1).

Stimulation of dopaminergic pathways may give rise to an early antidepressant response, and ECT gives rise to an acute increase in levels of dopamine and its metabolites and an increase in baseline levels following chronic administration. This may be a factor in its rapid onset of antidepressant effect.

The factors that influence speed of response include frequency of administration, electrode

---

Box 1.   ECT in emergencies

ECT works well in patients with psychosis or psychomotor retardation

ECT acts rapidly

Bilateral high-dose therapy three times a week is probably fastest but also causes most cognitive side-effects

Twice weekly high-dose unilateral treatment is slower but gives an adequate response with fewer cognitive side-effects

ECT is safe in most situations

---

placement and electrical dose administered. There is a general consensus that the side-effects of ECT administered more frequently than three times a week outweigh any benefits, even in extreme emergencies. Multiple induction of fits has also been abandoned. The question of whether to give ECT two or three times a week is more difficult. Speed of response is more rapid with ECT treatment three times a week (Shapira *et al*, 1998), but cognitive effects are more severe and there is no difference in final outcome. A three-times-a-week schedule is therefore only indicated in situations where rapid response is particularly crucial. Since treatments early in a treatment course seem to give rise to a proportionally greater degree of improvement than later treatments (Segman *et al*, 1995), there may be logic in giving three treatments in the first week and then reverting to a twice weekly schedule.

There is evidence that bilateral therapy works more quickly than unilateral therapy given an equivalent electrical dose (Sackeim *et al*, 1993). However, the cognitive side-effects of bilateral therapy are more severe. Where unilateral ECT is used, it now appears clear that the 'Lancaster' unilateral electrode position (as demonstrated on old ECT wallcharts) does not achieve sufficiently wide separation of the electrodes. Electrode placement should be in the d'Elia position (d'Elia, 1970) as demonstrated in the *Official Video Teaching Pack* of the Royal College of Psychiatrists' Special Committee on ECT (1994).

The electrical dose necessary to induce a generalised seizure varies considerably between patients (Sackeim *et al*, 1987). There is evidence that it is not the absolute electrical dose administered, but the dose above seizure threshold which is important (Sackeim *et al*, 1993), not only in producing a

response, but also in determining the speed of response. Dose titration can be used to determine the seizure threshold. This can be done using a variety of different protocols depending on the type of machine used (Lock, 1995). Sackeim *et al* (1993) showed, in a double-blind placebo-controlled trial, that for both unilateral and bilateral treatment, high-dose therapy resulted in a significantly quicker antidepressant response. In this study, low dose was close to seizure threshold and high dose was 2.5 times seizure threshold. High-dose therapy also resulted in significantly greater cognitive side-effects. There is little evidence regarding speed of response for even higher electrical doses. Low-dose unilateral therapy not only results in a significantly poorer early response but also in an overall poor response and despite reduced cognitive side-effects cannot therefore be recommended.

Evidence regarding seizure length is equivocal. Some patients appear to do well despite short seizures, but others do not. Every effort should be made to achieve adequate seizure length (at least 20 seconds) in the emergency situation. In addition, care should be taken to ensure that a seizure occurs at every treatment. This may be a particular problem when patients are being treated with large doses of benzodiazepines for agitation or violence. Long-acting benzodiazepines should be avoided if possible when ECT is being administered. Neuroleptics are generally proconvulsant and therefore better in this situation. Where a hypnotic is required during an emergency course of ECT, we recommend a short-acting hypnotic such as zolpidem (mean half-life 2.4 hours) which is unlikely to affect seizure threshold the following morning. If anticonvulsants are being used as mood stabilisers or to augment antidepressant effect, they may need to be discontinued while the ECT is in progress. It should be remembered, however, that the relapse rate is high following ECT and that it may be prudent to recommence these agents as soon as a course is completed. If, despite these measures, adequate fits cannot be induced, caffeine augmentation may be used (Lurie & Coffey, 1990).

Since emergency situations are more common where there is coexisting physical illness, safety of treatment is an important factor. However, with advances in the practise of ECT, it is increasingly possible to treat patients effectively and safely in virtually every situation. The American Psychiatric Association (1990) Task Force on ECT Report and the Royal College of Psychiatrists' *ECT Handbook* (Royal College of Psychiatrists, 1995) cite no 'absolute contraindications' to ECT. In particular, it has been shown that ECT can be used relatively safely in the elderly, in patients with cardiac abnormalities and even during pregnancy.

In summary, ECT is a rapid effective treatment for all forms of depression, but particularly in the emergency situations of psychosis and psychomotor retardation. It is safe for most patients, including the elderly. Maximum speed of response can be obtained using treatment three times a week, bilateral electrode placement and high-dose electrical stimulation, but this schedule gives rise to greater cognitive side-effects than more conservative schedules. We therefore only recommend this in dire emergencies, for instance when patients are dehydrated, stuporose or extremely suicidal. In less pressing situations we concur with the suggestion of Lock (1995) that unilateral ECT in a dose of 100–200% above seizure threshold should be used or, where staff are relatively inexperienced, bilateral ECT in a dose of 50–100% above seizure threshold.

Antidepressant pharmacotherapy

Speed of onset

Most antidepressant medications increase the activity of the serotonergic or the noradrenergic systems in the brain. They frequently also have effects on other transmitter systems. There is a widely held belief that these agents have a time lag of two weeks before they have an effect which is greater than placebo. However, this is based on clinical trials which often do not make repeated early measurements (and there is a dearth of reliable instruments to do this task) and in which an initial improvement in some patients may be masked by a number of non-responders. Various methods of analysis have been employed to attempt to overcome this problem and have been used in attempting to determine which treatments, if any, have an advantage in terms of speed of action. This issue has been well reviewed in a publication by the National Institute of Mental Health (1995). Various pharmacological mechanisms have been suggested which may contribute to delay in onset of antidepressant efficacy. β-Adrenoceptor down-regulation occurs in most cases after 2–4 weeks, a time lag which roughly corresponds to the observed onset of action of antidepressant treatments. It has been suggested that this down-regulation may be accelerated by a simultaneous action on both serotonergic and noradrenergic systems (Baron *et al*, 1988). A second suggested mechanism is auto-inhibition by presynaptic 5-HT_{1a} autoreceptors which only down-regulate after chronic treatment with serotonergic agents (Blier *et al*, 1988). This is the basis of strategies such as the use of the 5-HT_{1a} antagonist pindolol to accelerate response. It is now known that there are several other changes in

receptor sensitivity which occur with chronic antidepressant therapy and it seems unlikely that a single mechanism is involved.

Dopamine release or inhibition of its reuptake may result in an early response and may be a factor in the action of ECT and venlafaxine, which at high doses blocks dopamine reuptake. Psychostimulants such as amphetamine or methylphenidate give rise to a transient elevation of mood in a high proportion of patients with depression but there is no evidence that they are effective antidepressants and we would not recommend their use. Similarly L-dopa has proved ineffective apart from promoting a degree of psychomotor activation.

Tricyclic antidepressants (TCAs) have traditionally been the mainstay of acute antidepressant therapy. Claims of a rapid onset of action may often be due to a reduction in the Hamilton Rating Scale for Depression (HAM–D; Hamilton, 1960) score due to sedation. None the less, this side-effect may be particularly useful in agitated depression. The speed of action of TCAs may, however, be reduced if side-effects necessitate slow titration to an adequate dose. They should be used with extreme care in patients at risk of suicide, because of their toxicity in overdose.

It has been claimed that clomipramine has a rapid onset of action, particularly when administered intravenously. The rationale behind this is to avoid the extensive first-pass metabolism, which occurs with TCAs, and thereby achieve an adequate concentration more quickly. Closer examination of the evidence reveals that early oral administration of high doses may well achieve the same aim. Three double-blind trials of intravenous versus oral clomipramine have shown no differences in either response or side-effects. In one of these, patients received two doses of clomipramine (150 mg then 200 mg 24 hours later). Continuous treatment was not initiated for five more days (Pollock et al, 1989). The HAM-D score, five days after pulse-loading, had dropped by a mean of 35%, but with a marked variation in response between individuals. Relatively high concentrations of antidepressant were achieved in this study at an early stage, which may be the crucial factor. Genuine double-blind placebo-controlled trials of intravenous clomipramine are clearly difficult since the immediate side-effects will make it apparent which treatment is being taken and thereby unblind patients. The only recent study to attempt this involved only 16 adolescents and did not adequately address this issue (Sallee *et al*, 1989).

Similar claims have been made of an early response to venlafaxine which has, in common with clomipramine, a combined serotonergic and nor-adrenergic action. It also gives rise to early down-regulation of β-adrenoceptors and, at high dose, dopamine reuptake inhibition. Evidence suggests that a rapid response may only occur when the dose is rapidly escalated. In hospitalised patients with melancholic depression, the response to venlafaxine with doses rapidly escalating to 375 mg/day over five days was compared with the response to imipramine 200 mg (reached over five days; Benkert *et al*, 1996). The response was significantly faster as judged by the HDRS but not by the Montgomery–Åsberg Depression Rating Scale (MADRS; Montgomery & Åsberg, 1979). Another study compared venlafaxine with placebo in hospitalised patients with melancholic depression. High doses of venlafaxine averaging 350 mg/day were used. Venlafaxine provided significantly greater improvement in the MADRS scores after four days and in the HDRS scores after one week than did placebo. It also seems likely that the improvement was clinically significant (Guelfi *et al*, 1995). Further trials in out-patients also demonstrate a consistent early response using a number of different methods of analysis (Derivan *et al*, 1995). This early response may make clomipramine and venlafaxine good candidates in emergencies, especially when ECT is not being considered. Rapid escalation to high dose seems necessary for a rapid response and this is more likely to be tolerated with venlafaxine. However, overall efficacy data should also be considered (see Box 2).

There is no consistent evidence of a rapid response to selective serotonin reuptake inhibitors (SSRIs) or any other of the newer antidepressants.

Efficacy

While SSRIs are generally safer in overdose than TCAs, it has been argued that decreased effectiveness

---

in cases of severe depression may increase the rate of suicide by other means. Individual studies of efficacy give conflicting results. However, several recent meta-analyses have been conducted to examine the data as a whole. Interestingly, different results have been found depending on whether the analysis looks at severe depression (as measured by the HAM–D) or in-patient depression. This is important since the group of patients with severe depression as measured by rating scales is not necessarily the same group as in-patients, in whom there tend to be particularly high rates of melancholia and suicidality (Stage *et al*, 1998). In severe depression, Anderson & Tomenson (1994) found no advantage of TCAs as a group or of any individual TCAs, compared with SSRIs. However, a meta-analysis of 25 in-patient studies with a total of 1377 patients (Anderson, 1998) showed an advantage of TCAs over SSRIs. Looking at individual TCAs compared with all SSRIs, only amitriptyline showed a significantly greater efficacy than SSRIs, with the result for clomipramine being equivocal. One possible reason for the TCA–SSRI difference is the combined serotonergic and noradrenergic activity of amitriptyline and clomipramine. However, the lack of a clear superiority for clomipramine raises the possibility that it is the 5-HT$_2$ blocking properties of amitriptyline (Cusack *et al*, 1994) which confer a benefit in this group of patients. A definitive meta-analysis of the efficacy in in-patients of newer antidepressants such as venlafaxine or mirtazepine is not yet available.

Tolerability

In in-patient studies, meta-analysis showed a significantly higher discontinuation rate due to adverse effects for TCAs compared with SSRIs. Drop-out rates due to treatment failure were equivalent (Anderson, 1998). In out-patients, discontinuation due to side-effects is modestly but significantly more common with TCAs than SSRIs (Martin *et al*, 1997). These data come almost exclusively from short-term controlled trials in which the drop-out rate is probably much less than in the naturalistic clinical setting in the longer term.

Impulsivity

The reported inverse relationship between indices of central serotonin (5-HT) function and indices of impulsivity in human subjects suggests the possibility that enhancement of 5-HT activity with SSRIs and related drugs reduces impulsive behaviour. This may reduce anger, irritability and suicidality in patients with depression. Although several open studies suggest that SSRIs may be useful in

---

> **Box 2.   Antidepressants in emergencies**
>
> **Clomipramine and venlafaxine appear to induce an early antidepressant response when high doses are reached early in treatment**
>
> **Pulse loading may make early high-dose clomipramine more tolerable but there is no clear advantage of the intravenous route**
>
> **The mechanism of this early response is not clear; action on both noradrenergic and serotonergic systems may reduce the number of non-responders**
>
> **Both have proven efficacy in severe depression**

controlling anger attacks in subgroups of patients with depression in whom this is a problem, the only double-blind placebo-controlled trial so far conducted showed no significant difference between placebo and either active agent, and no difference between sertraline and imipramine (Fava *et al*, 1997). Therefore, the superiority of SSRIs in managing impulsive anger is not demonstrated. Likewise, there is no direct evidence that SSRIs specifically reduce the likelihood of impulsive suicide or parasuicide.

Combinations

The possible biological explanations for delay in antidepressant onset have led to at least two clinical strategies. Evidence that the combination of desipramine and fluoxetine leads to a rapid down-regulation of β-adrenoceptors led to a trial of these agents clinically and the suggestion that there was an early clinical response (Nelson *et al*, 1991). This has not yet been demonstrated in a double-blind trial. The combination has also been tried in treatment-resistant depression with equivocal results. There are inherent difficulties in the co-prescription of TCAs and SSRIs as the latter may inhibit tricyclic metabolism giving rise to large increases in TCA blood levels (Nemeroff *et al*, 1996). Pharmacodynamic interactions may also be a problem. If this strategy is to be used effectively in the acute situation, close monitoring of side-effects and TCA blood levels is necessary. The net effect of this combination may be mimicked by the use of antidepressants with combined serotonergic and noradrenergic activity, without the problem of unpredictable interactions.

Augmentation of SSRIs with pindolol has been suggested as a way of overcoming 5-HT$_{1a}$-mediated autoinhibition (Artigas *et al*, 1996). This has shown promising results in open label studies but placebo-controlled trials are currently conflicting. There is evidence that beta-blockers may actually cause depression (Avorn *et al*, 1986). This strategy cannot currently be recommended in emergency situations.

Special situations

Psychotic depression

In the Epidemiologic Catchment Area (ECA) Study (Johnson *et al*, 1991), 14% of subjects who met criteria for major depression had a history of psychotic features. Psychotic symptoms may increase the distress of depression and the risk of suicide may be greater in psychotic than non-psychotic depression (Roose *et al*, 1983). Prompt, effective treatment is therefore necessary. As discussed previously, in true emergencies, ECT is usually the treatment of choice because of its demonstrated speed of action. There has been no published double-blind study comparing ECT and combination antidepressant/antipsychotic treatment prospectively. A meta-analysis of individual studies published from 1959 to 1988 (Parker *et al*, 1992) found ECT to be superior to the combination of antidepressant and antipsychotic medications but different ECT schedules were compared with several different combinations, dosages and durations of medication and the speed of onset was not compared.

Most clinicians would agree that antipsychotics are useful in reducing the acute distress of psychotic depression. There is also good evidence of an advantage in terms of overall response. Several studies have demonstrated a response to the combination of a TCA and a neuroleptic agent after there had been no response to a TCA alone. Spiker *et al* (1985) compared the combination of amitriptyline and perphenazine, amitriptyline alone and perphenazine alone in the treatment of patients with psychotic depression over a five-week period. Seventy-eight per cent of 18 patients treated with the combination responded in contrast to 41% of 17 patients treated with amitriptyline and 19% of 16 patients treated with perphenazine. Seven of the 13 patients who failed to respond to perphenazine were not psychotic at the completion of the study but were still depressed. Atypical antipsychotics, which include central D$_2$-like and 5-HT$_2$ receptor antagonist properties should, in theory, be of therapeutic value in patients with psychotic and depressive symptoms. However, despite encouraging case studies, no double-blind trial has been carried out.

It has been suggested that particularly high doses of neuroleptics may be necessary in psychotic depression. In an open study (Nelson *et al*, 1986), there was a significantly better outcome in a small group of patients taking the equivalent of 45 mg/day perphenazine compared with patients taking less than 32 mg/day. However, we would suggest that higher doses be reserved for treatment-resistant, not emergency, cases.

We would suggest that antipsychotic medication should be used in most cases of acute psychotic depression. When antipsychotic agents are used, care should be taken to monitor for the possible side-effect of akathisia, which has been shown to increase violence (Crowner *et al*, 1990) and possibly also suicide (Sachdev & Loneragan, 1991). This may be a particular problem if antipsychotics are used in combination with serotonergic agents. Care should also be taken when neuroleptics are co-prescribed with antidepressants which inhibit the metabolism of the neuroleptics by the hepatic cytochrome P450 enzyme system. All the SSRIs except fluvoxamine and citalopram are potent inhibitors of cytochrome P450 2D6. Plasma levels of haloperidol have been found to be elevated following the addition of fluoxetine. Fluvoxamine is a potent inhibitor of cytochrome P450 1A2 and has been associated with increased serum concentrations of haloperidol and clozapine (Nemeroff *et al*, 1996).

Retardation and stupor

ECT works particularly well in this situation, especially where patients are unable to take oral medication. Particular attention should be paid to hydration and to the avoidance of complications such as chest infection, dental sepsis, decubitus ulcers and deep vein thrombosis. Intravenous fluids may be necessary.

Where stupor occurs, a history of development of this from a state of psychomotor retardation is often available. If no such history is available, the diagnosis should be reviewed regularly. The differential diagnosis in cases of stupor includes schizophrenia, hysteria and organic causes.

Suicidality

Fawcett *et al* (1990), in a controlled follow-up study of suicide in major affective disorder, reported the following risk factors for suicide within one year: anxiety, panic, insomnia, anhedonia, loss of concentration and alcohol misuse; and for suicide after one year: parasuicide and hopelessness. In addition, patients with stated intent are almost certainly at increased risk and the early morning may be a particularly risky time.

Three points are important when considering treatment. First, clinical experience suggests that early reduction in psychomotor retardation, in severe depression, may give patients the motivation which allows them to act on suicidal impulses or plans. Extreme vigilance should therefore be exercised in this early phase of treatment. Second, as mentioned above, akathisia should be carefully looked for.

Finally, it should be emphasised that studies have, in the past, shown that patients with a history of depression who have committed suicide have often been taking inadequate doses of antidepressants (Myers & Neal, 1978). We would emphasise the importance of identifying patients at risk of suicide and treating vigorously. A recent review confirms the beneficial effect of ECT on suicidality, in the short

term (Prudic & Sackeim, 1999). If antidepressants are used, an adequate dose should be reached early in the course of treatment (see Box 3).

Bipolar depression

Although bipolar depression is a frequent clinical problem, double-blind studies of its treatment are scarce. There is evidence that antidepressants induce mania and also that they may contribute to cycle acceleration in approximately one-quarter of patients (Altshuler *et al*, 1995). Therefore, in non-urgent situations it is usually best to avoid anti-depressants, particularly in high doses. Fluoxetine may be particularly problematic because of its long half-life. Depending on the history it may be possible to contain disturbance with symptomatic treatment while treating with a mood stabiliser. However, in cases of psychomotor retardation, psychosis, suicidality or extreme distress, some form of treatment is necessary. There is preliminary evidence that carbamazepine, sodium valproate, lamotrigine and gabapentin have an antidepressant effect (Post *et al*, 1996).

There is no clear evidence regarding rates of ECT-precipitated mania. ECT may be a good alternative in severe bipolar depression since it is also effective in treating mania. If mania is precipitated, many clinicians simply continue the course of ECT. However, we would advocate caution in the use of ECT since the overall effect on outcome is not known and there is not currently good evidence regarding the effect of ECT on cycle length.

It should also be remembered that depression during mania (dysphoric mania) may be a particularly serious situation since the risk of suicide appears to be much higher (Dilsaver *et al*, 1994). Antidepressants are not likely to be helpful in this

---

Box 3   Risk factors for suicide in depressive illness

Inadequate treatment

Anxiety, panic, insomnia, anhedonia, loss of concentration, alcohol misuse

Parasuicide, hopelessness

Akathisia

Activation early in treatment

situation and lithium appears to be substantially less effective than sodium valproate (Swann *et al*, 1997), which may be the treatment of choice.

Behavioural disturbance

The management of the acutely disturbed patient has been well reviewed by Macpherson *et al* (1998). Little has been written specifically on the issue of the acutely disturbed or violent depressed patient, but the principles of management are essentially the same. The two main classes of agents used as adjuncts to antidepressant therapy are neuroleptics and benzodiazepines. When a course of ECT is being prescribed, long-acting benzodiazepines may interfere with treatment and are therefore best avoided. There is no evidence that short-acting benzodiazepines cause behavioural disinhibition in agitated depression and they are often useful adjuncts to treatment. Neuroleptics are certainly indicated where there is psychosis.

Conclusions

Although many factors may give rise to a degree of urgency in treating depression, a relatively small range of treatments is appropriate. We have reviewed these in particular with regard to their efficacy in severe depression and their speed of action.

ECT remains the treatment of choice in many emergency situations and research is increasingly refining its practice and safety. Antidepressant medication is limited by a therapeutic delay but this may be overcome by early use of high doses and agents with a broad spectrum of pharmacological efficacy. The use of adjunctive medication such as benzodiazepines and neuroleptics may be beneficial, but careful monitoring for interactions and adverse effects is particularly important.

References

Altshuler, L. L., Post, R. M., Leverich, G. S., *et al* (1995) Antidepressant-induced mania and cycle acceleration: a controversy revisited. *American Journal of Psychiatry*, **152**, 1130–1138.

American Psychiatric Association (1990) *The Practice of ECT: Recommendations for Treatment, Training and Privileging.* Washington, DC: American Psychiatric Press.

Anderson, I. M. (1998) SSRIs versus tricyclic antidepressants in depressed in-patients: a meta-analysis of efficacy and tolerability. *Depression and Anxiety*, suppl. 7, 11–17.

—— & Tomenson, B. (1994) The efficacy of selective serotonin re-uptake inhibitors in depression: a meta-analysis of studies against tricyclic antidepressants. *Journal of Psychopharmacology*, **8**, 238–249.

Artigas, F., Romero, L., de Montigny, C., *et al* (1996) Acceleration of the effect of selected antidepressant drugs in major depression by 5-HT$_{1a}$ antagonists. *Trends in Neurosciences*, **19**, 378–383.

Avorn, B., Everitt, D. & Weiss, S. (1986) Increased antidepressant use in patients prescribed beta blockers. *Journal of the American Medical Association*, **255**, 357–360.

Baron, B. M., Ogden, A. M., Siegel, B. W., *et al* (1988) Rapid down regulation of β-adrenoceptors by co-administration of desipramine and fluoxetine. *European Journal of Pharmacology*, **154**, 125–134.

Benkert, O., Grunder, G., Wetzel, H., *et al* (1996) A randomized, double-blind comparison of a rapidly escalating dose of venlafaxine and imipramine in inpatients with major depression and melancholia. *Journal of Psychiatric Research*, **30**, 441–451.

Blier, P., de Montigny, C. & Chaput, Y. (1988) Electrophysiological assessment of the effects of antidepressant treatments on the efficacy of 5-HT neurotransmission. *Clinical Neuropharmacology*, **11**, S1–S10.

Buchan, H., Johnstone, E., McPherson, K., *et al* (1992) Who benefits from electroconvulsive therapy? Combined results of the Leicester and Northwick Park trials. *British Journal of Psychiatry*, **160**, 355–359.

Crowner, M. L., Douyon, R., Convit, A., *et al* (1990) Akathisia and violence. *Psychopharmacology Bulletin*, **26**, 115–117.

Cusack, B., Nelson, A. & Richelson, E. (1994) Binding of antidepressants to human brain receptors: focus on newer generation compounds. *Psychopharmacology*, **114**, 559–565.

Derivan, A., Entsuah, A. R. & Kikta, D. (1995) Venlafaxine: measuring the onset of antidepressant action. *Psychopharmacology Bulletin*, **31**, 439–447.

Dilsaver, S. C., Chen, Y. W., Swann, A. C., *et al* (1994) Suicidality in patients with pure and depressive mania. *American Journal of Psychiatry*, **151**, 1312–1315.

d'Elia, G. (1970) Unilateral electroconvulsive therapy. *Acta Psychiatrica Scandanavica*, **215** (suppl.), 5–98.

Fava, M., Nierenberg, A. A., Quitkin, F. M., *et al* (1997) A preliminary study on the efficacy of sertraline and imipramine on anger attacks in atypical depression and dysthymia. *Psychopharmacology Bulletin*, **33**, 101–103.

Fawcett, J., Scheftner, W. A., Fogg, L., *et al* (1990) Time-related predictors of suicide in major affective disorder. *American Journal of Psychiatry*, **147**, 1189–1194.

Guelfi, J. D., White, C., Hackett, D., *et al* (1995) Effectiveness of venlafaxine in patients hospitalized for major depression and melancholia. *Journal of Clinical Psychiatry*, **56**, 450–458.

Hamilton, M. (1960) A rating scale for depression. *Journal of Neurology, Neurosurgery and Psychiatry*, **23**, 56–62.

Johnson, J., Horwath, E. & Weissman, M. (1991) The validity of major depression with psychotic features based on a community study. *Archives of General Psychiatry*, **48**, 1075–1081.

Lock, T. (1995) Stimulus dosing. In *The ECT Handbook: The Second Report of the Royal College of Psychiatrists Special Committee on ECT* (Council Report CR39), pp. 72–87. London: Royal College of Psychiatrists.

Lurie, S. & Coffey, C. (1990) Caffeine-modified electroconvulsive therapy in depressed in-patients with medical illness. *Journal of Clinical Psychiatry*, **51**, 154–157.

Macpherson, R., Anstee, B. & Dix, R. (1998) Guidelines for management of patients with acutely disturbance. In *Acute Psychosis, Schizophrenia and Comorbid Disorders. Recent Topics from Advances in Psychiatric Treatment. Volume 1* (ed. A. Lee), pp. 7–11. London: Gaskell.

Martin, R. M., Hilton, S. R., Kerry, S. M., *et al* (1997) General practitioners' perceptions of the tolerability of anti-depressant drugs: a comparison of selective serotonin reuptake inhibitors and tricyclic antidepressants. *British Medical Journal*, **314**, 646–651.

Montgomery, S. A. & Åsberg, M. (1979) A new depression scale designed to be sensitive to change. *British Journal of Psychiatry*, **134**, 382–389.

Myers, D. H. & Neal, C. D. (1978) Suicide in psychiatric patients. *British Journal of Psychiatry*, **133**, 38–44.

National Institute of Mental Health (1995) Antidepressants. Can we determine how quickly they work? *Psychopharmacology Bulletin*, **31**, 21–55.

Nelson, J. C., Price, L. H. & Jatlow, P. I. (1986) Neuroleptic dose and desipramine concentrations during combined treatment of unipolar delusional depression. *American Journal of Psychiatry*, **143**, 1151–1154.

——, Mazure, C. M., Bowers, M. B., Jr, *et al* (1991) A preliminary, open study of the combination of fluoxetine and desipramine for rapid treatment of major depression. *Archives of General Psychiatry*, **48**, 303–307.

Nemeroff, C., DeVane, C. & Pollock, B. (1996) Newer antidepressants and the cytochrome P450 system. *American Journal of Psychiatry*, **153**, 311–320.

Parker, G. (1996) On lightening up: improvement trajectories in recovery from depression. *Advances in Psychiatric Treatment*, **2**, 186–193.

——, Roy, K., Hadzi-Pavlovic, D., *et al* (1992) Psychotic (delusional) depression: A meta-analysis of physical treatments. *Journal of Affective Disorders*, **24**, 17–24.

Pollock, B. G., Perel, J. M., Nathan, R. S., *et al* (1989) Acute antidepressant effect following pulse loading with intravenous and oral clomipramine. *Archives of General Psychiatry*, **46**, 29–35.

Post, R. M., Uhde, T. W., Rubinow, D. R., *et al* (1987) Differential time course of antidepressant effects after sleep deprivation, ECT, and carbamazepine: clinical and theoretical implications. *Psychiatry Research*, **22**, 11–19.

——, Ketter, T. A., Denicoff, K., *et al* (1996) The place of anticonvulsant therapy in bipolar illness. *Psychopharmacology*, **128**, 115–129.

Prudic, J. & Sackeim, H. A. (1999) Electroconvulsive therapy and suicide risk. *Journal of Clinical Psychiatry*, **60** (suppl. 2), 104–110.

Rodger, C. R., Scott, A. I. F. & Whalley, L. J. (1994) Is there a delay in the onset of the antidepressant effect of electroconvulsive therapy? *British Journal of Psychiatry*, **164**, 106–109.

Roose, S., Glassman, A., Walsh, B., *et al* (1983) Depression, delusions, and suicide. *American Journal of Psychiatry*, **140**, 1159–1162.

Royal College of Psychiatrists' Special Committee on ECT (1994) *Official Video Teaching Pack of the Royal College of Psychiatrists' Special Committee on ECT.* London: Gaskell.

—— (1995) *The ECT Handbook: The Second Report of the Royal College of Psychiatrists Special Committee on ECT* (Council Report CR39). London: Royal College of Psychiatrists.

Sachdev, P. & Loneragan, C. (1991) The present status of akathisia. *Journal of Nervous and Mental Disease*, **179**, 381–391.

Sackeim, H., Decina, P., Prohovnik, I., *et al* (1987) Seizure threshold in electroconvulsive therapy. Effects of sex, age, electrode placement, and number of treatments. *Archives of General Psychiatry*, **44**, 355–360.

——, Prudic, J., Devanand, D. P., *et al* (1993) Effects of stimulus intensity and electrode placement on the efficacy and cognitive effects of electroconvulsive therapy. *New England Journal of Medicine*, **328**, 839–846.

Sallee, F. R., Pollock, B. G., Perel, J. M., *et al* (1989) Intravenous pulse loading of clomipramine in adolescents with depression. *Psychopharmacology Bulletin*, **25**, 114–118.

Segman, R. H., Shapira, B., Gorfine, M., *et al* (1995) Onset and time course of antidepressant action: psychopharmacological implications of a controlled trial of electroconvulsive therapy. *Psychopharmacology*, **119**, 440–448.

Shapira, B., Tubi, N., Drexler, H., *et al* (1998) Cost and benefit in the choice of ECT schedule. Twice versus three times weekly ECT. *British Journal of Psychiatry*, **172**, 44–48.

Sobin, C., Prudic, J., Devanand, D. P., *et al* (1996) Who responds to electroconvulsive therapy? A comparison of effective and ineffective forms of treatment. *British Journal of Psychiatry*, **169**, 322–328.

Spiker, D. G., Weiss, J. C., Dealy, R. S., *et al* (1985) The pharmacological treatment of delusional depression. *American Journal of Psychiatry*, **142**, 430–436.

Stage, K. B., Bech, P., Gram, L. F., *et al* (1998) Are in-patient depressives more often of the melancholic subtype? *Acta Psychiatrica Scandinavica*, **98**, 432–436.

Swann, A. C., Bowden, C. L., Morris, D., *et al* (1997) Depression during mania. Treatment response to lithium or divalproex. *Archives of General Psychiatry*, **54**, 37–42.

Toxicity of newer versus older antidepressants

John A. Henry

Of all the controversies over the different medications used in psychiatry, there is probably least dispute about the effectiveness of antidepressants in controlling depressive illness. However, the choice of which antidepressant to use is bedevilled by the spectre of potential toxicity from adverse effects, interactions and overdose. The unwanted effects may vary from mild and tolerable to potentially lethal. At one time it was relatively easy to become familiar with the problems surrounding the original two main groups of antidepressants – the tricyclic antidepressants (TCAs) and the monoamine oxidase inhibitors (MAOIs). Recent years have seen the introduction of a number of newer drugs, with a wide range of chemical structures and differing pharmacological activities. They also have a new spectrum of adverse effects and interactions. It is worth reviewing the major differences between old and new antidepressants, and to identify the areas in which clinical caution must be exercised in order to avoid pitfalls and maximise clinical benefit.

Adverse effects

No drug is free from adverse effects. Those of the TCAs are well known, and can constitute relative contraindications for a number of different individuals and illnesses. The most important limitations are prostatic obstruction, narrow-angle glaucoma and some cardiac conditions. Most of the TCAs are contraindicated within three months of a myocardial infarction or in patients under treatment for heart failure. These drugs are also more likely to cause postural hypotension in the elderly. However, the newer drugs also produce adverse effects, which may limit their use in certain circumstances (see Table 1). Lofepramine can be considered an atypical tricyclic drug and has milder anticholinergic effects than the other TCAs. The most common adverse

effects caused by the different antidepressants are compared in Table 2. Other toxic effects are uncommon. Rashes occur with most drugs, including fluoxetine, and liver damage can occur with the TCAs and lofepramine.

Adherence

A major issue concerning adverse effects of antidepressants is their effect on adherence, which may limit the effectiveness of the treatment and thus prolong the depression, leaving the individual at risk of suicide. In addition the unused tablets are available for overdose. One evaluation of patients seen in general practice, attending psychiatric out-patient clinics and participating in antidepressant drug trials revealed that 32–64% of non-adhering patients defaulted because of side-effects, and some took no medication because they anticipated side-effects (Johnson, 1986). The potential of different antidepressants to cause side-effects varies greatly. However, tolerance of many of the adverse effects of antidepressants occurs. The anticholinergic effects of TCAs can be diminished by starting at a lower than therapeutic dose. Tolerance to nausea caused by selective serotonin reuptake inhibitors (SSRIs) soon occurs. The tolerability of SSRIs and TCAs in terms of adverse events has been compared in meta-analyses and these have been reviewed elsewhere (Anderson, this issue, 45–51).

Interactions

While drug interactions are liable to occur with all antidepressants, some groups of drug are more prone to interactions than others. The 'cheese' interaction with the older MAOIs is very well known, and consists

Table 1.   Adverse effects of antidepressants

Antidepressant	Adverse effects
Tricyclics	Dry mouth, blurred vision, constipation, urinary retention, drowsiness, postural hypotension
Monoamine oxidase inhibitors	Dry mouth, blurred vision, constipation, urinary retention, drowsiness (sometimes insomnia), tremor, dizziness, weakness, fatigue, gastrointestinal problems
Moclobemide	Insomnia, dizziness, nausea, headache, restlessness, agitation, confusion
Selective serotonin reuptake inhibitors	
Citalopram	Nausea, sweating, tremor, drowsiness, dry mouth
Fluoxetine	Nausea, headache, nervousness, insomnia, anxiety, dizziness, weakness
Fluvoxamine	Nausea, vomiting, drowsiness, diarrhoea, agitation, tremor, hypokinesia, asthenia
Paroxetine	Constipation, insomnia, dry mouth, tremor, weakness, sweating, nausea, drowsiness, headache
Sertraline	Dry mouth, nausea, diarrhoea, tremor, sweating, dyspepsia, ejaculatory delay
Atypical antidepressants	
Nefazodone	Weakness, dry mouth, nausea, dizziness, drowsiness
Venlafaxine	Nausea, headache, drowsiness, insomnia, dry mouth, dizziness, constipation, weakness, nervousness
Mirtazapine	Increased appetite, weight gain, drowsiness
Reboxetine	Insomnia, sweating, dizziness, tachycardia, postural hypotension, paraesthesia, dry mouth, dysuria, urinary retention, impotence, constipation

of a hypertensive crisis provoked by certain foods and drugs. This interaction is much less likely to occur with the newer selective inhibitor of monoamine oxidase A, moclobemide, and restriction of diet is not required provided that the patient does not indulge in binges of contraindicated foods. Some of the SSRIs may increase the adverse effects of lithium, especially fluoxetine, and although the TCAs are normally well tolerated with lithium there may rarely be myoclonus and seizures.

Since many of the newer drugs are serotonergic, the possibility of provoking a serotonin syndrome by simultaneously prescribing drugs with a serotonergic mode of action (the five SSRIs, clomipramine, mirtazapine, nefazodone and venlafaxine) needs to be considered carefully. In most cases this involves introducing the drug gradually by titrating the dose upwards and telling the patient not to take any further doses if they experience any untoward symptoms. The syndrome presents as progressive restlessness, hyperreflexia, shivering, tremor and sweating due to an excess of serotonin at a synaptic level. Agitation, confusion and hypomanic behaviour may occur. The pupils are usually widely dilated. If muscle spasms are severe or the patient develops a pyrexia, urgent medical attention will be required. Drugs such as propranolol or cyproheptadine may be used for their antiserotonergic effect (Brown *et al*, 1996). In extreme cases paralysis with muscle relaxants and mechanical ventilation may be required. Since the syndrome includes muscle stiffness and rigidity, restlessness,

agitation and a raised temperature, it needs to be considered in the differential diagnosis of neuroleptic malignant syndrome (Sternbach, 1991).

Another type of interaction which must be taken into account is the oxidative enzyme inhibiting properties of the SSRIs. Several of these drugs have the capacity to inhibit hepatic metabolism of drugs which the patient may be receiving. The plasma level of some TCAs may be raised by this mechanism. SSRIs such as fluvoxamine and sertraline can prolong the prothrombin time by inhibiting the metabolism of warfarin. Paroxetine also prolongs prothrombin time, but in addition may further increase the tendency to bleeding; the reason for this is not fully established. This drug should, therefore, be used with extreme caution in any patient taking warfarin.

Changing between antidepressants

Quite frequently the antidepressant first chosen does not produce the desired effect, and treatment needs to be changed to another drug. When introducing a new drug, the question of antidepressant–antidepressant interactions must be considered. This problem is compounded by the long elimination half-lives of some antidepressants, and the time taken for the pharmacological effect to disappear, which is particularly notable in the case of the older MAOIs. One exception is moclobemide, which in

Table 2.   Comparison of common adverse effects of different antidepressant drugs

Drug	Anticholin-ergic effect	Sedation	Stimulant effect	Nausea	Convulsant effect	Cardiac effects[1]	Toxicity in overdose
Tricyclic antidepressants							
Amitriptyline	+++	+++	0	+	++	+++	+++
Amoxapine	+++	+	0	0	+++	+	+++
Clomipramine	++	+	0	+	++	++	++
Desipramine	+	+	0	+	+	++	++
Dothiepin	++	++	0	0	++	++	+++
Doxepin	++	++	0	0	++	++	++
Imipramine	+++	++	0	+	++	++	+++
Lofepramine	+	+	0	0	0	+	0
Nortriptyline	++	++	0	+	+	++	++
Protriptyline	++	+	0	++	+	+	++
Trimipramine	+++	++	0	0	+	++	++
Monoamine oxidase inhibitors (MAOIs)							
Iproniazid	0	0	++	+	0	0	++
Isocarboxazid	0	0	+	+	0	+	++
Phenelzine	0	0	+	+	0	0	++
Tranylcypromine	0	0	+++	+	0	0	++
Reversible inhibitor of monoamine oxidase A (RIMA)							
Moclobemide	0	0	+	+	0	0	+
Selective serotonin reuptake inhibitors (SSRIs)							
Citalopram	0	0	0	++	0	+	+
Fluvoxamine	0	+	0	+++	+	0	0
Fluoxetine	0	+	++	0	0	0	0
Paroxetine	0	+	0	+	0	0	0
Sertraline	0	0	0	++	0	0	0
Atypical drugs							
Maprotiline	++	++	0	+	+++	++	+++
Mianserin	0	+++	0	0	0	0	0
Mirtazapine	0	+	+	0	0	0	0
Nefazodone	0	0	0	++	0	0	++
Reboxetine	++	0	0	0	+	+	0
Trazodone	0	++	0	+++	0	+	+
Venlafaxine	0	0	0	++	++	0	++
Viloxazine	+	+	0	++	0	0	0

1. Safety of administration in patients with heart problems (angina, arrhythmias, etc.). +++, very strong; ++, strong; +, low; 0, low or absent.

most cases requires no treatment-free interval when introducing a new drug, because its persistence in the body is short. Thus, the time factor deserves close consideration, particularly when changing antidepressants, especially with drugs such as fluoxetine, which has a long persistence in the body (up to 35 days; a seven-day interval is usually sufficient for other SSRIs, trazodone, nefazodone, reboxetine and venlafaxine) and the older MAOIs (interactions may occur up to 14 days after discontinuation).

Undertreatment

An important problem, especially in the field of general practice, is the danger of underdosing in order to reduce adverse effects. While there is no doubt that most adverse effects are dose-dependent and therefore will be reduced by prescribing a lower dose of drug, it is also apparent that this may prevent therapeutic levels of the drug from being reached, thus resulting in treatment failure. Sub-therapeutic dosing, particularly with the older TCAs, is liable to prejudice treatment outcome (Thompson & Thompson, 1989). A recent survey of 500 general practices in the UK based on over 70 000 anti-depressant prescriptions has shown that 61% were for amitriptyline, dothiepin and clomipramine, and that of these only 13.4% were prescribed at effective therapeutic doses (defined as 125 mg/day or more; Donoghue, 1994).

Fatal toxicity from antidepressant overdose

A number of studies have shown that drugs and drug groups can be ranked in terms of the number of deaths per million prescriptions (see Henry *et al*, 1995). When such a 'fatal toxicity index' is constructed, the older TCAs are the most lethal in overdose, the MAOIs have intermediate toxicity, and the newer drugs, which include the SSRIs, have lowest toxicity in overdose. Two of the older tricyclic drugs, amitriptyline and dothiepin, were associated with 81.6% of all antidepressant overdose deaths in Britain. These figures suggest that the older TCAs are more likely to prove fatal in overdose than most of the newer drugs. Although there are several sources of bias in these data, the figures correlate with clinical impressions of overdose toxicity and with animal studies of lethality of antidepressants (Molcho & Stanley, 1992; Kelvin & Hakansson, 1989). There is sufficient evidence to implicate several of the older tricyclic drugs in fatal toxicity of antidepressants.

Overdose of TCAs can lead to anticholinergic effects, such as tachycardia, hallucinations and mydriasis; other pharmacological properties can cause brisk reflexes, coma and convulsions, but the most serious effects are due to the quinidine-like effects of the tricyclic drugs, which can lead to hypotension and cardiac arrhythmias and may be responsible for a fatal outcome. Both the older and newer MAOIs in overdose can produce a severe serotonergic syndrome which may progress over 12–18 hours, leading to fatal hyperthermia unless treated. Other antidepressants in overdose gener-ally produce milder symptoms, and the outcome is rarely fatal; however, deaths from probable cardiotoxicity of citalopram have been reported (Öström *et al*, 1996).

Choice of medication clearly involves consider-ing the consequences of prescribing. Every doctor prescribing the older TCAs is confronted with the possibility that the treatment itself may prove the ultimate instrument of suicide (Meredith, 1995;

Smith, 1995). Safety in overdose should be a matter for concern. A change in prescribing habits could have an important public health impact and would help contribute to the 'Health of the Nation' strategy (Department of Health, 1994; Freemantle *et al*, 1994).

Conclusions

The Defeat Depression campaign launched in 1992 by the Royal College of Psychiatrists and the Royal College of General Practitioners aimed at improving the diagnosis and treatment of depression has resulted in a steady increase in the numbers of antidepressant presciptions in recent years. While antidepressants are demonstrably effective in controlling depressive illness, they must be prescribed with care, for three main reasons: they can produce adverse effects; they may interact with other medication; and they may cause morbidity or mortality in overdose. The most notable problem about adverse effects is that they may hinder adherence or lead to sub-therapeutic prescribing and thus defeat the object of treatment. Some interactions are potentially serious, and prescribers need to be aware of potential pitfalls. The older drugs have the obvious advantage of being well tried, while it takes time for experience and familiarity to develop with the newer drugs. The older drugs suffer from the limitation of adverse effects such as sedation and anticholinergic effects. Several of the newer drugs can cause initial nausea and their list of potential interactions is longer and more complex. Most of the newer antidepressants are relatively safe in overdose, but the older TCAs are demonstrably more toxic and are significantly more likely to prove fatal in overdose than other antidepressants. The prescribing psychiatrist needs to keep these considerations in mind in order to optimise treatment for a disease which is eminently treatable yet potentially lethal. Today's psychiatrist needs to be more of a physician and pharmacologist than his predecessor.

References

Anderson, I. (1999) Lessons to be learnt from meta-analyses of newer versus older antidepressants. In *Affective and Non-Psychotic Disorders. Recent Topics from Advances in Psychiatric Treatment, Volume 2*. pp. London: Gaskell.

Brown, T. M., Skop, B. P. & Mareth, T. R. (1996) Pathophysiology and management of the serotonin syndrome. *Annals of Pharmacotherapy*, **30**, 529–533.

Donoghue, J. M. (1994) The prescribing of antidepressants in general practice: The use of PACT data. *Postgraduate Medical Journal*, **70** (suppl. 2), S23–S24.

Freemantle, N., House, A., Song, F., *et al* (1994) Prescribing selective serotonin reuptake inhibitors as strategy for prevention of suicide. *British Medical Journal*, **309**, 250–253.

Department of Health (1994) *Health of the Nation: Suicide Prevention – The Challenge Confronted*. London: The Stationery Office.

Henry, J. A., Alexander, C. A. & Sener, E. K. (1995). Relative mortality from overdose of antidepressants. *British Medical Journal*, **310**, 221–224.

Johnson, D. A. W. (1986) Non-compliance with antidepressant therapy: An underestimated problem. *Internal Medicine*, **11** (suppl.), 14–17.

Kelvin, A. S. & Hakansson, S. (1989) Comparative acute toxicity of paroxetine and other antidepressants. *Acta Psychiatrica Scandinavica*, **80**, 31–33.

Meredith, T. (1995) Epidemiology of poisoning. *Medicine*, **23**, 1–3.

Molcho, A. & Stanley, M. (1992) Antidepressants and suicide risk: Issues of chemical and behavioural toxicity. *Journal of Clinical Pharmacology*, **12** (suppl. 2), S13–S18.

Öström, M., Eriksson, A., Thorson, J., *et al* (1996) Fatal overdose with citalopram. *Lancet*, **348**, 339–340.

Smith, T. (1995) Differences between general practices in hospital admission rates for self-inflicted injury and self-poisoning: Influence of socioeconomic factors. *British Journal of General Practice*, **45**, 458–462.

Sternbach, H. (1991) The serotonin syndrome. *American Journal of Psychiatry*, **148**, 705–713.

Thompson, C. & Thompson, C. M. (1989) The prescribing of antidepressants in general practice. II: A placebo-controlled trial of low-dose dothiepin. *Human Psychopharmacology*, **4**, 191–204.

Lessons to be learnt from meta-analyses of newer versus older antidepressants

Ian Anderson

Meta-analysis is the use of statistical techniques to analyse the findings of many individual analyses (Glass, 1977). It covers all aspects of the review process involving formulating relevant research questions, searching the literature, assessing the quality of studies and choosing relevant ones, extracting and combining the data (for reviews see Henry & Wilson, 1992; Wilson & Henry, 1992). Meta-analysis as part of a systematic review has advantages over a narrative review but there are problems in applying it in practice (Box 1).

The methodologies of meta-analyses themselves are frequently poor and should be examined critically before conclusions are accepted (Box 2). Interpretation requires an understanding of the summary measures used in order to combine studies.

Box 1. Adavantages and problems with meta-analysis

Advantages
Systematic review of evidence
Increased power to detect differences
Provides an estimate of the size of effect and confidence interval
Possibility of analysing subgroups not achievable in single study

Problems
Difficulty in identifying all relevant studies
Comparability of studies to be combined (e.g. diagnostic issues)
Quality of studies to be combined (e.g. methodology, completeness of data)
Publication bias
Statistical heterogeneity among studies (some controversy over whether pooling is then appropriate)

Box 2. How to assess the quality of a meta-analysis

The question should be answerable from the studies selected
The search should be explained and comprehensive
Selection criteria for studies should be described and be appropriate to the question
The statistical method should be explained and be appropriate
Pooling should be variance-weighted (larger studies with smaller variance are given more weight)
Results should be expressed with confidence intervals
Heterogeneity of studies should be assessed and taken into account in calculating the results
A sensitivity analysis should be undertaken, if possible, by examining better quality studies separately or by using alternative methods of analysis
Publication bias should be considered, for example with a funnel plot (see Wilson & Henry, 1992)

For continuous data a standardised difference (or effect size) can be calculated for each study (the difference in scores from the two treatments divided by the standard deviation; Hedges & Olkin, 1985). For events (e.g. response v. non-response) the odds ratio (Altman, 1991) or, better, the risk ratio (or relative risk; Sinclair & Bracken, 1994) is usually calculated. The odds ratio is the number of occurrences divided by the number of non-occurrences, and the risk is number of occurrences divided by the total number; the latter is better understood by clinicians. The odds ratio (relative risk) is the ratio of the odds (risks) in the treatment group compared with controls. It is also possible to calculate the absolute risk difference which is the difference between the risk in the treatment and control groups. This is useful to calculate the number of patients that would have to be treated with the new treatment for one patient to gain benefit. This is also called the number needed to treat and is simply the reciprocal of the risk difference (e.g. a risk difference of 0.25 gives a number needed to treat of 1/0.25=4).

Meta-analyses of newer versus older antidepressants

Meta-analysis is particularly relevant in comparative studies of antidepressants in which the power to detect differences between treatments is usually low because of small patient numbers. The variety of antidepressants does, however, restrict the number of studies available for individual drugs. If groupings of antidepressants (e.g. selective serotonin reuptake inhibitors, SSRIs) are considered, then respectable numbers can be achieved but only at the expense of missing possible differences between individual drugs. The present review is restricted to double-blind, randomised, comparative studies of antidepressants in depressive illness based on a MEDLINE search supplemented by manual searching of review articles and literature provided by drug companies. With duplicated or updated meta-analyses I considered only the most informative study.

The major groupings of antidepressants are tricyclic antidepressants (TCAs), monoamine oxidase inhibitors (MAOIs), second-generation antidepressants and SSRIs. Some drugs are not easily classified. For example, lofepramine is a TCA that is often grouped with second-generation antidepressants related to issues of tolerability and safety, and so called 'fourth-generation' antidepressants (e.g. venlafaxine, nefazodone, mirtazapine) share properties with earlier antidepressants. In general, meta-analyses have concentrated on comparisons between a newer drug or drug class and first-generation TCAs, either as a class or individually. I did not find any meta-analyses comparing MAOIs with newer antidepressants, but there is a review and meta-analysis available which examines the efficacy of MAOIs compared with placebo and TCAs (Thase *et al*, 1995). Detailed consideration of the analysis is outside the the the scope of this article, but, using a somewhat different

methodology to that described above, the authors conclude that MAOIs are more effective than placebo in treating depression and appear effective for outpatients who had failed to respond to TCAs. In comparative studies MAOIs appear less effective than TCAs in in-patients but are more effective in out-patients with atypical depression.

Efficacy

The question of efficacy, central to any comparison of antidepressants, is not straightforward because of variation in the diagnosis, nature and treatment setting of depressive illness and the analysis and definition of response. These issues are beyond the scope of this chapter.

Second-generation antidepressants

The efficacy of second-generation antidepressants versus first-generation TCAs is often questioned. Unfortunately, meta-analyses addressing this question have been few and generally poorly conducted. Some studies looking at a range of comparisons have suggested that trazodone and/or mianserin may be less effective than TCAs (Moller & Haug, 1988; Kasper *et al*, 1992) whereas others have not (Davis *et al*, 1993; Workman & Short, 1993). Unfortunately little weight can be given to these analyses because of methodological problems, including the lack of confidence intervals.

Patten (1992) analysed comparative trials of trazodone against imipramine and concluded equal odds of responding to treatment (odds ratio 0.93, 95% confidence interval (95% CI) 0.64–1.36). Strict inclusion criteria meant that he could include only six out of 25 identified studies (302 patients) and the pooling was not variance-weighted. The recalculated, variance-weighted relative risk is 0.86 (95% CI 0.70–1.05). This indicates that trazodone is unlikely to be better than imipramine but may be significantly worse as the confidence interval encompasses a 5% advantage but a 30% disadvantage. A major problem with that study is potential selection bias, which makes final interpretation difficult.

In a good-quality study Kerihuel & Dreyfus (1991) found that patients responded better to lofepramine than to older TCAs and maprotiline (mostly imipramine or amitriptyline; odds ratio 1.4, 95% CI 1.2–1.8). They were able to use 24 out of 29 studies identified and verified the data of 602 of the total of 2040 patients using original case report forms. The recalculated relative risk is 1.13 (95% CI 1.04–1.22) suggesting that patients are 13% more likely to respond to lofepramine than to older TCAs, with a confidence interval of 4–22%. There are methodological caveats (e.g. pooling is not variance-weighted and selection bias is not investigated) but these data suggest that lofepramine is at least as effective as older TCAs, and the possibility that it has advantages is intriguing but difficult to understand. A re-analysis using the individual studies would be valuable.

SSRIs

The comparative efficacy of SSRIs has been extensively investigated. Song *et al* (1993) calculated standardised differences using the final Hamilton Depression Rating Scale (HAM–D; Hamilton, 1960) score, and assigned pooled standard deviations to incomplete studies to yield results from 49 of 63 identified studies. They do not produce a single pooled value, but analyse different subsets according to the version of the HAM–D scale used. These, in general, show no significant difference in efficacy (although studies using the standard, 17-item version of the HAM–D favour comparators). A major criticism of this study is the inclusion of second-generation antidepressants. Therefore, we analysed only studies against noradrenaline reuptake inhibitors with exclusion of TCA doses below 100 mg to lessen bias towards SSRIs (Anderson & Tomenson, 1994) and have subsequently updated this analysis (Anderson, 1999). We calculated a standardised change in HAM–D scores and assigned an estimated standard deviation to incomplete studies. In the updated meta-analysis 102 studies (10 706 patients) were included, with sensitivity analyses performed using studies which were placebo-controlled, those with complete data and larger studies to provide quality control. We checked for selection bias and corrected for heterogeneity. In the first meta-analysis we showed that SSRIs and TCAs were significantly better than placebo (effect sizes for both about 0.4, a difference in HAM–D response of three points). In the updated meta-analysis the relative effect size was –0.03 (95% CI –0.09 to 0.03) indicating that any true difference in efficacy is small. In a tentative subgroup analysis (not corrected for multiple comparisons) individual SSRIs did not differ significantly, but paroxetine and citalopram tended to perform less well than TCAs (relative effect sizes –0.12, 95% CI –0.24 to 0.01 and –0.14, 95% CI –0.31 to 0.03 respectively) indicating that they are unlikely to be superior to TCAs but could be less effective. When individual TCAs were considered amitriptyline was significantly more effective than SSRIs (effect size –0.14, 95% CI –0.25 to –0.03, *P*=0.012) with dothiepin tending to perform worse (effect size 0.12, 95% CI –0.03 to 0.27). TCAs were significantly better than SSRIs in in-patients

to a potentially clinically important extent (effect size –0.23, 95% CI –0.40 to –0.05). The funnel plot for in-patient studies was symmetrical but that for amitriptyline was not, indicating that for amitrityline selection bias could not be ruled out. In the earlier meta-analysis we had suggested that TCAs with dual action in inhibiting noradrenaline and serotonin reuptake might be more effective than TCAs, but in the updated meta-analysis clomipramine did not appear to have superior efficacy although the confidence interval was wide due to great heterogeneity between studies. However, if the in-patient studies are considered alone then it still remains possible that dual action does confer greater efficacy (Anderson, 1998).

Further meta-analyses for individual SSRIs available using drug company trial databases (Bech & Cialdella, 1992; Pande & Sayler, 1993*a*) do not add to the conclusions above.

Other antidepressants

Moclobemide is a reversible inhibitor of monoamine oxidase A. A meta-analysis using individual data on 1256 patients on the drug company's database (Angst & Stabl, 1992) unfortunately has poor methodology (no examination of heterogeneity between study sites, no explanation of pooling method, lumping together all comparators and lack of confidence intervals). It is possible to calculate an overall relative risk of 1.03 (95% CI 0.95–1.12) suggesting that between 5% fewer and 12% more patients respond on moclobemide compared with comparators. However, a further meta-analysis of the use of moclobemide in 12 studies (730 patients) against imipramine and clomipramine in in-patients is less favourable (Angst *et al*, 1995). Individual patient data are used but the Danish University Antidepressant Group (1993) study, which found clomipramine significantly more effective, appears to be excluded on the grounds of a low fixed moclobemide dose (400 mg/day) and one study against imipramine is single-blind. The results are again unsatisfactorily presented, but calculation of the relative risk shows that moclobemide is less effective than both TCAs (combined results 0.88 (95% CI 0.78–0.99)), although this is not significant taking clomipramine and imipramine individually. Excluding lower dose moclobemide and clomipramine patients leaves the result as 0.89 (95% CI 0.78–1.01). Therefore, even patients on effective doses of moclobemide have up to a 22% greater risk of not responding compared with those treated with clomipramine and imipramine, although similar efficacy is not quite excluded.

Finally, a meta-analysis of the serotonin and noradrenaline reuptake inhibitor, venlafaxine, is presented as part of a cost-effectiveness analysis

(Einarson *et al*, 1995). As presented it is unacceptable because it averages response rates for individual drugs in comparative and non-comparative studies. Sound search and inclusion criteria (including drug dose), however, allow a variance-weighted relative risk of 1.15 (95% CI 1.00–1.32) to be calculated from six studies (636 patients) of venlafaxine against imipramine, trazodone, maprotiline and fluoxetine, indicating that venlafaxine is unlikely to be less effective than comparators and could be up to 32% more effective. The comparator drugs are heterogeneous and numbers are small but, given the suggestion that dual-action TCAs may be more effective than SSRIs, they deserve further investigation.

Tolerability

Tolerability has been assessed by counting drop-outs in comparative studies (which may underestimate side-effect burden), apart from one meta-analysis which considered the percentage of patients experiencing side-effects (which may overestimate significant side-effects).

Second-generation antidepressants

Kerihuel & Dreyfus (1991) found that significantly fewer patients on lofepramine compared with those taking first-generation TCAs experienced at least one side-effect (53 *v.* 64%). The odds ratio was 0.6 (95% CI 0.5–0.7) and a recalculated relative risk gives 0.83 (95% CI 0.77–0.89) indicating a 17% reduction with a range of 11–23%. This did not translate into a significant difference in the total number of patients stopping treatment, although the confidence interval is fairly wide and does not exclude a lower rate on lofepramine (relative risk 0.93, 95% CI 0.79–1.09).

SSRIs

Song *et al* (1993) challenged the view that SSRIs were better tolerated than older antidepressants in their meta-analysis of 58 studies with 5518 patients. Total drop-outs (odds ratio 0.95, 95% CI 0.82–1.11) and those due to treatment failure were not significantly different, whereas those due to side-effects just missed significance (odds ratio 0.81, 95% CI 0.65–1.00). Criticisms about the inclusion of non-TCA antidepressants resulted in further meta-analyses. Originally we (Anderson & Tomenson, 1995) analysed 64 studies with 6012 patients which has subsequently been updated to 95 studies with 10 553 patients (Anderson, 1999) in which SSRIs were compared

only with TCAs. In the updated meta-analysis we found a 12% decrease in the relative risk of dropping out (0.88, 95% CI 0.83–0.93), with the relative risk of dropping out due to side-effects reduced by 27% (relative risk 0.73, 95% CI 0.76–0.80). These results did not appear to be due to selection bias and indicated that, overall, about 4% fewer patients dropped out on SSRIs compared with TCAs. Of interest, if the studies were divided into those of six weeks duration or less and those of greater than six weeks' duration (mostly 7–12 weeks) the advantage of SSRIs was greater in the longer studies (5.9% fewer drop-outs overall compared with 2.2%). Montgomery & Kasper (1995) analysed 67 studies of SSRIs versus TCAs (6852 patients) with the same result for drop-outs due to side-effects; unfortunately they did not analyse total drop-outs. The better tolerability of SSRIs might suggest that they have a particular advantage over TCAs in elderly patients. Menting *et al* (1996) concluded that SSRIs did have a tolerability advantage when the analysis was confined to four studies with better methodology but acknowledged that inclusion of more studies changed the result. Mittmann *et al* (1998) and I (Anderson, 1999) could not demonstrate an advantage of SSRIs when all ten available studies were included. The drop-out rate due to side-effects appears higher in the elderly than in adults (about 22% *v.* 15%) with a non-significant difference between SSRIs and TCAs in our updated meta-analysis (Anderson, 1999; relative risk 0.91, 95% CI 0.74–1.11). SSRIs may therefore have an advantage over TCAs but it appears unlikely to be greater than in adults and has yet to be conclusively shown.

Hotopf *et al* (1997) have recently analysed the overall discontinuation rate from 92 studies comparing SSRIs with TCAs (75 studies) or second-generation antidepressants (17 studies). They divided the TCAs into older TCAs (imipramine and amitriptyline) and newer groups (all the rest). Their finding for imipramine and amitriptyline (51 studies) reinforces our earlier results (relative risk 0.88, 95% CI 0.82–0.94) but they go on to suggest that the 'newer TCAs' (24 studies) may be better tolerated on the grounds that the relative risk for this group considered separately failed to reach significance (relative risk 0.92, 95% CI 0.81–1.03). Statistically this is an unwarranted conclusion, although it may be true that some TCAs are better tolerated than others (e.g. dothiepin – see below). A limitation of this study is the failure to look separately at drop-outs due to side-effects given that only about half of all drop-outs are for this reason (Anderson & Tomenson, 1995; Anderson, 1999).

My conclusion is that fewer people discontinue treatment on SSRIs compared with TCAs and that this can be attributed to less severe side-effects, but the absolute risk reduction is small (2–6%) which is of uncertain significance; however the suggestion that the difference increases with duration of treatment may have important implications when considering the whole recommended treatment period for antidepressants of at least six months and often much longer. While we did not find statistically significant differences between SSRIs, individual results showed that for all SSRIs (apart from fluvoxamine) there was a significant advantage over TCAs for drop-outs due to side-effects and a similar pattern for total drop-outs (Anderson, 1999). This is in agreement with a meta-analysis of comparative studies of SSRIs (Edwards & Anderson, 1999) and with naturalistic cohort data using prescription event monitoring (Mackay *et al*, 1997). Therefore there is consistent data that fluvoxamine is less well tolerated than other SSRIs and may have little advantage over TCAs.

Pande & Sayler (1993*b*) looked at drop-outs in comparative trials with fluoxetine from the drug company database and found similar results.

As a twist in the tail, Donovan (1993) listed seven double-blind trials of dothiepin against SSRIs involving 619 patients. He provided sufficient data to calculate the relative risks for drop-outs due to side-effects (0.48, 95% CI 0.26–0.89), showing a large advantage to dothiepin, and for total drop-outs (0.77, 95% CI 0.57–1.04), which also favours dothiepin. I found identical results in my meta-analysis with an absolute risk difference of 8.9% favouring dothiepin for side-effect related drop-outs (Anderson, 1999).

These studies are mostly small with no guarantee that they are without selection bias, but they question whether all TCAs should be assumed to be equally likely to produce side-effects.

In the study by Hotopf *et al* (1997) the relative tolerability of SSRIs compared with second-generation antidepressants was analysed in 17 studies (1168 patients) by measuring total drop-out rate. The relative risk was was 1.02 (95% CI 0.78–1.35) showing no significant difference in tolerability with statistical homogeneity between studies although the confidence interval is fairly wide. As the drugs differed widely in pharmacology I looked separately at the seven studies comparing with mianserin (relative risk 1.06, 95% CI 0.78–1.45), which gave the same result. There was, however, a trend for fluoxetine to be favoured in three studies against trazodone (relative risk 0.61, 95% CI 0.36–1.03). The limitation of only analysing total drop-outs is discussed above and the results are from a relatively small number of studies. Therefore, while the results do not allow us to conclude that there is any difference in the tolerability of second-generation antidepressants and SSRIs, our confidence that they are in fact equally well tolerated is low.

Suicide risk

An important issue was addressed by Beasley *et al* (1991) following case reports that fluoxetine might cause patients to become suicidal. From drug company data they analysed 12 studies (1450 patients), used sound methodology and reported on the incidence (risk) difference (differences between drugs in absolute percentages). Suicidal acts (0.3%) and the emergence of substantial suicidal ideation (3%) were infrequent and there were no differences between fluoxetine and either placebo or TCAs. The narrow confidence intervals make it unlikely that fluoxetine promotes suicide although they do not rule out that up to 3–4% fewer patients develop substantial suicidal ideation on fluoxetine compared with placebo (incidence difference –1.5, 95% CI –3.3–0.3) or TCAs (–1.8, 95% CI –4.0–0.4). A limitation is the exclusion of patients with an initial substantial suicide risk from most studies.

Lessons to be learnt

General points: first, distrust claims for any antidepressant based on one or two studies (unless it is a 'mega-trial') as selection bias is likely; second, unless there are confidence intervals around any outcome measure, the clinical relevance is uncertain (see Box 3).

Box 3. Lessons to be learnt from the meta-analyses of newer versus older antidepressants

Distrust conclusions based on non-systematic reviews or single small studies

Clinical relevance can only be assessed if confidence intervals are given

SSRIs and lofepramine are as effective as older TCAs in the short-term treatment of depression

SSRIs and lofepramine have side-effect advantages over older TCAs. Short-term adherence may only be marginally better but this may increase with longer duration of treatment

Fluoxetine is no more likely than TCAs or placebo to cause suicidal ideation or actions in short-term use

Meta-analysis has shed limited light on the efficacy or tolerability of second-generation anti-depressants (Box 4). A meta-analysis of trazodone allows only modest confidence that it is as effective as imipramine. In contrast, lofepramine is at least equally as effective as older TCAs and is less likely to cause side-effects, although it remains uncertain that this results in better overall compliance.

For the SSRIs taken as a group there have been sufficient studies to conclude that they are as effective as older TCAs in treating depression. However the question of reduced efficacy in in-patients and against amitriptyline deserves further investigation. With regard to tolerability, significantly fewer patients stop treatment because of side-effects with SSRIs than with older TCAs. This probably accounts for fewer overall drop-outs on SSRIs, but only by four patients in 100 treated. The tolerability of SSRIs compared with second-generation antidepressants is uncertain, but there is no good evidence that they are better tolerated. When cost effectiveness analyses are carried out great caution is needed in choosing which figures to use for relative drop-outs and duration of treatment also needs to be taken into account.

Group findings for SSRIs and for TCAs may not hold for individual compounds. Evidence is accumulating that fluvoxamine is less well tolerated than other SSRIs and dothiepin appears to be tolerated at least as well as SSRIs. This accords with clinical impression and further investigation of these issues would be useful.

Fluoxetine and TCAs do not promote suicide in the short term in patients with depression who start with low suicide risk. Exceptions in individual cases are, however, not ruled out.

These meta-analyses are consistent with the interesting possibility that drugs inhibiting both serotonin and noradrenaline reuptake (e.g. clomipramine and venlafaxine) may have superior efficacy to single reuptake inhibitors.

There is less confidence that SSRIs and moclobemide are as effective as the older TCAs in in-patients, and TCAs (especially amitriptyline) probably remain first-line treatment for these patients.

Conclusions

Meta-analysis is useful and can raise new research questions as well as addressing current ones. It has been applied in only a limited fashion to comparative studies of antidepressants. Proposed short-term advantages to individual drugs (e.g. response of anxiety symptoms to SSRIs, speed of onset of antidepressant response with venlafaxine) and issues related to longer term treatment such as relapse prevention, tolerability and adherence should be subjected to meta-analysis. To achieve this, registration and comprehensive data recording from randomised controlled studies, such as by the Cochrane Collaboration (Godlee, 1994), is to be encouraged.

Box 4. Controversial issues

Efficacy of second-generation antidepressants (except lofepramine) compared with older TCAs

Relative tolerability of individual SSRIs (fluvoxamine is worse) and older TCAs (is dothiepin better?)

Magnitude and clinical importance of better tolerability of SSRIs over older TCAs in medium- to long-term use

Greater efficacy of amitriptyline and dual serotonin and noradrenaline reuptake inhibitors (clomipramine, venlafaxine) compared with SSRIs

Efficacy of newer antidepressants in in-patients

References

Altman, D. G. (1991) *Practical Statistics for Medical Research.* London & New York: Chapman and Hall.

Anderson, I. M. (1998) SSRIs versus tricyclic antidepressants in depressed in-patients: a meta-analysis of efficacy and tolerability. *Depression & Anxiety,* **7** (suppl. 1), 11–17.

—— (1999) Selective serotonin reuptake inhibitors versus tricyclic antidepressants: a meta-analysis of efficacy and tolerability. *Journal of Affective Disorders,* in press.

——— & Tomenson, B. M. (1994) The efficacy of selective serotonin reuptake inhibitors in depression: A meta-analysis of studies against tricyclic antidepressants. *Journal of Psychopharmacology,* **8**, 238–249.

—— & —— (1995) Treatment discontinuation with selective serotonin reuptake inhibitors compared to tricyclic antidepressants: A meta-analysis. *British Medical Journal,* **310**, 1433–1438.

Angst, J. & Stabl, M. (1992) Efficacy of moclobemide in different patient groups: A meta-analysis of studies. *Psychopharmacology,* suppl. 106, S109–S113.

——, Amrein, R. & Stabl, M. (1995) Moclobemide and tricyclic antidepressants in severe depression: Meta-analysis and prospective studies. *Journal of Clinical Psychopharmacology,* suppl. 15, 16S–23S.

Beasley, C. M., Dornseif, B. E., Bosomworth, J. C., *et al* (1991) Fluoxetine and suicide: A meta-analysis of controlled trials of treatment for depression. *British Medical Journal*, **303**, 685–692.

Bech, P. & Cialdella, P. (1992) Citalopram in depression – meta-analysis of intended and unintended effects. *International Clinical Psychopharmacology*, **6** (suppl. 5), 45–54.

Danish University Antidepressant Group (1993) Moclobemide. A reversible MAO-A-inhibitor showing weaker antidepressant effect than clomipramine in a controlled multicentre study. *Journal of Affective Disorders*, **28**, 105–116.

Davis, J. M., Wang, Z. & Janicak, P. G. (1993) A quantitative analysis of clincal drug trials for the treatment of affective disorders. *Psychopharmacology Bulletin*, **29**, 175–181.

Donovan, S. (1993) The efficacy and tolerability of dothiepin versus serotonin specific reuptake inhibitors in the treatment of depression. *European Neuropsychopharmacology*, **3**, 331–332.

Edwards, J. G. & Anderson, I. M. (1999) Systematic review and guide to selection of selective serotonin reuptake inhibitors. *Drugs*, **57**, 507–533.

Einarson, T. R., Arikian, S., Sweeney, S., et al (1995) A model to evaluate the cost-effectiveness of oral therapies in the management of patients with major depression. *Clinical Therapeutics*, **17**, 136–153.

Glass, G. V. (1977) Integrating findings: The meta-analysis of research. *Review of Research in Education*, **5**, 351–379.

Godlee, F. (1994) The Cochrane Collaboration. *British Medical Journal*, **309**, 969–970.

Hamilton, M. (1960) A rating scale for depression. *Journal of Neurology, Neurosurgery and Psychiatry*, **23**, 56–63.

Hedges, L. V. & Olkin, I. (1985) *Statistical Methods for Meta-Analysis*. Orlando, FL: Academic Press.

Henry, D. A. & Wilson, A. (1992) Meta-analysis. 1: An assessment of its aims, validity and reliability. *Medical Journal of Australia*, **156**, 31–38.

Hotopf, M., Hardy, R. & Lewis, G. (1997) Discontinuation rates of SSRIs and tricyclic antidepressants: a meta-analysis and investigation of heterogeneity. *British Journal of Psychiatry*, **170**, 120–127.

Kasper, S., Fuger, J. & Moller, H.-J. (1992) Comparative efficacy of antidepressants. *Drugs*, **43**, 11–23.

Kerihuel, J. C. & Dreyfus, J. F. (1991) Meta-analyses of the efficacy and tolerability of the tricyclic antidepressant lofepramine. *Journal of International Medical Research*, **19**, 183–201.

Mackay, F. J., Dunn, N. R., Wilton, L. V., et al (1997) A comparison of fluvoxamine, fluoxetine, sertraline and paroxetine examined by observational cohort studies. *Pharmacoepidemiology and Drug Safety*, **6**, 235–246

Menting, J. E., Honig, A., Verhey, F. R., et al (1996) Selective serotonin reuptake inhibitors (SSRIs) in the treatment of elderly depressed patients: a qualitative analysis of the literature on their efficacy and side-effects. *International Clinical Psychopharmacology*, **11**, 165–175.

Mittmann, N., Herrman, N., Einarson, T. R., et al (1998) The efficacy, safety and tolerability of antidepressants in late life depression: a meta-analysis. *Journal of Affective Disorders*, **46**, 191–217.

Moller, H. J. & Haug, G. (1988) Secondary and meta-analysis of the efficacy of non-tricyclic antidepressants. *Pharmaco-psychiatry*, **21**, 363–364.

Montgomery, S. A. & Kasper, S. (1995) Comparison of compliance between serotonin reuptake inhibitors and tricyclic antidepressants: A meta-analysis. *International Clinical Psychopharmacology*, **9** (suppl. 4), 33–40.

Pande, A. C. & Sayler, M. E. (1993a) Fluoxetine – a clinical and research update: Severity of depression and response to fluoxetine. *International Clinical Psychopharmacology*, **8**, 243–245.

—— & —— (1993b) Adverse events and treatment discontinuations in fluoxetine clinical trials. *International Clinical Psychopharmacology*, **8**, 267–269.

Patten, S. B. (1992) The comparative efficacy of trazodone and imipramine in the treatment of depression. *Canadian Medical Association Journal*, **146**, 1177–1182.

Sinclair, J. C. & Bracken, M. B. (1994) Clinically useful measures of effect in binary analyses of randomized trials. *Journal of Clinical Epidemiology*, **47**, 881–889.

Song, F., Freemantle, N., Sheldon, T. A., et al (1993) Selective serotonin reuptake inhibitors: Meta-analysis of efficacy and acceptability. *British Medical Journal*, **306**, 683–687.

Thase, M. E., Trivedi, M. H. & Rush, A. J. (1995) MAOIs in the contemporary treatment of depression. *Neuropsycho-pharmacology*, **12**, 185–219.

Wilson, A. & Henry, D. A. (1992) Meta-analysis. Part 2: Assessing the quality of published meta-analyses. *Medical Journal of Australia*, **156**, 173–187.

Workman, E. A. & Short, D. D. (1993) Atypical antidepressants versus imipramine in the treatment of major depression: A meta-analysis. *Journal of Clinical Psychiatry*, **54**, 5–12.

Pharmacological management of treatment-resistant depression

P. J. Cowen

The management of patients with depression who have failed to respond to antidepressant medication is a common problem in general and old age psychiatry. It has been estimated that about 20–30% of patients with major depression fail to respond to treatment with a single antidepressant drug given in adequate dosage for an appropriate period of time. At the current time there are many possible ways to pursue pharmacological treatment, but few controlled trials to help us choose between the various options. In addition there are few clinical predictors to help match patients to an appropriate treatment.

Definition

The definition of treatment-resistant depression is somewhat arbitrary, but in pharmacological terms there is the presumption that the depressive syndrome has not responded to an adequate trial (in terms of dose and duration) of at least one effective medication. It may be useful to identify different stages of resistant depression depending on the nature of treatments that have been un-successfully deployed (Box 1; Thase & Rush, 1997). Some patients may present with chronic untreated depression that has failed to remit spontaneously. Such patients can respond well to pharmacotherapy, although there is disagreement about whether remission rates are lower than in patients with depression with more acute presentation (Kupfer & Frank, 1996).

Assessment

Patients with depression are often now referred to psychiatrists after some considerable period of illness and after a number of different drug treatments have been tried. It is important to confirm the diagnosis of major depression and exclude possible general medical disorders. Some medical treatments may themselves precipitate or perpetuate depression; for example, recent epidemiological studies have drawn attention to excess rates of depression and suicide in patients taking calcium channel antagonists (Lindberg *et al*, 1998). Psychiatric comorbidity, for example substance misuse, can also worsen the outcome of depressive disorder.

The assessment should attempt to establish how long the depression has been present, its nature and course and the treatments that have been used. Often, patients will have improved to some extent and this may influence whether or not major changes in management are needed. It is helpful to try to establish how far psychosocial and personality factors may have played a role in the onset and maintenance of the depression. For this purpose it is usually necessary to interview an

---

Box 1. Stages of treatment resistance in depression (adapted from Thase & Rush, 1997)

Stage 1   Failure of at least one adequate trial of one major class of antidepressant

Stage 2   Stage 1 plus failure to respond to adequate trial of antidepressant from a different class

Stage 3   Stage 2 plus failure to respond to lithium augmentation

Stage 4   Stage 3 plus failure to respond to monoamine oxidase inhibitor

Stage 5   Stage 4 plus failure to respond to electroconvulsive therapy

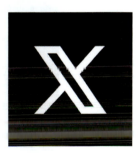
...ese factors does
...ug treatment, it

...res

...in the general
...assurance and
...onic depression
...pessimistic and
...to outline the
...ve exercise in
...l experience to
...c options while
...in treatment
...day activities
...ies can be useful
...ievements and
...king patterns.

...ntidepressants
...low doses and
...creased to 150–
...where tolerance
...be obtained by
...to 300 mg of
...a monitoring of
...t higher doses
...ularly if there
...tic interactions
...using high doses
...ectrocardiogram
...istory of cardiac
...medication that

...hat higher doses
...tive serotonin
...o have relatively
...this, if tolerance
...SRI can produce
...larly in patients
...(Fava *et al*, 1994).

...*ils*

...e antidepressant
...o try a different
...d studies of this

---

approach treat patients in an open, sequential way with a different class of antidepressant; clearly this cannot control for the placebo effect or the possibility of spontaneous remission. There is reasonable evidence that switching to another class of anti-depressant can produce benefit in about 50% of patients unresponsive to an initial medication.

If a patient has not responded to one kind of antidepressant, it would seem sensible to switch to an antidepressant with different pharmacological properties – this is my practice. However, it must be acknowledged that open studies have shown equally good response rates when patients who failed to respond to one SSRI were switched to another (Thase & Rush, 1997).

In the broad range of patients with depression, currently marketed antidepressants have roughly equal efficacy. However, there is evidence from meta-analyses that drugs that produce potent potentiation of both serotonin and noradrenaline (amitriptyline, clomipramine and venlafaxine) may be more effective than SSRIs in patients with severe depressive symptoms (Anderson, this issue, 45–51). This suggests that one of the former drugs should be tried at some point in patients unresponsive to initial medication (Poirer & Boyer, 1999).

Monoamine oxidase inhibitors

The use of non-selective irreversible monoamine oxidase inhibitors (MAOIs) in patients resistant to TCAs and other antidepressants has some support from controlled trials. For example, Nolen *et al* (1988) studied 21 patients who had failed to respond to treatment with imipramine, fluvoxamine or oxprotiline. The subjects were randomly allocated to double-blind treatment with nomifensine (a dopamine and noradrenaline reuptake inhibitor, later withdrawn because of rare autoimmune reactions) or the MAOI tranylcypromine. Of 11 patients receiving tranylcypromine, five responded with a 50% decrease in their score on the Hamilton Rating Scale for Depression (HAM–D; Hamilton, 1967). In a subsequent cross-over, five of eight non-responders to nomifensine responded to tranyl-cypromine. Eight of the 10 patients who responded to tranylcypromine maintained their response for at least six months.

There is also evidence that patients with certain clinical features may have a preferential response to MAOIs. For example, patients with symptoms of atypical depression (see Box 2) have a significantly higher response rate to phenelzine (about 70%) than imipramine (about 45%) (Quitkin *et al*, 1989).

Although MAOIs are undoubtedly useful drugs in treatment-resistant depression, their liability to produce dietary and drug interactions makes their use unlikely until most other options have been exhausted. The reversible type-A MAOI, moclobemide, is relatively free from tyramine interactions at standard doses and is better tolerated than conventional MAOIs. However, there is only limited evidence for its usefulness in resistant depression.

Stabl *et al* (1995) compared moclobemide (450 mg daily) with a combination of moclobemide and thioridazine in the treatment of 78 depressed in-patients who had failed to respond to at least two previous trials of antidepressants. Overall, about 75% of the patients showed a useful clinical response (50% decrease in HAM–D score) with no difference between the two treatment regimes. Thus, moclobemide can be worth trying in treatment-resistant patients but if it proves ineffective a switch to a conventional MAOI may still be warranted (Cowen, 1998).

A key issue for successful treatment with MAOIs is the use of adequate doses. For example, some patients may require up to 90 mg a day of phenelzine or 60 mg a day of tranylcypromine. With higher doses it is wise to monitor blood pressure for the development of postural hypotension.

Augmentation strategies

A problem in switching antidepressant preparations is that withdrawal of the first compound may not be straightforward. Patients may have gained some limited benefit from the treatment, for example, in terms of improved sleep or reduced tension, and this will be lost. In addition, if the first medication is stopped quickly, withdrawal symptoms may result. Alternatively, gradual tapering of the dose makes the change-over in medication rather protracted, which may not be easily tolerated by a despairing patient with depression. For this reason, in patients unresponsive to first-line medication, it may be more appropriate to add a second compound to the primary antidepressant, in the hope of producing an additive or even synergistic effect. The major disadvantage of this

procedure is that the risk of adverse effects through drug interaction is increased.

Antipsychotic drugs

Naturalistic studies have shown that patients with depressive psychosis have low response rates to treatment with TCAs alone but may respond well when antipsychotic drugs are combined with a TCA. In a double-blind, random allocation study of 51 in-patients with depressive psychosis, Spiker *et al* (1985) found that the response rate (final HAM–D <7) to amitriptyline alone was 41%, while that to perphenazine alone was 19%. However, patients receiving combined treatment with these drugs had a significantly higher response rate (78%) than either of the other two groups.

Most of the reports of the drug treatment of depressive psychosis have involved TCAs. However, in an open study Rothschild *et al* (1993) found that the combination of fluoxetine (up to 40 mg daily) and perphenazine (up to 35 mg daily) produced a 73% response rate (reduction in HAM–D rating of at least 50%) in 30 patients with DSM–III–R (American Psychiatric Association, 1987) depressive psychosis.

It therefore appears that a combination of SSRIs and antipsychotic drugs may be effective in depressive psychosis. However, in the above study 14 patients developed tremor and two experienced akathisia. SSRIs can cause extrapyramidal movement disorders and may potentiate the extrapyramidal effects of antipsychotic drugs through both pharmacodynamic and pharmacokinetic interactions (Young & Cowen, 1994).

There is interest in the role of new antipyschotic agents such as risperidone and clozapine in depressive psychosis, and a number of positive case reports and series have appeared. However, a controlled trial found that risperidone monotherapy was significantly less effective than a combination of amitriptyline and haloperidol in patients with psychotic depression (Muller-Siecheneder *et al*, 1998).

Antipsychotic drugs are also used occasionally in patients who do not have depressive psychosis but who are anxious and agitated. With conventional antipsychotic agents there is little indication of a specific antidepressant effect in this situation. However, a preliminary report of a placebo-controlled trial (Tollefson *et al*, 1998) suggested that the addition of olanzapine (median dose 10 mg daily) to patients with major depression who had not responded to fluoxetine did result in significant improvements in depression ratings. There are also anecdotal accounts of the use of low-dose risperidone to augment the effect of SSRI treatment in partial responders (Ostroff & Nelson, 1999).

> **Box 2. Clinical predictors of response to conventional MAOIs**
>
> (a) **Atypical depression – mood reactivity, overeating, oversleeping, overwhelming fatigue, rejection sensitivity**
>
> (b) **Bipolar depression with anergia and hypersomnia**

Lithium

Lithium given alone has modest antidepressant properties in patients with bipolar disorder, but other depressed patients show little response. There is now, however, good evidence from uncontrolled and controlled trials that lithium added to ineffective antidepressant treatment can produce useful clinical improvement in patients with major depression. Whether this effect of lithium is a true potentiation (augmentation) of the primary antidepressant compound or simply represents an additive antidepressant effect of its own is debatable.

Uncontrolled trials have reported that lithium addition is followed by a rapid onset of antidepressant effect (within 48 hours) in a high proportion of subjects (60–70%). Double-blind, placebo-controlled trials confirm that lithium is effective, but shows a more gradual onset of action over 2–3 weeks in about 40–50% of patients with depression (Cowen, 1998).

Lithium appears to be effective in improving antidepressant response when added to different kinds of primary antidepressant treatment, including TCAs, SSRIs and MAOIs (Johnson, 1991). Caution is needed when using lithium together with SSRIs because both treatments combine to potentiate brain 5-HT function leading to a risk of 5-HT neurotoxicity. This combination, however, does not seem to have greater therapeutic efficacy than other lithium–antidepressant combinations, despite the marked increase in brain 5-HT function that it produces (Katona *et al*, 1995). On the basis of open studies it has been suggested that the combination of lithium with an MAOI may be particularly helpful in treatment-resistant depression (Price *et al*, 1985).

The plasma level of lithium required to produce an antidepressant effect in treatment-resistant patients has not been clearly established, but levels of 0.5–0.8 mmol/l are usually adequate. It is usually best to initiate lithium treatment at a low dose, for example 200–400 mg daily, particularly where patients are taking serotonergic antidepressants such as SSRIs and MAOIs.

Triiodothyronine

Several open studies have indicated that the addition of triiodothyronine to ineffective TCA treatment can bring about a good clinical response, and this has been supported in three out of four controlled studies. In the most recent controlled investigation, Joffe *et al* (1993) studied 50 out-patients with unipolar, non-psychotic major depression. They had failed to respond to five weeks' treatment with a TCA (daily dose 2.5 mg/kg) after which they were randomly allocated to double-blind addition of lithium carbonate, triiodothyronine (37.5 µg/day)

or placebo for two weeks. At the end of treatment 10 of 17 patients treated with triiodothyronine had responded (50% reduction in HAM–D with final HAM–D score <10). A similar response rate (nine of 17 patients) was noted in patients receiving lithium, while only three of 16 subjects responded to placebo.

The data suggest that addition of triiodothyronine is a useful means of augmenting TCA treatment in patients with depression. In the UK, triiodothyronine is available as a 20 µg tablet (equivalent to about 100 µg thyroxine). When added to TCAs this dose is usually well tolerated; however, caution should be used in patients with cardiovascular disease. If this dose is unsuccessful but tolerance is good there is the option of increasing to 40 µg. At the higher dose symptoms of tachycardia, sweating, hot flushes and anxiety may be experienced. There are at present no comparative data to show that triiodothyronine can augment the action of other classes of antidepressant drugs, but in clinical practice such combinations are sometimes used.

L-Tryptophan

There is evidence from controlled trials that the addition of L-tryptophan can improve the therapeutic effect of MAOI treatment. However, there are no controlled trials to indicate that L-tryptophan can reliably produce therapeutic benefit in patients who have failed to respond to MAOIs or TCAs. Nevertheless, the use of L-tryptophan has been recommended to supplement the 5-HT potentiating effects of lithium–MAOI and lithium–clomipramine combinations (Barker *et al*, 1987; Hale *et al*, 1987).

L-tryptophan has been associated with the development of the eosinophilia myalgic syndrome, a severe connective tissue disease that can have a fatal outcome. Subsequent studies have shown that eosinophilia myalgic syndrome was almost certainly caused by a contaminant that occurred in the production of L-tryptophan from a single manufacturing source (Slutsker *et al*, 1990). In the UK it remains possible to prescribe L-tryptophan, in combination with other antidepressant drugs, for patients with chronic treatment-resistant depression. It should be noted, however, that the combination of L-tryptophan with MAOIs can lead to 5-HT neurotoxicity, so caution is needed. In addition L-tryptophan given with SSRIs can also result in 5-HT toxicity, so this combination is not recommended (Sternbach, 1991).

Combining TCAs and MAOIs

The combination of TCAs and MAOIs has been in use since the 1960s when the efficacy of this regime was first strongly advocated. Although the combination of MAOIs and TCAs is reported to be hazardous, the risks of significant interaction can be minimised if reasonable precautions are taken. These include avoiding imipramine and clomipramine, and starting the drugs together at low dose or adding the MAOI cautiously to established TCA treatment (see Chalmers & Cowen, 1990).

In patients not selected for treatment resistance the combination of MAOIs and TCAs does not appear to confer additional therapeutic benefit over either drug used alone. However, Sethna (1974) carried out an open study of MAOI–TCA treatment in 12 patients with depression who had failed to respond to either TCAs or MAOIs given separately (or electroconvulsive therapy (ECT) in 10 cases). At follow-up periods of 7–24 months, nine subjects were reported to be without significant depressive symptomatology. Most of these subjects had chronic non-melancholic depression with prominent anxiety symptoms.

In addition to these series, case reports continue to appear where it seems well documented that a patient has failed to respond to either a TCA or an MAOI given alone, but achieves a good clinical response when both drugs are used together (Tyrer & Murphy, 1990). Therefore, although controlled evidence is lacking, it seems likely that individual patients with refractory depression are helped by MAOI–TCA combinations. Generally, the adverse effects of the combination are no worse than with either drug alone, although weight gain and postural hypotension may be more troublesome. Conversely, if an MAOI is given with a TCA such as amitriptyline or trimipramine, MAOI-induced insomnia may be prevented.

There is less information about the combination of other antidepressants with MAOIs. However, trazodone in doses of 50–150 mg is fairly commonly used to treat MAOI-induced insomnia and is generally well-tolerated (Nierenberg & Keck, 1989).

Combining TCAs and SSRIs

Some open case series have suggested that combining TCA and SSRI treatment may be helpful in refractory depression. For example, in a retrospective chart review, Weilburg *et al* (1989) reported a positive response (defined as improvement noted by both patient and clinician) in 22 of 25 out-patients with depression when fluoxetine was added to ongoing TCA treatment. This study does not clarify whether or not the improvement was due to the fluoxetine alone or the combination of fluoxetine with the TCA. However, in eight patients the therapeutic response was lost when the TCA was withdrawn, and restored when it was recommenced.

Subsequently, Weilburg *et al* (1991), in a similar study, found resolution of depression in 13 of 20 out-patients in whom nortriptyline or desipramine added to ineffective fluoxetine treatment. One patient worsened with severe agitation. Finally, Seth *et al* (1992) reported remarkable improvement in eight elderly patients with chronic refractory depression who received an SSRI–TCA combination (usually sertraline and nortriptyline). Some patients received concomitant lithium treatment.

The only prospective study of TCA–SSRI treatment was carried out by Fava *et al* (1994) who treated 41 out-patients suffering with depression who had failed to achieve a 50% reduction in HAM–D scores in response to a standard dose of fluoxetine (20 mg daily). Subjects were randomly allocated to three different groups: (a) high-dose fluoxetine (40–60 mg daily); (b) the addition of desipramine (25–50 mg daily); or (c) lithium. Taking response as a final HAM–D score (at five weeks) of <7, the most effective treatment was high-dose fluoxetine (53% response rate) while lithium and desipramine augmentation appeared of similar efficacy (response rates of 29% and 25%, respectively). However, the plasma levels of lithium obtained in this study were low and probably sub-therapeutic.

Taken together the controlled evidence for the efficacy of TCA–SSRI combinations is not compelling. In addition there are numerous case reports of adverse reactions with agitation and, rarely, seizures. These reactions are generally associated with marked elevations in plasma TCA levels because SSRIs are potent inhibitors of the cytochrome P450 system by which TCAs are metabolised. While some SSRIs, for example, citalopram and sertraline, may be less likely to produce this effect, the use of low doses of TCAs in conjunction with plasma monitoring is advisable if combination treatment is used (Taylor, 1995). Another option may be to use treatment with a single drug such as clomipramine or venlafaxine which produces potent 5-HT and noradrenaline reuptake inhibition.

Another drug commonly used in combination with SSRIs is trazodone. Although there are some uncontrolled data suggesting that trazodone can augment the antidepressant effects of SSRIs (Weilburg *et al*, 1991), the usual reason for employing this combination is that the hypnotic effect of trazodone can amelioriate SSRI-induced sleep disturbance. Low doses of trazodone (50–150 mg) are usually sufficient and the combination is generally well tolerated, although there are rare reports of symptoms suggestive of serotonin toxicity.

Pindolol

Repeated administration of a number of antidepressant drugs, particularly SSRIs and MAOIs, desensitises inhibitory 5-HT_{1A} autoreceptors on 5-

HT cell bodies. It has been suggested that this effect contributes to the antidepressant effect of such drugs by freeing 5-HT cell bodies from feedback control and thereby facilitating the release of 5-HT from nerve terminals (Blier & de Montigny, 1994).

Based on this idea, Artigas *et al* (1994) proposed that the addition of a 5-HT$_{1A}$ receptor antagonist to the medication of patients who had not responded to conventional antidepressants, particularly SSRIs, might produce a therapeutic effect. Because there are at present no selective 5-HT$_{1A}$ receptor antagonists available for clinical use, these authors employed pindolol, a β-adrenoceptor antagonist with 5-HT$_{1A}$ receptor antagonist properties.

Pindolol (2.5 mg three times daily) was added to the drug treatment of seven patients with major depression who had been resistant to multiple medication trials. Five subjects were currently taking an SSRI (four paroxetine, one fluvoxamine) while one received imipramine and one phenelzine. All subjects showed a decrease in HAM–D score of at least 50% after a week of pindolol addition and in five, HAM–D scores were less than eight, indicating full remission (Artigas *et al*, 1994).

Subsequently, Blier & Bergeron (1995) reported on the addition of pindolol to 18 patients with major depression who had failed to respond to treatment with an antidepressant together with the addition of another treatment, usually lithium. Pindolol (2.5 mg three times daily) was added to paroxetine (eight subjects), sertraline (five subjects), fluoxetine (three subjects) and moclobemide (two subjects). Overall, pindolol produced a significant improvement in depressive symptoms after one week. By two weeks all the patients, except those on sertraline, had a HAM–D score of 10 or less showing a good clinical improvement. Despite the intriguing results from open studies a recent large placebo-controlled study of pindolol addition to ineffective SSRI treatment showed no benefit over placebo (Perez *et al*, 1999).

Pindolol addition is generally well tolerated, although careful clinical screening is needed to exclude patients with asthma or cardiac conduction disturbances. In open studies pindolol addition has been associated with irritability and one patient developed mania.

ECT

Among the indications for ECT is that of failure to respond to adequate antidepressant drug treatment. Trials of ECT typically report high response rates (about 80%), but patients who are unresponsive to drug treatment are not usually considered as a separate group.

Prudic *et al* (1990) studied the effect of previous antidepressant drug treatment on the response of 53 patients who received bilateral ECT. They found that among those who had received adequate pharmacotherapy (a TCA at a dose of at least 200 mg daily for at least four weeks) the response rate to ECT (defined as a 60% reduction in HAM–D score) was 50%. In contrast, the response rate of patients who had not received adequate drug treatment was significantly greater (86%). The presence of medication resistance, therefore, decreases the likelihood that a patient will respond to ECT. Nevertheless, at least half of such subjects are likely to experience significant improvement.

Another point that needs to be considered is the outcome after ECT. Sackeim *et al* (1990) followed 58 patients who responded to ECT and found that one year post-treatment, 50% had relapsed. The relapse rate in patients who had received adequate drug treatment prior to ECT was significantly higher than in those who had not (64 *v*. 32%). The relapse rate after ECT was only weakly influenced by whether or not patients received adequate antidepressant drug treatment post-ECT.

The practical point from this is that if patients have been unresponsive to a particular medication prior to ECT, continuing with this medication after successful ECT treatment may not provide effective prophylaxis. Therefore consideration should be given to using another class of antidepressant or perhaps lithium prophylaxis if this has not been tried previously. Development of appropriate continuation therapy after ECT is a research priority.

ECT can be used at any point in the treatment of resistant depression. Clinical features that will encourage earlier use include severe depression with high acute suicidal risk, depressive psychosis and pronounced psychomotor features, especially where fluid intake is compromised.

Bipolar depression

The management of bipolar depression is outside the scope of this article, but it is worth noting that it poses additional problems to those encountered in the treatment of resistant unipolar depression. Among these problems are the possibility of induction of mania or rapid cycling by antidepressant drugs. Where patients are having what appears to be a rapidly relapsing depressive illness it is important to establish whether or not the clinical picture is, in fact, rapid cycling with periods of mild hypomania interspersed with depression (Hurowitz & Liebowitz, 1993). Recording of daily moods by the patient can be helpful in clarifying the diagnosis. If rapid cycling is confirmed, withdrawal of antidepressant treatment and the institution of mood stabilising medication can be a useful strategy.

In the treatment of bipolar illness the primary aim is that of mood stabilisation, and there is scope for the use of mood stabilising agents such as carbamazepine in depressive spells (Cowen, 1998). Indeed, a recent placebo-controlled study showed the efficacy of the anticonvulsant drug, lamotrogine, as a monotherapy in patients with bipolar disorder with depression (Calabrese *et al*, 1999). The clinical impression is that antidepressant drugs often seem somewhat less effective in bipolar depression, although bipolar depression with features of anergia and hypersomnia may respond better to MAOIs than to TCAs (Himmelhoch *et al*, 1991).

Conclusion

General and old age psychiatrists need to have confidence in their ability to manage the pharmacological aspects of treatment-resistant depression. It is important to retain the belief that ultimately the patient can recover, because it continues to be the case that even several years of severe depression can be followed by clinical remission (Mueller *et al*, 1996). At the same time it is necessary to recognise (and acknowledge to the patient) the limitations and discomforts of contemporary drug treatments.

Patients are usually aware that miracles are not on offer but do appreciate a practitioner who systematically follows a carefully explained treatment plan. A stepwise approach organised along the lines suggested in this review is shown in Box 3. It is always helpful to have in mind what the next step will be if the current treatment regime fails. Thase & Rush (1997) warn that it is important for the clinician not to become demoralised or frustrated by a patient's lack of response and point out that even where promising pharmacological options appear to be limited, supportive psychological treatment has an important, life-sustaining function (Holmes, 1995).

References

American Psychiatric Association (1987) *Diagnostic and Statistical Manual of Mental Disorders* (3rd edn, revised)(DSM–III–R). Washington, DC: APA.

Anderson, I. (1999) Lessons to be learnt from meta-analyses of newer versus older antidepressants. *Affective and Non-Psychotic Disorders. Recent Topics from Advances in Psychiatric Treatment*, Volume 2 (ed A. Lee), pp. 45–51. London: Gaskell.

Artigas, F., Perez, V. & Alvarez, E. (1994) Pindolol induces a rapid improvement of depressed patients treated with serotonin reuptake inhibitors. *Archives of General Psychiatry*, **51**, 248–251.

Barker, W. A., Scott, J. & Eccelston, D. (1987) The Newcastle Chronic Depression Study: results of a treatment regime. *International Clinical Psychopharmacology*, **2**, 261–272.

Blier, P. & de Montigny, C. (1994) Current advances and trends in the treatment of depression. *Trends in Pharmacological Sciences*, **15**, 220–226.

Blier, P. & Bergeron, R. (1995) Effectiveness of pindolol with selective antidepressant drugs in the treatment of major depression. *Journal of Clinical Psychopharmacology*, **15**, 217–222.

Calabrese, J. R., Bowden, C. L., Sachs, A. S., *et al* (1999) A Double-blind placebo-controlled study of lamotrogine monotherapy in out-patients with bipolar depression. *Journal of Clinical Psychiatry*, **60**, 79–88.

Chalmers, J. S. & Cowen, P. J. (1990) Drug treatment of tricyclic resistant depression. *International Review of Psychiatry*, **2**, 239–248.

Cowen, P. J. (1998) Treatments for resistant depression. In *The Management of Depression* (ed. S. Checkley), pp. 234–251. London: Blackwell.

Fava, M., Rosenbaum, J. F., McGrath, P. J., *et al* (1994) Lithium and tricyclic augmentation of fluoxetine treatment for major depression: a double-blind controlled study. *American Journal of Psychiatry*, **151**, 1372–1374.

Hale, A. S., Procter, A. W. & Bridges, P. K. (1987) Clomipramine, tryptophan and lithium in combination for resistant endogenous depression: seven case studies. *British Journal of Psychiatry*, **151**, 213–217.

Hamilton, M. (1967) Development of a rating scale for primary depressive illness. *British Journal of Social and Clinical Psychology*, **6**, 278–296.

Himmelhoch, J. M., Thase, M. E., Mallinger, A. G., *et al* (1991) Tranylcypromine versus imipramine in anergic bipolar depression. *American Journal of Psychiatry*, **148**, 910–916.

Holmes, J. (1995) Supportive psychotherapy. The search for positive meanings. *British Journal of Psychiatry*, **167**, 439–445.

Hurowitz, G. I. & Liebowitz, M. R. (1993) Antidepressant-induced rapid cycling: six case reports. *Journal of Clinical Psychopharmacology*, **13**, 52–56.

Box 3. Approach for pharmacological treatment of resistant depression

(a) Adjust treatment to maximum therapeutic dose dependent on tolerance (add antipsychotic drug if depressive psychosis)

(b) Switch antidepressant (e.g. TCA for SSRI and vice versa)

(c) Augment with lithium

(d) Augment with triiodothyronine

(e) MAOI (can continue with lithium)

(f) Other combinations (e.g. MAOI + TCA, lithium + MAOI + L - t r y p t o p h a n , lithium + clomipramine + L-tryptophan)

ECT can be used at any stage, depending on clinical features and the need for quick response

Joffe, R. T., Singer, W., Levitt, A. J., *et al* (1993) A placebo-controlled comparison of lithium and triiodothyronine augmentation of tricyclic antidepressants in unipolar refractory depression. *Archives of General Psychiatry*, **50**, 387–393.

Johnson, F. N. (1991) Lithium augmentation therapy for depression. *Reviews in Contemporary Pharmacotherapy*, **2**, 3–52.

Katona, C. L. E., Abou-Saleh, M. T., Harrison, D. A., *et al* (1995) Placebo-controlled trial of lithium augmentation of fluoxetine and lofepramine. *British Journal of Psychiatry*, **166**, 80–86.

Kupfer, D.J. & Frank, E. (1996) Maintenance therapy for chronic depression. *Archives of General Psychiatry*, **53**, 775–776.

Lindberg, G., Bingefors, K., Ranstam, J., *et al* (1998) Use of calcium channel blockers and risk of suicide: ecological findings confirmed in population based cohort study. *British Medical Journal*, **316**, 741–745.

Mueller, T. J., Keller, M. B., Leon, A. C., *et al* (1996) Recovery after 5 years of unremitting major depressive disorder. *Archives of General Psychiatry*, **53**, 794–799.

Muller-Siecheneder, F., Muller, M. J., Hillert, A., *et al* (1998) Risperidone versus haloperidol and amitriptyline in the treatment of patients with a combined psychotic and depressive syndrome. *Journal of Clinical Psychopharmacology*, **18**, 111–120.

Nierenberg, A. A. & Keck, P. E. (1989) Management of monoamine oxidase inhibitor-associated insomnia with trazodone. *Journal of Clinical Psychopharmacology*, **9**, 45–54.

Nolen, W. A., Van de Putte, J. J., Dijken, W. A., *et al* (1988) Treatment strategy in depression. II. MAO inhibitors in depression resistant tricyclic antidepressants: two controlled cross-over studies with tranylcypromine versus 1-5-hydroxytryptophan and nomifensine. *Acta Psychiatrica Scandinavica*, **78**, 676–683.

Ostroff, R. B. & Nelson, C. (1999) Risperidone augmentation of selective serotonin reuptake inhibitors in major depression. *Journal of Clinical Psychiatry*, **60**, 256–259.

Perez, V., Soler, J., Puigdemont, D., *et al* (1999) A double-blind, randomised, placebo-controlled trial of pindolol augmentation in depressive patients resistant to serotonin reuptake inhibitors. *Archives of General Psychiatry*, **56**, 375–379.

Poirer, M.-F. & Boyer, P. (1999) Venlafaxine and paroxetine in treatment-resistant depression. Double-blind, randomised comparison. *British Journal of Psychiatry*, **175**, 12–16.

Preskorn, S. H. (1993) Pharmacokinetics of antidepressants: Why and how are they relevant to treatment? *Journal of Clinical Psychiatry*, **54** (suppl. 9), 14–34.

Price, L. H., Charney, D. S. & Heninger, G. R. (1985) Efficacy of lithium–tranylcypromine treatment in refractory depression. *American Journal of Psychiatry*, **142**, 619–623.

Prudic, J., Sackeim, H. A. & Devanand, D. P. (1990) Medication resistance and clinical response to electroconvulsive therapy. *Psychiatry Research*, **31**, 287–296.

Quitkin, F. M., McGrath, P. J., Stewart, J. W., *et al* (1989) Phenelzine and imipramine in mood reactive depressives. *Archives of General Psychiatry*, **46**, 787–793.

Rothschild, A. J., Samson, J. A., Bessette, M. P., *et al* (1993) Efficacy of the combination of fluoxetine and perphenazine in the treatment of psychotic depression. *Journal of Clinical Psychiatry*, **54**, 338–342.

Sackeim, H. A., Prudic, J., Devenand, D. P., *et al* (1990) The impact of medication resistance and continuation of pharmacotherapy on relapse following response to electroconvulsive therapy in major depression. *Journal of Clinical Psychopharmacology*, **10**, 96–104.

Seth, R., Jennings, A. L., Bindman, J., *et al* (1992) Combination treatment with noradrenaline and serotonin reuptake inhibitors in resistant depression. *British Journal of Psychiatry*, **161**, 562–565.

Sethna, E. R. (1974) A study of refractory cases of depressive illnesses and the response to combined antidepressant treatment. *British Journal of Psychiatry*, **124**, 265–272.

Slutsker, L., Hoesly, F. C., Miller, L., *et al* (1990) Eosinophilia-myalgia syndrome associated with exposure to tryptophan from a single manufacturer. *Journal of the American Medical Association*, **264**, 213–217.

Spiker, D. G., Weiss, J. C. & Dealy, R. S. (1985) The pharmacological treatment of delusional depression. *American Journal of Psychiatry*, **142**, 430–436.

Stabl, M., Kasas, A., Blajev, B., *et al* (1995) A double-blind comparison of moclobemide and thioridazine versus moclobemide and placebo in the treatment of refractory severe depression. *Journal of Clinical Psychopharmacology*, **15** (suppl. 2), 41S–45S.

Sternbach, H. (1991) The serotonin syndrome. *American Journal of Psychiatry*, **148**, 705–713.

Taylor, D. (1995) Selective serotonin reuptake inhibitors and tricyclic antidepressants in combination: interactions and therapeutic uses. *British Journal of Psychiatry*, **167**, 575–580.

Thase, M. E. & Rush, A. J. (1997) When at first you don't succeed: sequential strategies for antidepressant non-responders. *Journal of Clinical Psychiatry*, **58** (suppl. 13), 23–29.

Tollefson, G. D., Shelton, R., Tohen, M., *et al* (1998) Efficacy of olanzapine, fluoxetine and combination therapy in treatment-resistant major depressive disorder without psychotic features. *11th ECNP Congress Abstracts*, 1122.

Tyrer, P. & Murphy, S. (1990) Efficacy of combined antidepressant therapy in resistant neurotic disorder. *British Journal of Psychiatry*, **156**, 115–118.

Weilburg, J. B., Rosenbaum, J. F., Biderman, J., *et al* (1989) Fluoxetine added to non-MAOI antidepressants converts non-responders to responders: a preliminary report. *Journal of Clinical Psychiatry*, **50**, 447–449.

—, —, Meltzer-Brody, S., *et al* (1991) Tricyclic augmentation of fluoxetine. *Annals of Clinical Psychiatry*, **3**, 209–213.

Young, A. H. & Cowen, P. J. (1994) Antidepressant drugs. In *Side-Effects of Drugs Annual, Vol. 17* (eds J. K. Aronson & C. J. Van Boxtel), pp. 16–25. Amsterdam: Elsevier.

Prevention of relapse and recurrence of depression: newer versus older antidepressants

J. Guy Edwards

In a 17- to 19-year follow-up study it was shown that patients admitted to the Maudsley Hospital, London (whose index episode marked their first psychiatric contact), had a 50% chance of readmission during their lifetime; those with previous admissions had a similar chance of readmission within three years. Less than one-fifth of the patients had remained well, and over one-third suffered severe chronic distress and handicap or had died unnaturally (Lee & Murray, 1988). Similar gloomy pictures were reported in a 15-year follow-up study of patients in London and Sydney (Kiloh *et al*, 1988) and an 11-year follow-up study of patients in Montreal (Lehmann *et al*, 1988). As a result of such findings, much emphasis is now placed on the importance of continuation and maintenance treatment of depression.

Continuation treatment is given to help consolidate recovery from an episode of depression and to prevent relapse, whereas maintenance (prophylactic) treatment is given to help prevent a recurrence of depression. A relapse is a worsening of an ongoing or recently treated episode, whereas a recurrence is a new episode of depression. When there is a long interval between episodes the distinction is easier to make, but when the interval is short the distinction is to a certain extent arbitrary and may not reflect underlying pathogenic processes. There is agreement among researchers that 4–6 months' remission (during which time the patient's affective state returns to its premorbid level) should occur before a further depressive episode is regarded as a recurrence.

Many trials of continuation and maintenance treatment have been carried out. Over the years, larger numbers of patients have been included in trials and the methodology has improved. The placebo-controlled studies undertaken up to 1997 are shown in Table 1. It is difficult to make meaningful comparisons between older and newer antidepressants because of differences in the patients included in trials of older and newer compounds and differences in methodology. However, the studies included patients who met conventional diagnostic criteria, such as those in DSM–III–R (American Psychiatric Association, 1987) and who had defined scores on rating scales for depression. Most subjects included were responders to open treatment with the drug being investigated, or those who had responded during a controlled trial of shorter term (acute) treatment with the drug. Relapse or recurrence was defined as a worsening or return of depression with a predetermined increase in a score on a rating scale. However, there are a number of methodological difficulties that have to be taken into account in the interpretation of the results of long-term trials (Box 1).

Notwithstanding these difficulties, the studies suggest that about 60% (range 22–76%) of those who respond to an antidepressant and are then switched to placebo remain in remission for up to two or three years. If instead the patients continue with the

---

Box 1. Methodological problems in studies of long-term treatment

Difficulties in defining remission, relapse and recurrence
Small sample sizes
Matching on all variables, including number of previous episodes of affective disorder
Effect of previous treatment
Effect of concomitant treatment
Drop-outs
Difficulty in tracing patients
Difficulty in obtaining accurate follow-up data

Table 1. Placebo-controlled studies of antidepressants in the prevention of relapse and recurrence of depression

Study	Age range (months)	Duration of study	Antidepressants	Patients, n	Relapses or recurrences, n (%)	
Montgomery et al, 1988	ns	12	Fluoxetine 40 mg	88	23	(26)
			Placebo	94	54	(57)
Georgotas et al, 1989	>55	12	Nortriptyline[1]	13	7	(54)
			Phenelzine[2]	15	2	(13)
			Placebo	23	15	(65)
Rouillon et al, 1989	18–78	12	Maprotiline 75 mg	385	62	(16)
			Maprotiline 37.5 mg	382	92	(24)
			Placebo	374	131	(35)
Frank et al, 1990	21–65	36	Imipramine mean 200 mg	28	6	(21)
			Imipramine+IPT	25	6	(24)
			Placebo	23	18	(78)
Robinson et al, 1991	>18	24	Phenelzine 45 mg	12	4	(33)
			Phenelzine 60 mg	19	5	(26)
			Placebo	16	13	(81)
Doogan & Caillard, 1992	18–70	11	Sertraline 50–200 mg	184	24	(13)
			Placebo	105	48	(46)
Kupfer et al, 1992	21–65	24	Imipramine mean 200 mg	11	1	(9)
			Placebo	9	6	(67)
Old Age Depression Interest Group, 1993	>60	24	Dothiepin 75 mg	33	10	(30)
			Placebo	36	20	(56)
Montgomery & Dunbar, 1993	23–65	12	Paroxetine 20–30 mg	68	11	(16)
			Placebo	67	29	(43)
Montgomery et al, 1993	18–70	24	Citalopram 20 mg	48	4	(8)
			Citalopram 40 mg	57	7	(12)
			Placebo	42	13	(31)
Anton et al, 1994	ns	12	Nefazodone 100–600 mg	139	12	(9)
			Imipramine 50–300 mg	66	5	(8)
			Placebo	71	18	(25)
Robert & Montgomery, 1995	19–70	6	Citalopram 20–60 mg	150	21	(14)
			Placebo	74	18	(24)
Total			Antidepressant	1723	302	(18)
			Placebo	934	383	(41)

1. Dose adjusted to maintain plasma nortriptyline levels at 190–648 mmol/l. 2. Dose adjusted to maintain plasma platelet inhibition at >70%. IPT, interpersonal therapy; ns, not specified.

treatment to which they have responded, they have overall a 20–25% better chance of maintaining their improvement. Some of the studies referred to also revealed advantages of antidepressant over placebo in the time to onset of relapse or recurrence and in the depression scores of those who did not relapse. The studies cited are important in showing the efficacy of continuation and prophylactic treatment, but there is a paucity of knowledge on variables which may predict benefit for individual patients.

Which antidepressant?

Few long-term comparative studies have been carried out and most of these were comparisons of tricyclic antidepressants (TCAs) and lithium. The choice of drug in long-term treatment, therefore, has to be based on the results of short-term trials, epidemiological studies of untoward effects, pharmacological experiments and impressions gleaned from studies of continuation and maintenance treatment.

Therapeutic effects

Meta analyses have shown that there are no significant differences in effectiveness of different types of antidepressants during short-term treatment (Anderson, this volume), although data from some individual trials suggest that selective serotonin reuptake inhibitors (SSRIs) other than fluvoxamine could be less effective than TCAs in the treatment of severely melancholic in-patients (Anderson, this issue). As there are insufficient data on long-term treatment (merely hints of a possible lower relapse rate on SSRIs than TCAs), there is no good reason based on effectiveness for choosing one antidepressant rather than another for maintenance treatment.

Adverse effects

The choice of antidepressant (or antidepressant class) for continuation or prophylactic treatment is therefore based on its tolerability (which is related to the adverse effect profile), toxicity in overdose and cost. Many unwanted effects of both new and old drugs have been reported, but only those that occupy a dominant place in the new-versus-old antidepressant debate will be discussed here. Conspicuous among these are anticholinergic and anti-α-adrenoceptor effects and sedation.

There are problems in comparing drugs because of difficulties in defining common effects (which are often identical to the symptoms of depression) and because of differences between studies in the way adverse effects are elicited, recorded and related to treatment. Notwithstanding these problems, the newer antidepressants have been shown to cause less sedation and autonomic effects than older TCAs. Thus, they produce fewer anticholinergic effects, such as decreased salivary flow and gastrointestinal mobility, which lead to dental caries and constipation, respectively, and less anti-α-adrenoceptor effects, which may result in postural hypotension (causing falls and injuries). Accidents may also be caused by over-sedation. On the other hand, the newer drugs cause other effects, such as gastrointestinal symptoms and central nervous system excitatory effects in the case of SSRIs (see Henry, this volume). In the case of both older and newer antidepressants adaptation to unwanted effects, such as sedation and nausea, may occur.

Adherence

These various reactions influence adherence, which in turn may have an effect on relapse and recurrence. Meta-analyses of adherence with continuation and maintenance treatment have not been carried out, although comments in reports of trials of long-term treatment with TCAs and newer antidepressants imply that both types of drugs are well tolerated. Clinicians are therefore influenced in their choice of drugs by the results of meta-analyses of short-term

treatment. These show, for example, no difference between SSRIs and tricyclics in drop-outs due to inefficacy, but a small significant difference (4.4–4.7%) in drop-outs due to side-effects (Anderson & Tomenson, 1995; Montgomery & Kasper, 1995; Anderson, this volume).

Much is made of this difference but more important is the overall drop-out rate, as it is often difficult to be sure exactly why patients stop their treatment. Drug-induced dysphoria (a side-effect) may be misinterpreted as lack of effectiveness, while patients may not tolerate side-effects that they would otherwise accept, or drop out for other reasons, due to their depression failing to respond to treatment. Overall drop-out rates in meta-analyses do not show a significant difference between SSRIs and TCAs.

It is possible that overviews obscure differences between individual drugs. For instance, in a comparative trial there were 10% less drop-outs due to inefficacy and side-effects during treatment with paroxetine than imipramine (Dunbar *et al*, 1991), whereas in a small meta-analysis there were 9.6% less drop-outs due to adverse effects during treatment with dothiepin than SSRIs (Donovan *et al*, 1993).

Meta-analyses focus on trials in which highly selected patients are included. It is not known whether the apparent advantage of SSRIs also exists in the real world of general practice where most patients with depression are treated, or whether there is a lower discontinuation rate during longer term treatment when adaptation to adverse effects might be expected to occur. Nor is it known whether the advantage would be upheld in populations of patients given better information and reassurance about side-effects, which is known to improve adherence.

Behavioural effects

The older TCAs (and some other antidepressants, e.g. mianserin, trazodone) have been shown to cause more impairment than the newer antidepressants (including lofepramine) in laboratory tests of cognitive and psychomotor function (Hindmarch *et al*, 1992). The older tricyclics have also been shown to cause impairment in driving tests, whereas SSRIs, reversible inhibitors of monoamine oxidase A (RIMAs) and nefazodone cause little or no impairment (Louwerens *et al*, 1986; Ramaekers *et al*, 1994; Robbe & O'Hanlon, 1995; van Laar *et al*, 1995). Although these findings support the use of the newer drugs for long-term treatment, the predictive validity of psychomotor tests has been questioned (Parrott, 1987; Freeman & O'Hanlon, 1995). Many skilled tasks can be performed without undue effort and with spare processing capacity left available, and it has been suggested that information-processing tasks are measures of competence (potential) rather than actual performance (Parrott, 1991).

Furthermore, most of the investigations were carried out after short-term administration of drugs (sometimes in single doses), rather than during longer term treatment, when adaptation may occur. Adaptation to the effects of TCAs on driving has, in fact, been demonstrated (Ramaekers *et al*, 1994; Robbe & O'Hanlon, 1995; Van Laar *et al*, 1995). Perhaps these considerations explain why TCAs were found in the body fluids of only 0.2% of people who died in traffic accidents, compared with alcohol in 35% and other drugs liable to affect the central nervous system in 7.4% (Everest *et al*, 1989).

Consistent with the observations that older TCAs cause psychomotor impairment is the finding that elderly drivers treated with these drugs have an increased risk of vehicle crashes in which injuries are sustained, and that there is a relationship between the risk and dose of drug (Ray *et al*, 1992; Leveille *et al*, 1994). This suggests that the drugs contribute to the accidents, although inability to control for all potentially confounding variables does not allow for definite conclusions to be reached.

The extent to which antidepressants cause or contribute to road traffic and other accidents is not known. Nevertheless, the aforementioned concerns should be taken into account in the choice of drug for long-term treatment. Although the risk may be greater when treatment is first introduced, it should also be considered when the dose is increased or when antidepressants are taken with other substances that affect cognition and psychomotor performance. For patients thought to be at high risk of accidents, including those who experience persistent sedation when taking TCAs or drug combinations, it is sensible to err on the side of safety and prescribe non-sedative antidepressants.

Drug interactions

The more receptors and enzymes affected by a drug, the greater the number of potential interactions. Thus, older monoamine oxidase inhibitors (MAOIs) and TCAs cause more interactions than newer drugs, such as RIMAs and SSRIs. However, SSRIs interact with other drugs that affect serotonergic transmission and they inhibit hepatic enzymes involved in the metabolism of a wide range of other compounds. Fluoxetine and paroxetine, for instance, are powerful inhibitors of CYP2D6, a specific cytochrome P450 isoenzyme which catalyses the metabolism of many other drugs. Concurrent treatment with SSRIs may lead to increased plasma concentrations of these drugs (Spina & Perucca,

1994; Edwards, 1995). However, the evidence for some interactions is weak; many are of more theoretical than practical interest; and similar numbers of potentially hazardous interactions occur with SSRIs as with TCAs (Edwards, 1995; Henry, this volume). Such interactions can be avoided by the careful choice of drugs.

Lethality in overdose

Antidepressants introduced before 1970 have a higher fatal toxicity index (the number of deaths due to overdose per million prescriptions) than those introduced more recently (Henry *et al*, 1995; Henry, this volume). Despite the limitations of the methodology (especially uncertainty over the cause of death; the quantities of drugs and other substances taken; and the medical condition of the patients), the results show that death due to overdose of antidepressants is more likely to occur if older drugs are taken. This is consistent with the known cardiotoxic effects of older TCAs and the relative freedom from these effects of the newer anti-depressants.

On the strength of these observations, it has been recommended that the newer antidepressants should be used routinely as first-line treatment of depression. However, the risk of death from overdose has to be seen in perspective. Only about 4% of all suicides are due to overdose of single antidepressants (Office of Population Censuses and Surveys, 1975–1992) and it is not known what proportion of these are taken during treatment (when choice is more relevant).

Furthermore, different suicide rates among patients prescribed different antidepressants may be influenced by their doctors' perception of suicidal risk. It has been shown, for instance, that amitriptyline is prescribed more often for patients with severe depression and depression associated with severe insomnia, which in turn could be associated with an increased propensity for suicide (Isacsson *et al*, 1994). Also, patients treated with TCAs may not be at greater overall risk of suicide (by any method) than those treated with less toxic drugs, as those who have their minds set firmly on killing themselves will choose a method of doing so. In keeping with this are two other findings: first, deaths due to self-poisoning in England and Wales have decreased since safer antidepressants have been more widely used, while those due to more violent methods have increased (Office of Population Censuses and Surveys, 1975–1992); second, the incidence of suicide by any method during treatment with the newer and older antidepressants in general practice is similar (Jick *et al*, 1995).

There is need for more epidemiological research. Until the results of this are available, it is advisable to avoid, or reduce access to, the older antidepressants that are more lethal in overdose in patients at high risk of suicide.

Relative costs and benefits

Purchasers of health care who have limited budgets have to weigh the direct and indirect costs of expensive new treatments against the benefits. A balanced view (Box 2) suggests that the benefits of the newer over older antidepressants may not be as clearly defined or as large as some believe. New drugs are expensive (Table 2). If there were a total shift in prescribing to SSRIs, in England alone the cost to the National Health Service at 1995 prices and consumption volumes would be almost £350 million per annum more than treating the same patients with amitriptyline. The purchases that can be made from this additional cost are often overlooked. They include, for instance, the purchase of 2.8 million days of in-patient treatment, 6.9 million days of day patient treatment or 4.1 million out-patient attendances per year for patients with mental health problems (calculated at 1994/95 costs). As an alternative, almost 22 million hours of community psychiatric nurse time could be bought. Outside psychiatry, the additional costs of SSRIs would allow for the purchase of a wide variety of operations ranging from about 12 000 heart or bone marrow transplants to 770 000 D & Cs.

Opinions on the advantages and disadvantages of the newer and older drugs are polarised, but there is

---

Box 2.   Advantages and disadvantages of SSRIs compared with older TCAs and related antidepressants

Advantages
Tolerance: 3.4–4.9% fewer drop-outs from trials due to side-effects
Unwanted effects: less sedation; less anticholinergic effects; less weight gain; possibly fewer accidents
Toxicity in overdose: less likely to be lethal

Disadvantages
Unwanted effects: more gastrointestinal side-effects; long-term toxicity unknown
Cost: more expensive

Comments
Tolerance: no significant difference in overall drop-out rate; not known whether advantage exists in routine clinical practice
Unwanted effects: more epidemiological data are needed
Toxicity in overdose: suicide rate by any method among patients treated with different antidepressants is similar
Cost: extra expense means less money available for other areas of medical care

---

little place for dogmatism. The most objective view is that based on scientific evidence, rather than on frustration with the relative lack of effectiveness of antidepressants in general, novelty and hype.

Table 2.   National Health Service prescriptions for antidepressants and their costs in England in 1995

Antidepressants	Prescription items (x10³)	Net ingredient cost (£ x10³)	Average cost per prescription (£)
TCAs and related antidepressants	8610.9	36 439.4	4.23
Amitriptyline	2461.7	1890.0	0.77
Imipramine	437.1	438.9	1.00
Dothiepin	3308.3	13 963.0	4.22
Selective serotonin reuptake inhibitors	3793.9	103 230.9	27.21
Total for all antidepressants	13 227.2	146 832.9	11.10

Drug classification as in British National Formulary (1994). Data refer to all NHS prescriptions dispensed by community pharmacists and dispensing doctors. The net ingredient costs are the costs of drugs before discounts; they do not include dispensing costs or fees. The data are published with permission of the Statistics Division of the NHS Executive.

References

American Psychiatric Association (1987) Diagnostic and Statistical Manual of Mental Disorders (3rd edn, rev)(DSM–III–R). Washington, DC: APA.

Anderson, I. & Tomenson, B. M. (1995) Treatment discontinuation with selective serotonin reuptake inhibitors compared with tricyclic antidepressants: A meta-analysis. *British Medical Journal*, **310**, 1433–1438.

Anton, S. F., Robinson, D. S., Roberts, D. L., *et al* (1994) Long-term treatment of depression with nefazodone. *Psychopharmacology Bulletin*, **30**, 165–169.

British National Formulary (1994) *British National Formulary*. Number 28. London: British Medical Association and the Royal Pharmaceutical Society of Great Britain.

Donovan, S., McGrady, H., Pownall, R., *et al* (1993) The efficacy and tolerability of dothiepin and three selective serotonin reuptake inhibitors in the treatment of major depression: A review of double-blind studies. *Current Therapeutic Research*, **54**, 275–288.

Doogan, D. P. & Caillard, V. (1992) Sertraline in the prevention of depression. *British Journal of Psychiatry*, **160**, 217–222.

Dunbar, G. C., Cohn, J. B., Fabre, L. F., *et al* (1991) A comparison of paroxetine, imipramine and placebo in depressed out-patients. *British Journal of Psychiatry*, **159**, 394–398.

Edwards, J. G. (1995) Drug choice in depression. Selective serotonin reuptake inhibitors or tricyclic antidepressants? *CNS Drugs*, **4**, 141–159.

Everest, J. T., Tunbridge, R. J. & Widdop, B. (1989). *The Incidence of Drugs in Road Accident Fatalities* (TRRL Research Report 202). Crowthorne: Transport and Road Research Laboratory.

Frank, E., Kupfer, D. J., Perel, J. M., *et al* (1990) Three-year outcomes for maintenance therapies in recurrent depression. *Archives of General Psychiatry*, **47**, 1093–1099.

Freeman, H. L. & O'Hanlon, J. E. (1995) Acute and subacute effects of antidepressants on performance. *Journal of Drug Development and Clinical Practice*, **7**, 7–20.

Georgotas, A., McCue, R. E. & Cooper, T. B. (1989) A placebo-controlled comparison of nortriptyline and phenelzine in maintenance therapy of elderly depressed patients. *Archives of General Psychiatry*, **46**, 783–786.

Henry, J. A., Alexander, C. A. & Sener, E. K. (1995) Relative mortality from overdose of antidepressants. *British Medical Journal*, **310**, 221–224.

Hindmarch, I., Alford, C., Barwell, F., *et al* (1992) Measuring the side effects of psychotropics: the behavioural toxicity of antidepressants. *Journal of Psychopharmacology*, **6**, 198–203.

Isacsson, G., Redfors, I., Wasserman, D., *et al* (1994) Choice of antidepressants: questionnaire survey of psychiatrists and general practitioners in two areas of Sweden. *British Medical Journal*, **309**, 1546–1549.

Jick, S. S., Dean, A. D. & Jick, H. (1995) Antidepressants and suicide. *British Medical Journal*, **310**, 215–218.

Kiloh, L. G., Andrews, G. & Neilson, M. (1988) The long-term outcome of depressive illness. *British Journal of Psychiatry*, **153**, 752–757.

Kupfer, D. J., Frank, E., Perel, J. M., *et al* (1992) Five-year outcome for maintenance therapies in recurrent depression. *Archives of General Psychiatry*, **49**, 769–773.

Lee, A. S. & Murray, R. M. (1988) The long-term outcome of Maudsley depressives. *British Journal of Psychiatry*, **153**, 741–751.

Lehmann, H. E., Fenton, F. R. & Deutsch, M., *et al* (1988) An 11-year follow up study of 110 depressed patients. *Acta Psychiatrica Scandinavica*, **78**, 57–65.

Leveille, S. G., Buchner, D. M., Koepsell, T. D., *et al* (1994) Psychoactive medications and injurious motor vehicle collisions involving older drivers. *Epidemiology*, **5**, 591–598.

Louwerens, J. W., Brookhuis, K. A. & O'Hanlon, J. F. (1986) Several antidepressants' acute effects upon actual driving performance and subjective mental activation. In *Drugs and Driving* (eds J. F. O'Hanlon & J. J. de Gier), pp. 203-213. Philadelphia, PA: Taylor & Francis.

Montgomery, S. A. & Dunbar, G. (1993). Paroxetine is better than placebo in relapse prevention and the prophylaxis of recurrent depression. *International Clinical Psychopharmacology*, **8**, 189–195.

—— & Kasper, S. (1995) Comparison of compliance between serotonin reuptake inhibitors and tricyclic antidepressants: A meta-analysis. *International Clinical Psychopharmacology*, **9** (suppl. 4), 33–40.

—––, Dufour, H., Brion, S., *et al* (1988) The prophylactic efficacy of fluoxetine in unipolar depression. *British Journal of Psychiatry*, **153** (suppl. 3), 69–73.

—––, Rasmussen, J. G. C. & Tanghøj, P. (1993) A 24-week study of 20 mg citalopram, 40 mg citalopram, and placebo in the prevention of relapse of major depression. *International Clinical Psychopharmacology*, **8**, 181–188.

Office of Population Censuses and Surveys (1975–1992) *Mortality Statistics: Cause. Reviews of the Registrar General on Deaths by Cause, Sex and Age, in England and Wales*. London: HMSO.

Old Age Depression Interest Group (1993) How long should the elderly take antidepressants? A double-blind placebo-controlled study of continuation/prophylaxis therapy with dothiepin. *British Journal of Psychiatry*, **162**, 175–182.

Parrott, A. C. (1987) Assessment of psychological performance in applied situations. In *Human Psychopharmacology. Measures and Methods*, vol. 1 (eds I. Hindmarch & P. D. Stonier), pp. 93–112. Chichester: Wiley.

—— (1991) Performance tests in human psychopharmacology. 3: Construct validity and test interpretation. *Human Psychopharmacology*, **6**, 197–207.

Ramaekers, J. G., van Veggel, L. M. A. & O'Hanlon, J. F. (1994) A cross-study comparison of the effects of moclobemide and brofaromine on actual driving performance and estimated sleep. *Clinical Neuropharmacology*, **17** (suppl. 1), S9–S18.

Ray, W. A., Fought, R. L. & Decker, M. D. (1992) Psychoactive drugs and the risk of injurious motor vehicle crashes in elderly drivers. *American Journal of Epidemiology*, **136**, 873–883.

Robbe, H. W. J. & O'Hanlon, J. F. (1995) Acute and subchronic effects of paroxetine 20 and 40 mg on actual driving, psychomotor performance and subjective assessments in healthy volunteers. *European Neuropsychopharmacology*, **5**, 35–42.

Robert, P. H. & Montgomery, S. A. (1995) Citalopram in doses of 20–60 mg is effective in depression relapse prevention: A placebo-controlled six-month study. *International Clinical Psychopharmacology*, **10** (suppl. 1), 29–35.

Robinson, D. S., Lerfald, S. C., Bennet, B., *et al* (1991) Maintenance therapies in recurrent depression: New findings. *Psychopharmacology Bulletin*, **27**, 31–39.

Rouillon, F., Phillips, R., Serrurier, D., *et al* (1989) Prophylactic efficacy of maprotiline on relapses of unipolar depression. *Encephale*, **15**, 527–534.

Spina, E. & Perucca, E. (1994) Newer and older antidepressants. A comparative review of drug interactions. *CNS Drugs*, **2**, 479–497.

Van Laar, M. W., van Willgenburg, A. P. P. & Volkerts, E. R. (1995) Acute and subchronic effects of nefazodone and imipramine on highway driving, cognitive functions, and daytime sleepiness in healthy adult and elderly subjects. *Journal of Clinical Psychopharmacology*, **15**, 30–40.

Advances in the practice of electroconvulsive therapy

Toni Lock

The first electroconvulsive treatment was administered by Cerletti & Bini in 1938. The event was essentially an experiment, carried out like a military operation (Endler, 1988). The patient was stimulated three times, each time increasing the intensity of the stimulus before a generalised seizure was induced. He had been suffering from an acute psychosis with a poor prognosis, but responded to a course of 11 treatments and was discharged free of symptoms two months later. The first paper on electroconvulsive therapy (ECT) in English was published in the *Lancet* in 1939 (Kalinowski, 1939). At that time, somatic treatment alternatives for the severely ill in large mental institutions included lobotomy and insulin coma therapy. In comparison, unmodified ECT (albeit associated with a significant risk of serious physical morbidity) was predictable, efficient, quick and effective. It is understandable why the treatment became widely and fairly indiscriminately adopted before systematic objective evidence of its efficacy was collected.

The introduction of general anaesthesia and muscle relaxants reduced the risk of physical morbidity, and more recent improvements of anaesthetic procedures and patient monitoring have further improved the safety of ECT. The morbidity rate today (1 death per 50 000 treatments) is similar to that of general anaesthesia in minor surgical procedures (Kramer, 1985).

That ECT is safe and dramatically effective in some cases is not disputed by the medical profession or the lay public (Mind , 1988). Nevertheless, ECT continues to evoke strong feelings, because of its history of indiscriminate use, and because of an innate fear of the treatment itself – deliberate administration of electric shocks to the brain to induce epileptiform seizures. Given the considerable advances in antipsychotic and antidepressant drug treatment over the last 40 years, does ECT still have a place in contemporary psychiatry?

Research into ECT has focused on efficacy in specific syndromes, indications for treatment, mode of action and side-effects. The focus over the last 20 years has been on maximising the therapeutic response while minimising the cognitive side-effects of treatment. In general, ECT research has tended to generate questions faster than it has resolved them. The procedures of stimulus dosing and EEG monitoring are widely used in North American ECT clinics, but these concepts are new to many British psychiatrists, and their appropriateness for British ECT practice is debatable. Stimulus dosing is, however, not a recent invention– Cerletti & Bini stimulus-dosed their first patient.

This chapter provides an overview of the recent research and audit findings that have driven changes in British ECT practice since the first ECT audit report to the Royal College of Psychiatrists (Pippard & Ellam, 1981).

Indications

ECT tends to be reserved as a second-line treatment for patients who have failed to respond to an adequate trial of drugs, in particular antidepressant drugs for depressive illness. The treatment is used less frequently as a first-line intervention for:

(a) Patients who are unwilling or unable to tolerate the side-effects of effective drug treatment.
(b) Patients who have responded well to ECT in the past but not to antidepressants.
(c) Cases where a fast response to treatment is needed to relieve intense suffering or to save the life of the patient, because of either an immediate risk of suicide or death from other causes (e.g. deep melancholic syndromes, lethal catatonia and manic frenzy leading to exhaustion).

Empirical clinical and research evidence supports the efficacy of ECT in the treatment of a wide range of psychiatric disorders, including major depressive illness, mania, acute schizophreniform psychoses, catatonic states, neuroleptic malignant syndrome, postpuerperal psychosis, psychiatric disorders associated with epilepsy, spontaneous epileptic disorders *per se*, idiopathic Parkinson's disease, and drug-induced extrapyramidal disorders. For reviews of research data in relation to specific syndromes see *The Practical Administration of Electroconvulsive Therapy* (Royal College of Psychiatrists' ECT Sub-Committee of the Research Committee; Royal College of Psychiatrists' Special Committee on ECT, 1995) and the equivalent publication of the American Psychiatric Association (1990). There is remarkable consistency in the findings of open and controlled clinical trials which show the efficacy of ECT in depressive illness, mania and acute schizophreniform syndromes. Patients treated with ECT only or a combination of ECT and drugs (ECT plus antidepressants for depressive illness; ECT plus lithium for mania; ECT plus neuroleptics for schizophrenia) show a more rapid and complete response in the short term (i.e. the initial 4–6 weeks of treatment) than patients treated only with drugs or no specific drug therapy. ECT is particularly effective for severe depressive illness associated with psychotic delusions (Buchan *et al*, 1992). ECT is also effective in drug-resistant depression (Prudic *et al*, 1990) and schizophrenia (Taylor, 1990).

Most, if not all, ECT trials are, however, open to criticism on methodological grounds, which diminishes the weight that can be attached to the conclusions reached (Crow & Johnstone, 1986), and which contributes to ongoing doubts about

its efficacy. The issue not addressed by trials is whether ECT contributes a therapeutic effect which may be achieved by other means. For example, where ECT has been shown to be superior to drug treatment in depressive illness, mania and schizophrenia, control subjects may not have been treated with adequate doses of antipsychotic or antidepressant drugs; where ECT has been shown to be particularly effective in depressive illness associated with delusions, control subjects were not treated with an adequate combination of antidepressant and neuroleptic drugs; where ECT has been shown to bring about faster and more complete symptomatic relief from depressive illness, control subjects were not treated with the potent combination of antidepressants and lithium. Another issue which remains uncertain is whether there are any longer-term advantages of ECT over alternative drug treatments after the initial 4–6 weeks of treatment. The evidence is that the advantage of ECT (on its own or in combination with drugs) over drug-only treatment disappears after the initial treatment period.

Research attempts to define specific indicators for a good outcome to ECT have, to some extent, been complicated by the diagnostic process itself. For example, it is sometimes difficult to determine whether acute paranoid delusions are primary (i.e. part of a primary paranoid psychosis) or secondary (i.e. to a severe affective disorder) without the patient's psychiatric history. Paranoid delusions respond well to ECT, regardless of the primary diagnosis (Buchan *et al*, 1992). Endogenous affective symptoms (e.g. melancholic or manic type) respond well to ECT, regardless of whether primary (i.e. part of an affective disorder) or secondary (i.e. to schizophrenia). Similarly, marked alterations in psychomotor activity respond well to ECT, regardless of the primary diagnosis.

As with drug treatment, a sudden onset and short duration of illness is an indicator of good outcome. In the case of affective disorders, evidence of pre-morbid personality maladjustment and neurosis (e.g. hypochondriasis, somatisation and obsessive–compulsive symptoms) are indicative of a poor long-term prognosis, even if there is some short-term response to ECT.

The decision to offer ECT must rest with the practitioner and should be made after carefully weighing the comparative risks of ECT with those of drug treatments. As ECT is effective in drug-resistant depression and schizophrenia then – with hindsight – it is evident that a decision to withhold treatment in the first instance may mean that some patients and their carers may have to endure a more lengthy period of stress and hardship.

Box 1. Use of ECT

ECT is usually a second-line treatment, but may be a first-line treatment in some cases. Candidates for ECT include those displaying a combination of:

(a) Endogenous affective symptoms
(b) Acute (florid or type 1) schizophreniform symptoms
(c) Marked alterations in psychomotor activity

Clinical standards

The first ECT audit report to the Royal College of Psychiatrists (Pippard & Ellam, 1981) asserted that about one in three ECT clinics was ill-equipped, the staff poorly trained, and the treatment ineffective. Considerable improvements were made over the following decade (Pippard, 1992a,b), less so, however, in those aspects of treatment which are the direct responsibility of psychiatrists than those which are not (e.g. anaesthetic and nursing practices). Of particular concern was the finding that approximately one in four treatment applications was unlikely to result in therapeutically effective seizures. Furthermore, the standard of training and supervision of junior doctors was generally below that recommended by the Royal College of Psychiatrists (1977; Royal College of Psychiatrists' ECT Sub-Committee of the Research Committee, 1989), and most juniors did not use the ECT equipment competently. Some anaesthetists have a very low regard for disinterested, poorly skilled and poorly supervised trainees, whom they describe as 'button pushers' (Haddad & Benbow, 1993). ECT equipment was another cause for concern.

As a result of these findings the Special Committee on ECT of the Royal College of Psychiatrists was re-established and given a wide remit (Freeman, 1992). The Committee revised the existing ECT guidelines (Royal College of Psychiatrists' ECT Sub-Committee of the Research Committee, 1989) and the revised Guidelines (*The ECT Handbook. The Second Report of the Royal College of Psychiatrists' Special Committee on ECT*) were published in 1995 (Royal College of Psychiatrists' Special Committee on ECT, 1995). Recommendations related both to structures (e.g. the quality of ECT suites and equipment) and to procedures (e.g. the administration of electrical current, monitoring of seizure activity, management of anaesthesia and recovery, and the organisation, training and supervision of personnel). By late 1996, about 300 psychiatrists had attended one of the ECT revision courses run as part of the College's efforts towards continuing professional development. British and American ECT machines were reviewed, and a short-list of approved models was produced (Lock, 1995a; Robertson & Fergusson, 1996). A video teaching pack was produced and widely disseminated (Gearney, 1993; Lock, 1994; Duffett & Lelliot, 1998). A third revision of the ECT guidelines is planned for publication in 2000.

Have standards of practice improved as a result of the above College activity? The authors of the third College audit cycle of ECT (Duffett & Lelliott, 1998) concluded:

"20 Years of activity by the Royal College of Psychiatrists and three large-scale audits have been associated with only modest improvements in local practice."

One of the authors stated that, had he required it, he would have been reluctant to receive ECT in one out of every four clinics he visited. Using a schedule based on the 1995 recommendations, only one in three clinics were rated as meeting College standards. Fifty-nine per cent of clinics had upgraded their machines to one of the models in the College's short-list, but about one in 10 clinics were still using machines considered out of date in 1989. Only one in three clinics had clear treatment policies to help staff administer ECT effectively. Problems were also noted with respect to the ECT procedure itself – in particular monitoring of seizures and re-stimulation in the event of inadequate seizures – which would suggest that about one in five treatment applications was unlikely to result in therapeutically effective seizures. Overall, standards tended to be higher in clinics where the consultant had attended one of the College's revision courses and had read the 1995 Guidelines.

It has long been recognised that many consultants in charge of ECT clinics do not take their training and supervision responsibilities sufficiently seriously (Pippard & Ellam, 1981; Pippard, 1992a,b; Castle *et al*, 1994; Duffett & Lelliott, 1997, 1998). The 1998 College audit found that only 16% of ECT consultants attended their ECT clinic weekly, only 6% had sessional time for their ECT duties, and fewer than one in two ECT consultants had attended one of the College's ECT revision courses.

These findings are worrying given that most ECT in Britain is administered by the most junior and least experienced trainees, including general practitioner trainees. While many clinics had upgraded their ECT equipment, there seemed to be little advantage from using new expensive equipment without a commitment to understanding how it operates, and learning how to use it competently. More importantly still, the junior staff who administer the treatment need to be taught how to use equipment competently, how to monitor seizures properly and how to ensure that patients are adequately stimulated. The training and supervision duties of ECT consultants will be closely scrutinised in forthcoming College accreditation visits.

Mode of action of ECT

Exactly how or why ECT is effective in such a wide range of psychiatric disorders remains unclear.

Studies on animals using experimental paradigms mimicking a clinical course of treatment provide evidence of neurotransmitter receptor changes (up-regulation and down-regulation), which are thought to underlie the therapeutic effects of ECT and cognitive side-effects (Lehrer *et al*, 1986; Green & Nutt, 1987). A similar pattern of receptor alterations is seen with antidepressant drugs, and affects serotonin and noradrenalin receptors in particular.

Why, then, is ECT effective in the treatment of acute mania and schizophrenia where, according to the dopamine hypothesis for the mode of action of neuroleptic drugs, disturbed dopamine function would be assumed? ECT also appears to have an effect on brain regions (e.g. nucleus accumbens and substantia nigra) which are associated with disturbed dopamine function in acute psychosis (Lock & McCulloch, 1991). Thus, if ECT simultaneously exerts an antidepressant and antipsychotic effect through its action on noradrenalin, serotonin and dopamine function, its efficacy in patients manifesting a mixture of endogenous affective and acute psychotic symptoms would be explained in biological terms.

It has long been generally accepted that the induced convulsion is essential for the therapeutic effect of ECT, and that unwanted cognitive side-effects are related to the amount of electricity used to induce that convulsion (Ottosson, 1960). Surprisingly, studies comparing simulated ('sham') ECT[1] with real ECT for depressive illness have shown only small, albeit significant, differences between groups (Crow & Johnstone, 1986), and have failed to provide unequivocal evidence that the convulsion is the critical element of the treatment response; nor have these studies provided evidence that the convulsion is not important.

Sham ECT is a powerful antidepressant treatment, although not as powerful as real ECT. The word 'placebo' generally refers to an inert or harmless substance or treatment which nevertheless exerts a powerful therapeutic effect because of the patient's belief in them. A course of general anaesthetics is not a placebo intervention and it is therefore incorrect to conclude that ECT has a powerful 'placebo effect'; instead, a strong case can be made for the therapeutic efficacy of repeated general anaesthesia for depressive illness (Lock, 1995).

There is no objective evidence that ECT causes brain damage (Abrams, 1992). Prospective quantitative magnetic resonance imaging of the brain has found no evidence of structural brain damage after repeated courses of ECT (Scott *et al*, 1991).

---

1. The term *sham* ECT is used to describe an ECT procedure from which the electrical shock (and hence the induced convulsion) is deliberately omitted for research purposes. Sham subjects are given a general anaesthetic and muscle relaxant as per usual practice.

Patient preparation

A full explanation of ECT in language that patients and their families can understand is important to maintain good working relationships. It has been shown, however, that about one in three patients has "no idea" what treatment entails (Freeman & Kendell, 1986). Adequate physical preparation – comprising at least a recent physical examination and blood tests – is essential for safety reasons. Nevertheless, anaesthetists continue to encounter physically ill patients arriving inadequately prepared for treatment (Haddad & Benbow, 1993).

The task of obtaining consent is often delegated to junior medical staff, but it is the responsibility of the patient's responsible medical officer (RMO) to ensure that ECT is administered legally , in particular to determine whether there are grounds for compulsory treatment under the Mental Health Act where patients refuse treatment or – by virtue of their mental disturbance – are unable to give 'real' consent to treatment (Pippard & Taylor, 1995). Real consent assumes that the patient has made a valid decision to agree to treatment – that is, that a full explanation of ECT has been given and that the patient is capable of making a decision based on an understanding of the information. It is generally advisable to regard a patient as not consenting to treatment if real consent is in any way questionable. ECT may only be given without a patient's consent in two circumstances:

(a) Where urgent action is necessary to save the patient's life, or to prevent serious and immediate danger to self or other people.

(b) When a patient is detained under an order which permits compulsory treatment for 28 days or longer and where a doctor appointed by the Mental Health Act Commission certifies that ECT is necessary.

The nature and extent of the information which should be given is summarised in *ECT: A Factsheet for You and Your Family* (available from the Public Education Department of the Royal College of Psychiatrists) A verbal explanation should be supplemented with written or audio visual material.

Patients giving real consent are required to sign a consent form in the presence of a doctor who countersigns, as evidence that the correct procedure was undertaken. Failure to undertake the above procedure correctly could constitute legal liability on grounds of negligence, and treatment without consent could constitute battery. Consent is best regarded as an on-going process, for it can be withdrawn at any time, and ECT clinic staff are advised to be alert for the possibility that consenting patients may change their mind at the last minute.

Treatment schedules

A treatment schedule needs to encompass all the factors known to have an effect on clinical outcome (Shapira *et al*, 1991*a,b*). Flexibility is important with respect to maximising the therapeutic response and minimising cognitive side-effects. The main factors to consider are the type of ECT machine, electrode placement, seizure threshold, stimulus dose, and frequency of treatments.

ECT machines

Most ECT machines manufactured after 1981 deliver electrical stimulation in the form of brief (1–2 ms) square-wave pulses (Fig. 1). 'Brief-pulse' stimulation delivers only a fraction of the electrical energy of older ECT machines (which generated alternating

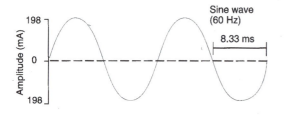
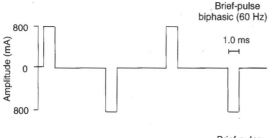
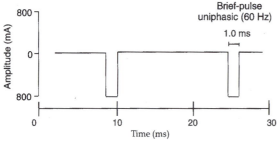

Fig. 1. Wave forms: sine-wave (alternating current; constant voltage) and biphasic and uniphasic brief pulses (constant current) (from Lock, 1995*a*).

Box 2. ECT machines

Constant-current ECT machines were recommended by the Department of Health and Social Security in 1982

All ECT machines with the exception of four short-listed models (British versions of Mecta's SR2 & JR2, Thymatron DG and Ectron series 5a models) must now be considered obsolete and replaced

The best selection for local use requires a general understanding of the merits and limitations of available equipment and of local ECT practice

sine-wave current) and it is highly efficient in the induction of seizures (Abrams, 1992). Brief-pulse current is also associated with less memory impairment than sine-wave ECT (Weiner *et al*,1986). Modern machines estimate the impedance of the patient's head and can be pre-set to deliver a fixed amount of charge. Such machines are termed *constant-current apparatus,* as they maintain current at a constant value by automatically adjusting output voltage to compensate for changes in impedance, and their use was recommended by the Department of Health and Social Security in 1982.

By 1998, almost all ECT clinics were equipped with brief-pulse constant-current machines: 59% with one of the four short-listed models and the remainder with under-powered ECT machines considered obsolete. A Scottish audit (Robertson & Fergusson, 1996) found that one in three clinics were using obsolete equipment.

Selecting an ECT machine is not an easy matter and it must be stressed that there is little advantage in purchasing new equipment without a commitment to understanding how it operates, and learning how to use it competently. Machines differ with respect to the characteristics of the stimulus generated, the means of controlling that stimulus and other features which may be built in. Some of these are important for safety reasons; some are useful but not essential, and others offer little if any practical advantage, despite claims to the contrary by the manufacturers. The best buy for local use requires a general understanding of the merits and limitations of available equipment – and of local ECT practice. For a comprehensive review of available equipment, see Lock (1995*a*) and Robertson & Fergusson (1996). Since the publication of these reviews and of the College's short-list of suitable machines, one company has recently introduced four versions of their new machine, the Spectrum – a fact which highlights the problem of keeping abreast with technological and research developments.

Electrode placement

In 1977, the Royal College of Psychiatrists recommended the use of brief-pulse equipment and unilateral electrode placement. By 1989 it was clear that the therapeutic efficacy of this combination was less than when using bilateral ECT and earlier sine-wave models. The cause of the problem was that the early Ectron (Series 2 and Series 3) constant-current machines were under-powered.

Recent American and Scandinavian research using more powerful brief-pulse machines has shown that therapeutic equivalence may be achieved with unilateral and bilateral electrode placement (Abrams *et al*, 1991).

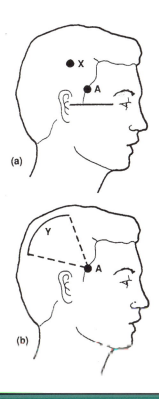

Fig. 2. (a) The Lancaster electrode placement positions for unilateral ECT: A=4 cm above the mid-point between the external auditory meatus and angle of the orbit; X=6 cm from A, and above the external auditory meatus. **(b)** The d'Elia electrode placement positions: A, as above; Y=on the mid-line, anywhere in the region of the occipito-parietal junction.

> **Box 3.   Treatment schedules**
>
> **The decision to use bilateral or unilateral ECT should be based on a risk–benefit analysis. Switch from bilateral to unilateral ECT if a patient develops troublesome cognitive side-effects. Switch from unilateral to bilateral ECT if the patient fails to improve and has no side-effects**
>
> **The unilateral use of brief pulse stimulation gives the least cognitive disturbance, while bilateral ECT with sine-wave stimulation gives the most**
>
> **Combining brief-pulse stimulation and bilateral electrode placement offers the best compromise of effective treatment and moderate memory disturbance**

Effective unilateral treatment is critically dependent on:
  (a) A stimulus dose which is at least 2.5 times the patient's seizure threshold.
  (b) Wide separation of the electrodes.

The 'Lancaster' unilateral electrode position (as demonstrated on the old ECT wallcharts; see Fig. 2a) does not achieve a sufficiently wide electrode separation, and the d'Elia electrode positions are recommended (as demonstrated in the *Official Video Teaching Pack of the Royal College of Psychiatrists' Special Committee on ECT*, 1994; see Fig. 2b). Doubts continue to be expressed about the therapeutic equivalency of unilateral and bilateral electrode placement (Sackeim *et al*, 1991), and small but statistically significant differences in seizure quality have been observed.

Flexibility with respect to electrode placement is important. The American Psychiatric Association Task Force on ECT (1990) recommended that the decision to use bilateral or unilateral ECT should be based on a risk benefit analysis for each patient. Bilateral ECT is recommended if the rate of response is most important (e.g. in the case of urgent treatment); unilateral ECT is recommended if minimising the risk of cognitive side-effects is most important. It may, furthermore, be advisable to switch from one to the other during a course of treatment. For example, if a patient develops troublesome cognitive side-effects with bilateral ECT, switching to unilateral ECT may help; similarly, if a patient fails to improve with unilateral

Table 1. Factors affecting seizure threshold	
Factor	Effect
Age (increasing)	↑
Anticonvulsants – concurrent or recent	↑
Baldness	↑
Barbiturates – concurrent or recent	↑
Benzodiazepines – concurrent or recent	↑
Bilateral electrode placement	↑
Bones (thick), e.g. Paget's disease	↑
Caffeine	↓
Carbon dioxide saturation of blood (low)	↓
Dehydration	↑
ECT – increasing no. of treatments	↑
ECT – previous course within last month	↑
Electrode contact with scalp (poor)	↑
Hyperventilation	↓
Methohexitone dose > 1.2 mg/kg	↑
Methohexitone and ketamine in half-doses	↓
Oxygen saturation of blood (low)	↑
Propofol	↑
Gender (male)	↑
Theophyllin	↓

↑, increase; ↓, decrease.

The absolute measurement of seizure threshold is heavily dependent on the type of ECT machine (Abrams, 1992), but regardless of which machine is used, a wide variation in seizure threshold has been observed in clinic populations (e.g. 17–800 mQ or more; Sackeim *et al*, 1987; using a Mecta SR1 machine), and a rise in seizure threshold (range 25–200%; mean 80%) has been noted during a course of ECT. Factors affecting seizure threshold are listed in Table 1). See Sackeim *et al* (1987, 1991) for the relative magnitude of these effects.

'Stimulus dosing' refers to the adjustment of the amount (or dose) of the electrical stimulus to the requirements of the patient at different points during the course of ECT. The consensus of the American Psychiatric Association Task Force on ECT (1990) is that the best results – in terms of maximising the therapeutic response to ECT while minimising cognitive side-effects – are achieved using a 'moderately suprathreshold treatment dose', that is, a dose which is 50–200% above seizure threshold. The exact percentage increase for bilateral and unilateral ECT is a subject of ongoing international debate: given the controversy, a figure of about 50% is suggested for bilateral ECT and at least 250% for unilateral ECT (Sackeim, 1991). In addition, the selected dose may need to be increased during a course of ECT to compensate for the rise in seizure threshold as the course of ECT progresses.

Individualised stimulus dosing using the above guidelines is dependent on knowing the patients's seizure threshold dose. Given the many factors which can, alone or in combination, affect seizure threshold, the most reliable assessment of seizure threshold is by empirical measurement – a procedure which has been termed 'dose titration', or 'seizure threshold titration'. This is done by applying a low charge stimulus, and restimulating the patient with an increased charge until a seizure is induced. Seizure threshold titration tables have been developed (see Table 2) for all the short-listed ECT machines, which simplifies the procedure (Lock, 1995*b*).

The practice of applying a fixed dose to all patients at every treatment session is still common in Britain (Pippard, 1992*a*). The problem with this approach

ECT and is not experiencing side-effects, switching to bilateral ECT may help.

Non-dominant (unilateral) ECT is associated with significantly fewer unwanted cognitive problems compared with bilateral ECT; patients reorientate faster, and experience less disturbance of objective retrograde and anterograde memory impairment, and weaker subjective autobiographical amnesia (Weiner *et al*, 1986). Electrode placement and stimulus waveform exert synergistic effects on cognitive function; the combination of unilateral ECT and brief-pulse stimulation is associated with the least cognitive disturbance, while the combination of bilateral ECT and sine-wave stimulation gives the most cognitive disturbance. Other combinations offer a compromise of effective treatment and mild memory disturbance (Weiner *et al*, 1986).

Seizure threshold and stimulus dosing

Seizure threshold refers to the minimum amount of electricity needed to induce a generalised cerebral seizure. The term 'dose' (of electricity) has crept into the literature as an alternative to the term 'amount'. Seizure threshold may be measured using a variety of units (e.g. volts, V; amps, A; coulombs, Q). The most valid measure is the coulomb, the unit of electrical charge[2].

---

2. The amount of charge in millicoulombs is calculated as follows: multiply current (in amps) by pulse width (in milliseconds) to get the electrical charge of one brief pulse in millicoulombs (mQ); multiply this figure by frequency (the number of pulses per second) and by the length of time that current flows (i.e. the duration of the stimulus in seconds). If the ECT machine produces biphasic brief-pulse current (all American models), this figure must be multiplied by 2. If the ECT machine produces uniphasic brief-pulse current (e.g. Ectron models), the multiplication factor is 1. Relevant parameters will be quoted in the manufacturer's instruction manual. (One millicoulomb (mQ) is equal to one-thousandth (1/1000) of a coulomb.)

is that if a fixed high dose is selected, a significant proportion of patients are likely to have relatively low seizure thresholds, and may therefore be at increased risk of cognitive side-effects; with a fixed low-dose schedule, patients with a relatively high seizure threshold are at risk of receiving a course of treatment characterised by poor seizures and a poor response.

Whether seizure threshold titration should be part of routine clinical practice is a contentious issue. The consensus of the Special Committee on ECT is that seizure threshold titration is useful if bilateral ECT is administered, because of the risks to memory function posed by inadvertent gross suprathreshold stimulation; and useful in the case of unilateral ECT because of the need to ensure that a sufficiently high stimulus is given to maximise the therapeutic response. Fixed high-dose schedules are considerably simpler to undertake than the alternative – dose titration – and are appropriate for unilateral ECT (Abrams *et al*, 1991). Stimulus dosing guidance for bilateral ECT, taking into consideration the three most important factors affecting seizure threshold (age, gender and concomitant medication), are given in Table 2, and are based on local experience using a Mecta SR2 'British version' machine. It is important to stress that absolute values (in mQ) may differ for other models, and users are referred to Lock (1995*c*) for specific guidance.

Frequency of treatment

ECT is usually administered twice weekly in Britain, and three times weekly in the USA, for treatment of depressive illness. This difference appears to be one of personal preference (Scott & Whalley, 1993). An alternative to switching from bilateral to unilateral electrode placement in cases where cognitive side-effects (in particular confusion) are troublesome is to reduce the frequency of treatments from twice to once a week (Benbow, 1995). It has been claimed, on the basis of empirical clinical experience, that daily treatments are indicated when a patient's mental state is seriously disturbed (e.g. uncontrolled manic excitement or catatonia). In the case of continuation (maintenance) ECT, the frequency of treatments should take into consideration the patient's clinical progress. Some patients' symptoms may relapse unless one treatment is administered per week, while others may remain asymptomatic with less frequent treatments.

Table 2. Stimulus dosing guidelines for Mecta SR2/JR2 British version machines			
Level	Seizure threshold dose, mQ	Treatment dose,mQ Bilateral	Unilateral
1	25	50	75
2	50	75	125
3	75	125	200
4	125	200	275
5	200	275	400
6	275	400	600

Starting levels: 1=female unilateral ECT; 2=male unilateral and female bilateral ECT; 3=male bilateral ECT. Start one level higher if patient: is over 65 years old; is taking the equivalent of 15 mg/day of diazepam; has received more than three ECT treatments within the previous three weeks. Start two levels higher if patient is taking carbamazepine or any other anticonvulsant, or if an anticonvulsant has been discontinued within the previous three weeks. If the first stimulation fails to elicit a generalised tonic–clonic convulsion lasting 15 seconds peripherally, re-stimulate the patient by increasing the stimulus dose by one level. If the second stimulation fails to induce an adequate seizure, re-stimulate the patient again and increase the stimulus to the next level, e.g. 50 mQ; no seizure, re-stimulate with 75 mQ; if still no adequate seizure, re-stimulate with 125 mQ. Approximately one in three patients respond to the first stimulation and one in 20 patients require three stimulations; the remainder require two stimulations at the first treatment session. From the second session onwards, increase the dose by one level when there is a significant (i.e. 20% or more) reduction in seizure length relative to seizure length at the previous treatment session.

Monitoring and restimulation

There are several causes of 'missed fits' (i.e. absence of peripheral seizure activity) and partial seizures (seizure involving only the face, one limb, or both limbs on the same side):

(a) Poor electrical contact.
(b) Total attenuation of muscle activity by muscle relaxant.
(c) Absence of cerebral seizure activity because the dose of the stimulus was below the patient's seizure threshold, thus failing to induce a generalised cerebral seizure.

Poor electrical contact can easily be excluded by routinely testing that static impedance values are within the recommended range for a given ECT machine before stimulating the patient. The routine use of the cuff technique has been recommended, as it provides the most reliable means of monitoring peripheral seizure activity (Royal College of Psychiatrists, 1989, 1995). This technique makes use of a blood pressure cuff, inflated to about 20 mmHg above systolic blood pressure, which is applied immediately before the muscle relaxant is administered. Muscle relaxant is therefore unable to pass beyond the inflated cuff, where peripheral seizure activity is better observed. This technique is well demonstrated in the official teaching video.

The most direct means of monitoring seizure activity induced by an ECT stimulus is by means of the electroencephalogram (EEG). American ECT machines offer built-in EEG monitoring, which is considered useful, but not essential, by the Special Committee on ECT of the Royal College of Psychiatrists.

The appropriate action to be taken in response to a missed or partial seizure will depend on its cause. If due to lack of cerebral seizure activity, then the strength of the stimulus needs to be increased; if due to poor electrical contact, then the electrodes should be prepared again and reapplied (and impedance should again be measured). When peripheral seizure activity is absent but cerebral seizure activity is confirmed by means of an EEG recording, then the operator needs to verify that the cerebral convulsion is adequate, and should also liaise with the anaesthetist, as a reduction in the dose of muscle relaxant may be appropriate at subsequent treatment sessions. (For a discussion on EEG monitoring, see Scott *et al* (1989)). Sample EEG recordings are also provided by the Royal College of Psychiatrists Special Committee on ECT (1995). Where built-in EEG recording is not available, the only means of differentiating between inadequate seizures due to absent cerebral activity and total attenuation of peripheral muscular activity by muscle relaxant is by using the cuff technique.

Conclusions

This review has attempted to examine the scientific rationale underlying recommended improvements in British ECT practice, in the light of the findings of the three audits comissioned by the Royal College of Psychiatrists (Pippard & Ellam, 1981; Pippard, 1992*a*; Duffett & Lelliott, 1998). The nature of ECT is that it is controversial, and research findings are generally inconclusive and open to debate. An attempt has been made throughout this paper to offer explanations based on the consensus opinion of both the Special Committee on ECT of the Royal College of Psychiatrists and the American Psychiatric Association Task Force on ECT. Where their views differ, the view of the Special Committee has been presented. Both bodies consider ECT to be a safe and effective procedure for which there exists an ongoing need. The caveat is that ECT must be properly and legally administered and that the decision to offer or withhold treatment should be based on a careful consideration of alternatives for a given patient, not on the basis of personal bias on the part of the practitioner.

The question we all need to ask ourselves is this: would we, if we were suffering from a severe schizoaffective disorder, consent to ECT treatment in our local ECT clinic?

References

Abrams, R. (1992) *Electroconvulsive Therapy* (2nd edn). Oxford: Oxford University Press.
——, Swartz, C. M. & Vedak, C. (1991) Antidepressant effects of high-dose right unilateral electroconvulsive therapy. *Archives of General Psychiatry*, **48**, 746–748.
American Psychiatric Association Task Force on ECT (1990) *The Practice of Electroconvulsive Therapy: Recommendations for Treatment, Training and Privileging*. Washington, DC: APA.
Benbow, S. (1995) ECT in the elderly patient. In *The ECT Handbook. The Second Report of the Royal College of Psychiatrists' Special Committee on ECT*. Council Report CR39, (ed. C. P. L. Freeman), p. 17. London: Royal College of Psychiatrists.
Buchan, H., Johnstone, E., McPherson, K., *et al* (1992) Who benefits from electroconvulsive therapy? Combined results of the Leicester and Northwich Park trials. *British Journal of Psychiatry*, **160**, 355–359.
Castle, D., Reeve, A., Ivinson, L., *et al* (1994) What do we think about our training? Report of a Working Party of the Collegiate Trainees Committee. *Psychiatric Bulletin*, **18**, 357–359.
Crow, T. J. & Johnstone, E. C. (1986) Controlled trials of electroconvulsive therapy. *Annals of the New York Academy of Sciences*, **462**, 12–29.
Duffett, R. & Lelliott, P. (1997) Junior doctors training in the theory and practice of electroconvulsive therapy. *Psychiatric Bulletin*, **21**, 563–565.
—— & —— (1998) Auditing electroconvulsive therapy. The third cycle. *British Journal of Psychiatry*, **172**, 401–405.
Endler, N. S. (1988) The origins of electroconvulsive therapy (ECT). *Convulsive Therapy*, **4**, 5–23.
Freeman, C. P. L. (1992) Special Committee on ECT. *Psychiatric Bulletin*, **16**, 121.
—— & Kendell, R. E. (1986) Patients' experiences of and attitudes to electroconvulsive therapy. *Annals of the New York Academy of Science*, **462**, 341–351.
Gearney, D. (1993) Electroconvulsive therapy: the official video of the Royal College of Psychiatrists' Special Committee on ECT, (videotape review). *Psychiatric Bulletin*, **17**, 702–703.
Green, R. A. & Nutt, D. J. (1987) Psychopharmacology of repeated services: possible relevance to the mechanism of action of electroconvulsive therapy. In *Handbook of Psychopharmacology* (eds I. L. Iversen, S. D. Iversen & S. M. Snyder), pp. 375–419. New York: Plenum Press.
Haddad, P. M. & Benbow, S. M. (1993) Electroconvulsive therapy – related knowledge among British anaesthetists. *Convulsive Therapy*, **9**, 101–107.
Kalinowski, L. B. (1939) Electro-convulsive therapy in schizophrenia. *Lancet*, ii, 1232–1233.
Kramer, B. A. (1985) Use of ECT in California, 1977–1983. *American Journal of Psychiatry*, **142**, 1190–1192.
Lehrer, B., Stanley, M., Altma, M., *et al* (1986) An annual model of electroconvulsive therapy-induced amnesia. *Annals of the New York Academy of Sciences*, **462**, 91–98.
Lock, T. (1994) *Electroconvulsive Therapy (ECT). Official Video Teaching Pack of the Royal College of Psychiatrists' Special Committee on ECT*. London: Royal College of Psychiatrists.
—— (1995*a*) Review of ECT machines. In *The ECT Handbook. The Second Report of the Royal College of Psychiatrists' Special Committee on ECT*. Council Report CR39, (ed. C. P. L. Freeman), pp. 122–148. London: Royal College of Psychiatrists.

—— (1995*b*) Stimulus dosing. In *The ECT Handbook. The Second Report of the Royal College of Psychiatrists' Special Committee on ECT*. Council Report CR39, (ed. C. P. L. Freeman), pp. 72–87. London: Royal College of Psychiatrists.

—— (1995*c*) Non-convulsive electrical shock treatment. In *The ECT Handbook. The Second Report of the Royal College of Psychiatrists' Special Committee on ECT*. Council Report CR39, (ed. C. P. L. Freeman), pp. 31–32. London: Royal College of Psychiatrists.

—— & McCulloch, J. (1991) Local cerebral glucose utilization after chronic elecroconvulsive shock: implications for the mode of action of electroconvulsive therapy. *Journal of Psychopharmacology*, **5**, 111–119.

Mind (1988) *ECT: Pros, Cons and Consequences (Special Report)*. London: Mind.

Ottosson, J. O. (ed.) (1960) Experimental studies of the mode of action of electroconvulsive therapy. *Acta Psychiatrica Scandinavica* (suppl. 145).

Pippard, J. (1992*a*) Audit of electroconvulsive treatment in two National Health Service regions. *British Journal of Psychiatry* **160**, 621–637.

—— (1992*b*) Auditing the administration of ECT. *Psychiatric Bulletin*, **16**, 59–62.

—— & Ellam, L. (1981) Electroconvulsive treatment in Great Britain. A report to the College. *British Journal of Psychiatry*, **139**, 563–568.

—— & Taylor, P. J. (1995) ECT, the law and consent to treatment. In *The ECT Handbook. The Second Report of the Royal College of Psychiatrists' Special Committee on ECT*. Council Report CR39, (ed. C. P. L. Freeman), pp. 97–102. London: Royal College of Psychiatrists.

Prudic, J., Sackeim, M. A. & Devenard, D. P. (1990) Medication resistance and clinical response to electroconvulsive therapy. *Psychiatric Research*, **31**, 287–296.

Robertson, C. & Fergusson, G. (1996) Electroconvulsive therapy machines. *Advances in Psychiatric Treatment*, **2**, 24–31.

Royal College of Psychiatrists (1977) Memorandum on the use of electroconvulsive therapy. *British Journal of Psychiatry*, **131**, 261–272.

Royal College of Psychiatrists' ECT Sub-Committee of the Research Committee (1989) *The Practical Administration of Electroconvulsive Therapy (ECT)*. London: Gaskell.

Royal College of Psychiatrists' Special Committee on ECT (1995) *The ECT Handbook. The Second Report of the Royal College of Psychiatrists' Special Committee on ECT*. Council Report CR39, (ed. C. P. L. Freeman). London: Royal College of Psychiatrists.

Sackeim, H. A. (1991) Optimizing unilateral electro-convulsive therapy. *Convulsive Therapy*, **7**, 201–212.

——, Decina, P., Prohovnik, I., *et al* (1987) Seizure threshold in electroconvulsive therapy; effects of sex, age, electrode placement, and number of treatments. *Archives of General Psychiatry*, **44**, 355–360.

——, Devanand, D. P. & Prudic, J. (1991) Stimulus intensity, seizure threshold and seizure duration: Impact on the efficacy and safety of electroconvulsive therapy. In *Psychiatric Clinics of North America: Electroconvulsive Therapy*, vol. 14, (ed. C. H. Kellner), pp. 803–843. Philadelphia, PA: Saunders.

Scott, A. I. F., Shering, P. A. & Dykes, S. (1989) Would monitoring by electroencephalogram improve the practice of electroconvulsive therapy? *British Journal of Psychiatry*, **154**, 853–857.

——, Turnbull, L. W., Blare, A., *et al* (1991) Electroconvulsive therapy and brain damage. *Lancet*, **338**, 264.

—— & Whalley, L. J. (1993) The onset and rate of the antidepressant effect of electroconvulsive therapy. A neglected topic of research. *British Journal of Psychiatry*, **162**, 725–732.

Shapira, B., Calev, A. & Lerer, B. (1991*a*) Optimal use of electroconvulsive therapy: choosing a tratment schedule. In *Psychiatric Clinics of North America*: *Electroconvulsive Therapy*, vol. 14, (ed. C. H. Kellner), pp. 935–946. Philadelphia, PA: Saunders.

——, Hadjez, J., Calev, A., *et al* (1991*b*) Schedule of ECT administration: implications for antidepressants efficacy and adverse effects. *Biological Psychiatry*, **1**, 257–259.

Taylor, P. J. (1990) Schizophrenia and ECT – a case for a change in prescription? In *Dilemmas and Difficulties in the Management of Psychiatric Patients* (eds K. Hawton & P. Cowan). Oxford: Oxford University Press.

Weiner, R. D., Rogers, H. J., Davidson, J. R. T., *et al* (1986) Effects of stimulus parameters on cognitive side-effects. *Annals of the New York Academy of Science*, **462**, 315–325.

Lithium therapy

I. N. Ferrier, S. P. Tyrer & A. J. Bell

Since the introduction of lithium therapy 30 years ago it has become a major weapon in psychiatrists' armamentarium. It is the drug of first choice for the prevention of recurrent mood disorders, and it is estimated that about one person in every thousand people in Britain receives lithium at any one time. It therefore behoves doctors to be familiar with its use (Drug and Therapeutics Bulletin, 1999). This chapter is not a comprehensive account of the pharmacology of lithium (for this the reader is referred to Johnson (1987) and Peet & Pratt (1993)) but concentrates on its clinical use in practice and some less well known, but important, phenomena.

Indications for use

Prevention of recurrent affective disorder

Lithium is the primary agent in the prophylaxis of bipolar affective disorder. Comparative trials have been carried out with other agents, most frequently with carbamazepine and sodium valproate, but no definite advantage has been shown with the alternative drugs except in complicated disorders (such as rapid cycling affective disorder), and lithium remains the first choice for initial treatment (Hopkins & Gelenberg, 1994; Schou, 1997). There is increasing evidence for the usefulness of anti-convulsants alone or in combination with lithium in poor outcome patients, but the details are outside the scope of this chapter.

There are few absolute contraindications to giving lithium, as dosage adjustment and careful monitoring normally allow patients who have compromised medical health to receive lithium. Relative contraindications include: administration during pregnancy, in particular the first trimester; variable renal function; second- or third-degree heart block; and conditions that cause electrolyte imbalance, in particular hyponatraemia.

The decision about when to institute lithium treatment in a patient with mood disorder depends upon the severity and frequency of previous episodes of illness, the effect that future episodes are likely to have on the patient's functioning, and family history of affective illness. As the onset of mania can be devastating to domestic and occupational life, the indications for treatment by lithium in bipolar disorder are stronger than in unipolar illness and if two discrete episodes of mania or depression occur within a three-year period, lithium should normally be given unless there are contra-indications (Grof et al, 1978). In patients with recurrent depression it is usual to consider lithium after three episodes of illness. However, the decision on when to start lithium depends above all on discussion with the patient of the risks involved of recurrence of illness and the impositions of lithium treatment. It may be advisable to give prophylactic lithium after only one manic episode when a further manic attack could have profound social and/or financial consequences.

Use in other conditions

Lithium is effective in acute mania (but there is a lag period of 5–7 days before major effects are shown). However, Swann et al (1997) found that even modest pre-treatment depressive symptoms predicted a poor antimanic response to lithium and a better response to valproate. Lithium is also effective in the augmentation of antidepressants in the treatment of resistant depression and in cluster headache. It inhibits DNA viruses (Amsterdam et al, 1996). Lithium reduces impulsive aggression in patients with organic brain damage (Tyrer, 1994) and has a licensed indication for aggression in those with learning disability. It has been used in the treatment of schizophrenia, particularly when affective symptoms are prominent, and may improve the response of patients with schizophrenia to neuroleptics.

Augmentation in depression

In patients who have been treated with adequate doses of antidepressants for at least a four-week period, in whom adherence is assured and in whom no or inadequate response has been obtained, addition of lithium has been shown to improve depression (De Montigny *et al*, 1983). Although initial studies suggested that the addition of lithium improved depression considerably within one week, later studies suggest that it may be necessary to give lithium for at least four weeks before assuming lack of response (Price *et al*, 1986). A meta-analysis of lithium augmentation has shown a significant but modest effect (Austin *et al*, 1991).

In a patient with a normal serum creatinine it is usual to add 400 mg of lithium at night to the existing antidepressant dose regime and measure serum lithium levels after one week. If this level is below 0.4 mmol/l, the dosage of lithium can be increased to 600 mg or 800 mg at night and the patient maintained on this dose. Lithium levels should be maintained within the therapeutic range of 0.4–0.8 mmol/l for at least four weeks before deciding on alternative treatments.

Lithium can be added to selective serotonin re-uptake inhibitors (SSRIs) and monoamine oxidase inhibitors (MAOIs) with improvement in depression. Isolated reports of the serotonergic syndrome (agitation, hyperpyrexia and myoclonus) have been documented. It is wise to keep the doses of SSRIs and lithium at the lower end of the recommended range.

On the basis of case reports and two retrospective studies (Small & Millstein, 1990) it has been suggested that lithium should be withdrawn before starting electroconvulsive therapy (ECT) in order to avoid neurotoxicity, and it should not be re-instated for several days following the last convulsive treatment.

Initiation of treatment

Before starting treatment a full medical history should be taken and appropriate investigations carried out. Examination should include measurement of body weight, blood pressure and, if there is any suggestion of cardiac symptoms or abnormality, an electrocardiogram should be performed. Serum thyroxine, thyroid stimulating hormone, serum creatinine and electrolyte analysis should be carried out in every case. It is not normally necessary to carry out creatinine clearance estimations unless there is evidence from the history or examination of impaired renal function.

Before starting treatment each patient should be given an information pamphlet about the use of lithium treatment and the reasons for monitoring its prescription. It is important to record administration of these instructions in the case notes and it may be advisable for the patient to endorse having received this information (see Box 1)(Birch *et al*, 1993).

Lithium preparations and treatment regime

Lithium is normally administered in tablet or capsule form but a syrup is available. The preparations most frequently used in the UK contain lithium carbonate. These preparations are available in 200 mg and 400 mg strengths and have comparable bioavailability. A slower release preparation containing lithium citrate is available and is preferred if nausea and early gastrointestinal symptoms are a problem.

It is usual to start lithium by giving a dosage of 0.15–0.20 mmol/kg/day (i.e. about 400–600 mg/day of lithium carbonate or 1000–1500 mg/day of lithium citrate for a person weighing 70 kg), and measuring serum lithium concentration one week later, when steady-state conditions have normally been reached. The dosage can then be adjusted to the desired steady-state concentration as there is a direct relationship between dose and serum lithium level. Thus, if a daily maintenance dose of 1200 mg of lithium per day produces a steady-state concentration of 0.9 mmol/l, a dosage of 800 mg will result in a concentration of 0.6 mmol/l.

Patients with acute mania require greater doses of lithium to maintain therapeutic serum lithium

Box 1. Tests before starting lithium treatment

Measure blood pressure
Electrocardiogram if any cardiac symptoms, particularly if patient is over 50 years old
Measure weight and serum thyroxine, TSH, creatinine and electrolytes
Give information leaflet regarding lithium treatment to patient

levels and a corresponding starting dose in a 70 kg patient with mania would be about 1000 mg of lithium carbonate. This dose should be given in divided doses in mania, although in prophylaxis a single night-time dose is preferred in order to increase adherence.

It is possible, but not usually necessary, to determine the dosage regime in an individual patient by using the serum lithium concentration measured after a single loading dose of lithium carbonate combined with prediction tables (Perry *et al*, 1986; Aronson & Reynolds, 1992).

The normal maintenance serum lithium range is between 0.5 and 0.8 mmol/l. Serum lithium concentrations lower than 0.4 mmol/l are not effective in the majority of patients; serum concentrations over 1.0 mmol/l are more likely to be accompanied by side-effects and render the patient liable to neurotoxicity.

In order to achieve standardisation of serum lithium levels, blood for serum lithium should be taken 12 hours after the last dose of the drug. In practice, intervals of between 11 and 14 hours between the dosage and venepuncture are acceptable, although if blood is taken more than an hour outside the 12-hour period the timing of the blood sample should be recorded.

Monitoring of lithium treatment

As the therapeutic ratio (serum level achieving therapeutic benefit : toxic serum lithium level) is low, it is essential to monitor serum lithium levels closely. The recommended range of serum lithium levels to achieve therapeutic efficacy varies according to the condition for which lithium is being given. For the prophylactic treatment of recurrent depression the dose of lithium should be adjusted to maintain a 12-hour serum lithium level of between 0.5 and 0.8 mmol/l. It has been shown in patients with bipolar disorder that the risk of relapse is reduced 2.6 times if lithium levels are maintained between 0.7–0.9 mmol/l, but adherence is poorer with this regime (Gelenberg *et al*, 1989). However, later studies have been less conclusive (Vestergaard *et al*, 1998).

For the acute treatment of mania retrospective evidence suggests that a serum lithium level of between 0.9 and 1.4 mmol/l is necessary (Prien *et al*, 1972), and once there is normalisation of mood the dosage of lithium can be reduced. Serum lithium monitoring should be carried out frequently over this period.

Once a patient is maintained on lithium, serum lithium levels should be determined immediately there is any suggestion of lithium toxicity or affective relapse. If the patient's mood remains euthymic,

lithium levels should normally be checked at one or two monthly intervals within the first six months of starting the drug, but if lithium levels are stable and the patient's insight is good the monitoring interval can be extended to six months (three months in elderly patients).

There is little consensus on these figures and scant evidence that checking lithium levels more frequently is helpful in the long run – some argue that monitoring of the side-effects and regular checks of renal function are all that is required (Aronson & Reynolds, 1992). However, adherence may be enhanced by informing the patient that lithium itself is to be measured and the intervals stated seem prudent from the medico-legal standpoint.

Serum creatinine and thyroid function tests should be carried out at least once a year in patients receiving lithium treatment.

Measurement of lithium

Most laboratories carry out lithium analysis by flame spectrophotometry. It is usual to carry out lithium analysis on serum so clotted blood should be used. A lithium ion selective analyser is now available which allows determination of lithium in whole blood within a minute (Birch *et al*, 1993). If this apparatus is available the patient and doctor can discuss the results of the blood tests and adherence can be enhanced.

Reasons for possible lithium inefficacy

Unsatisfactory response to lithium treatment may have causes other than ineffective serum lithium concentration. The diagnosis of affective illness may not be correct; the drug may not have been given for a sufficient length of time (it may be necessary to continue treatment for three months before any therapeutic effect is obtained), and there may be irregular tablet intake. The most common reason for failure of lithium treatment is non-adherence, and it should be emphasised to patients starting lithium that drug therapy is a long-term commitment. In patients with limited insight, in those who have disorganised and chaotic lifestyles (independent of their affective state) and in regular substance misusers, lithium should not normally be prescribed because of the likelihood of poor adherence.

It is wise to involve the patient's partner in discussions about lithium treatment and if there is concern about the patient's mental state or adherence with the drug regime, the partner should be given every encouragement to contact the clinician. It may be helpful to initiate a treatment plan where the patient agrees to comply with medication and monitoring is carried out for a set time (perhaps three years) with a full review being arranged at that time.

It has been reported that, in some patients, lithium becomes less effective over time (Post, 1993). Work from the same group suggests that there is reduced responsivity to lithium when the drug is re-administered after a discontinuation-induced relapse. However, a later larger study in patients with bipolar disorder who had discontinued lithium for a time showed no difference in efficacy between the first and second treatment periods (Tondo *et al*, 1997).

Early side-effects

Side-effects within the first five days of starting lithium treatment include thirst, abdominal discomfort, nausea, diarrhoea, a metallic taste, muscle weakness and fatigue. The frequency of these symptoms is related to serum lithium level, and ranges from 60% for thirst to 6% for diarrhoea at a mean serum lithium level of 0.7 mmol/l (Vestergaard *et al*, 1988). It is worthwhile warning the patient of these possibilities and stressing their transitory nature, so as to maximise adherence at a stage before any clinical benefit is seen.

Long-term side-effects

Lithium toxicity and neurotoxicity

The toxic effects of lithium salts on the central nervous system have been described for nearly a century (see Box 2). Toxic symptoms become increasingly common above serum levels of 1.2 mmol/l and occur in three main organ areas: cerebral, gastrointestinal and cerebellar. Early signs are of mental lassitude or malaise occurring with or without agitation. This can progress to a confused state with vomiting and/or diarrhoea, coarse tremor, Parkinsonism and cerebellar signs (ataxia and dysarthria). The final stages are characterised by general disturbances of consciousness and neuro-muscular function, seizures, coma and death. Long-term neurological defects (usually cerebellar) can result from acute lithium toxicity in about 10% of cases (Schou, 1984).

However, of concern to the clinician are the reports of clinically unpredictable cases of neurotoxicity occurring at therapeutic levels of lithium. The symptoms of lithium neurotoxicity at therapeutic levels are mostly neurological, and differ only in degree from those described in cases of toxicity with high levels. They can occur in both acute and chronic therapy and the most common presentation is one of an encephalopathy. Rarely focal neurological disturbances (sensory and motor nerve palsies), motor disturbances, psychotic episodes (paranoia and visual/auditory hallucinosis), and specific cognitive deficits can occur (Verdoux & Bourgeois, 1990; Sheean, 1993; Bell & Ferrier, 1995).

Factors leading to toxicity and neurotoxicity

There are general factors, affecting all patients, which will produce a rise in serum lithium level with consequent toxic symptoms. These are relatively predictable and can be guarded against by careful monitoring and patient information. They arise from:

(a) Increased intake of lithium – prescription or patient error.

(b) Increased retention of lithium
  (i) Sodium depletion, e.g. salt-free diets, vomiting and diarrhoeal illnesses, excessive sweating and dehydration
  (ii) Drug interactions, e.g. thiazide diuretics, most non-steroidal anti-inflammatory drugs (particularly indomethacin, ibuprofen, piroxicam, naproxen and phenylbutazone), and some antibiotics excreted by the kidney (erythromycin, metronidazole and tetracycline)
  (iii) Systemic illness – particularly cardiac failure, renal disease and any pyrexial or gastrointestinal disturbance.

Box 2. Side-effects and toxicity: key learning points

The diagnosis of lithium toxicity should be made on clinical grounds rather than on the basis of blood results

Hypothyroidism on lithium is common in women and requires active intervention. TSH is the most useful marker

Renal function is unimpaired in the absence of episodes of toxicity but requires frequent monitoring

Careful sympathetic assessment of side-effects increases adherence

There are also individual specific factors which reduce lithium tolerance and are associated with neurotoxicity at much lower serum levels.

Some individuals seem to have a cerebral vulnerability and/or sensitivity to lithium. There have been reports of neurotoxic symptoms at therapeutic lithium levels in patients with pre-treatment electroencephalogram (EEG) abnormalities (particularly temporal lobe epilepsy), schizophrenia or schizoaffective illnesses. Reversible neurotoxic reactions have also occurred in cases of previously unsuspected intracerebral pathology and in association with Parkinsonism and mild cognitive impairment in the elderly.

A separate category of subjects absorb more lithium intracellularly, probably as a result of inherited sodium pump deficiencies, and manifest by increased red blood cell (RBC) (and, by implication, intracerebral) lithium concentrations. Factors affecting this process are co-prescription of phenothiazines (particularly thioridazine), weight fluctuation and changes in mood.

More potent neuroleptics, for example butyrophenones, have been associated with a neuroleptic malignant syndrome (NMS) picture. Particularly ominous is the coexistence of NMS with lithium neurotoxicity which has been associated with permanent cerebellar damage at levels of 0.89 mmol/l (Verdoux & Bourgeois, 1990).

Recently there have been a number of reports of severe neurotoxicity, when calcium channel blockers have been added to lithium. The unpredictability of this interaction suggests that close monitoring of clinical state and levels is required, and particular caution is advised in the elderly. This interaction is less likely if lithium levels are maintained at or around 0.5 mmol/l (Wright & Jarrett, 1991).

Management

Treatment of lithium toxicity depends primarily on the clinical state of the patient but also on the duration of previous lithium exposure, serum lithium concentration, renal lithium clearance and the extent of dehydration (Tyrer, 1996). If there is evidence of a reduced level of consciousness, confusion or ataxia, lithium should be discontinued and blood taken for serum lithium, creatinine and electrolytes. Patients should be told that if they feel unwell they can stop the drug for 24–48 hours without hazard.

A serum level in the toxic range needs to be treated accordingly, but a therapeutic level does not exclude neurotoxicity. The diagnosis of lithium toxicity is made on clinical grounds rather than on the basis of blood results. Confirmatory investigations include: the EEG which shows increased theta and delta activity with diffuse slowing and background disorganisation; the RBC lithium level which normally should be less than 0.6 mmol/l; and the RBC/serum lithium ratio (normal range 0.3–0.5).

Fluid intake should be encouraged but if there is a progressive increase in serum lithium, hypernatraemia or hypotension, an intravenous line should be inserted and transfer arranged immediately to a medical unit. Haemodialysis may be required if the renal lithium clearance is below 7 ml/min, although the value of this procedure has been questioned (Swartz & Jones, 1994). Clinical improvement can take up to three weeks and is paralleled by improvement in the EEG.

Tremor

Tremor is common in patients taking lithium and it is important for physicians to be able to recognise the different forms and react accordingly. Tremor is one of the commoner reasons given by patients for discontinuing lithium.

Fine tremor

This occurs in about 15% of lithium-treated patients (Vestergaard *et al*, 1988). In most patients it is either transitory or sporadic (sometimes associated with anxiety) and balanced reassurance is helpful to the patient. It is usually seen in the outstretched hands and is rare elsewhere. In most cases the tremor does not interfere with function, but if so then reduction of the dose to achieve a level of 0.5 mmol/l is helpful in the majority of cases. If the problem is persistent then β-adrenergic blockade (with the usual care) is helpful to some.

Flapping or coarse tremor

This tremor is associated with impending or established toxicity Muscle fasciculation, myoclonus, cerebellar signs or athetoid movements may be ominous concurrent features. These tremors are widespread and are usually, but not always, accompanied by other symptoms of toxicity. The presence of dysarthia with coarse tremor should set alarm bells ringing.

Pill-rolling tremor

A significant percentage of older patients on lithium, usually those with long exposure, complicated histories and poor outcome, develop either a Parkinsonian-like picture with tremor as a predominant feature or a tardive dyskinesia-type syndrome. Subclinical movement disorder may also be revealed by specific testing in these and less disabled patients.

These clinical states may be associated with cognitive decline. Previous neuroleptic medication intake is commonly found in such patients. Anti-cholinergic drugs are ineffective. Reduction of the dose of any concomitant neuroleptic and lithium is recommended and should precede any attempt to use dopaminergic agonists.

Thyroid disorders

It is well established that lithium therapy is linked to hypothyroidism and goitre in some patients. There are reports of hyperthyroidism occurring in lithium-treated patients and some cases have resulted after the dose of lithium was reduced, suggesting overcompensation of thyroid function following lithium-induced impairment.

The frequency of lithium-induced hypothyroidism is unknown but current estimates put this risk at between 2 and 3%. As with hypothyroidism not induced by lithium treatment, this complication is found principally in middle-aged women – the female to male ratio of published reports is 9:1. The average duration of lithium therapy before the diagnosis of hypothyroidism is 18 months – there are, however, case reports of this occurring dramatically within a month of therapy.

Subtle changes in thyroid function occur frequently in patients who do not develop frank hypo-thyroidism. Serum thyroxine falls (although within the euthyroid range) and a slight rise in TSH is seen. However, these changes are transitory and values should return to normal after one year.

The presence of thyroid auto-antibodies is a strong indicator of the likelihood of developing frank hypothyroidism in patients taking lithium (Bochetta *et al*, 1992). These antibodies are found in about 10% of the normal population but the frequency of them rises steeply in women after the age of 45 years. Patients with auto-antibodies and/or raised TSH are at high risk of developing hypothyroidism and measurement of these before lithium treatment is started is recommended (Myers *et al*, 1985). There is growing evidence that lithium may induce thyroid-antibody formation (Wilson *et al*, 1991), most probably in those already predisposed (Lee *et al*, 1992).

Regular monitoring of thyroid function in lithium-treated patients is recommended. Current suggestions are that this should be done yearly in men and six-monthly in women. The possibility of clinical hypothyroidism should be borne in mind particularly when reviewing a patient who has had a depressive relapse despite adequate lithium levels.

Once hypothyroidism has been diagnosed (even on biochemical grounds) treatment of the condition

should be instigated rapidly. Most authors would agree that low/borderline T4 should be treated by thyroxine and some would argue that patients with normal T4 but significantly raised TSH (especially over 15 mU/l) should be treated particularly if auto-antibodies are present. Referral to a physician is not usually necessary but is recommended in complicated cases, for example some elderly patients and those with cardiovascular disease. Discontinuation of lithium therapy is an option but in most cases the psychiatric indication for continuing it is strong.

Goitre occurs in approximately 5% of lithium-treated patients – the frequency rises with length of treatment. Thyroid size has found to be increased in cigarette smokers (Bochetta *et al*, 1996). It is not usually associated with hypothyroidism – supported by the slight male preponderance of cases. It is not usually of clinical concern and no case of lithium-associated thyroid malignancy has been reported. If the goitre enlarges then either lithium should be stopped or a small dose of thyroxine given.

Metabolic and other disturbances

A significant percentage of patients on lithium develop polyuria and polydipsia; this is a nephrogenic diabetes insipidus-like syndrome mediated by lithium's effect on cyclic adenosine monophosphate (AMP) and the action of vasopressin. These effects are reversible and complications are avoided by maintaining an adequate fluid and salt intake. If polyuria is troublesome a reduction in lithium level to 0.5–0.7 mmol/l and/or a change to a single daily dose may be helpful (although this is a matter of dispute). Long-term impairment of renal concentrating ability and/or pathological change in the kidney is seen only in patients who have episodes of lithium toxicity (Schou, 1988).

Long-term lithium therapy may be associated with a slight rise in serum calcium (about 3% after adjustment for protein) and a slight increase in parathyroid hormone secretion. Ionised calcium remains unchanged. Surgically verified hyper-parathyroidism has been found in 2.7% of patients receiving lithium for over 15 years (Bendz *et al* 1996). Serum calcium should be monitored in patients receiving long-term lithium, especially if there is any suggestion of kidney stones or bone pain.

Weight gain is seen in about a third of patients on lithium, is more common in women, and is an important cause of non-adherence. The mechanism remains unclear (little effect of dose reduction has been noted). No clinically relevant changes in liver or endocrine function are reported with lithium but there are a few case reports of sexual dysfunction in men (Johnson, 1987).

A rise in the white cell count (predominantly neutrophils) and, to a lesser extent, platelet count is seen in patients on lithium. The rise in the white blood cell count can be 30–45%, but rises of such magnitude are usually transitory; a 10% increase in counts is more usual in long-term therapy.

Discontinuation of lithium

Discontinuation of lithium is associated with an increased likelihood of relapse of affective illness. Mania is more likely to occur than depression in bipolar patients but depression is the rule in unipolar illness. The risk of relapse is increased if the patient has been taking lithium for a short time; it has been shown that unless lithium is given for at least two years at a dosage to maintain a therapeutic serum lithium level, the risk of an affective relapse is greater than if no treatment was given for the condition (Goodwin, 1994). Unless lithium treatment is well supervised, control of affective disturbance is poor and explains why some have doubts about its effectiveness (Moncrieff, 1997). The danger of non-adherence leading to manic relapse may explain the increase in admissions for mania at a time when the use of lithium was increasing (Tyrer, 1987). There is increased mortality in this group (2½ times what would be expected (Muller-Oerlinghausen *et al*, 1996)). Unless adherence is assured, lithium should not be given.

If a decision is made to discontinue lithium the risks of this procedure should be discussed in detail with the patient beforehand. It is important to discuss the signs and symptoms of relapse with the patient and their carers, and to encourage them to seek help early. It is advisable to reduce the dose of lithium slowly, as reductions of between 20 and 50% led to an increased risk of manic relapse in bipolar patients (Tyrer *et al*, 1983). This risk is substantially reduced if discontinuation takes place very slowly over a 14-month period (Baldessarini *et al*, 1997).

References

Amsterdam, J. D., Maislin, G. & Hooper, M. B. (1996) Suppression of herpes simplex viral infections with oral lithium carbonate. *Pharmacotherapy*, **16**, 1070–1075.

Aronson, J. K. & Reynolds, D. J. M. (1992) Lithium. *British Medical Journal*, **305**, 1273–1276.

Austin, M. P., Souza, F. G. & Goodwin, G. M. (1991) Lithium augmentation in antidepressant-resistant patients. A quantitative analysis. *British Journal of Psychiatry*, **159**, 510–514.

Baldessarini, R. J., Tondo, L., Floris, G., *et al* (1997) Reduced morbidity after gradual discontinuation of lithium treatment for bipolar I and II disorders: a replication study. *American Journal of Psychiatry*, **154**, 551–553.

Bell, A. J. & Ferrier, I. N. (1995) Lithium – induced neurotoxicity at therapeutic levels – an aetiological review. *Lithium*, **5**, 181–186.

Bendz, H., Sjodin, I., Toss, G., *et al* (1996) Hyperparathyroidism and long-term lithium therapy: a cross-sectional study and the effect of lithium withdrawal. *Journal of Internal Medicine*, **240**, 357–365.

Birch, N. J., Grof, R, HuHin, R. P., *et al* (1993) Lithium prophylaxis: Proposed guidelines for good clinical practice. *Lithium*, **4**, 225–230.

Bochetta, A., Bernardi, F., Burrai, C., *et al* (1992) The course of thyroid abnormalities during lithium treatment: a two year follow-up study. *Acta Psychiatrica Scandinavica*, **86**, 38–41.

——, Cherchi, A., Loviselli, A., *et al* (1996) Six-year follow-up of thyroid function during lithium treatment. *Acta Psychiatrica Scandinavica*, **94**, 45–48.

De Montigny, C., Cournoyer, G., Morissette, R., *et al* (1983) Lithium carbonate addition to tricyclic antidepressant-resistant unipolar depression. *Archives of General Psychiatry*, **40**, 1327–1334.

Drug and Therapeutics Bulletin (1999) Using lithium safely. *Drug and Therapeutics Bulletin*, **37**, 22–24.

Gelenberg, A. J., Kane, J. M., Keller, M. B., *et al* (1989) Comparison of standard and low serum levels of lithium for maintenance treatment of bipolar disorder. *New England Journal of Medicine*, **321**, 1489–1493.

Goodwin, G. M. (1994) Recurrence of mania after lithium withdrawal. *British Journal of Psychiatry*, **164**, 149–152.

Grof, P., Zis, A. P., Goodwin, F. E., *et al* (1978) Patterns of recurrence in bipolar affective illness. *Scientific Proceedings of American Psychiatric Association*, **179**, 120.

Hopkins, H. S. & Gelenberg, A. J. (1994) Treatment of bipolar disorder; how far have we come? *Psychopharmacology Bulletin*, **30**, 27–38.

Johnson, R N. (1987) *Depression and Mania: Modern Lithium Therapy*. Oxford: IRL Press.

Lee, S., Chow, C. C., Wing, Y. K., *et al* (1992) Thyroid abnormalities during chronic lithium therapy in Hong Kong Chinese: a controlled study. *Journal of Affective Disorders*, **26**, 173–178.

Moncrieff, J. (1997) Lithium evidence reconsidered. *British Journal of Psychiatry*, **171**, 113–117.

Muller-Oerlinghausen, B., Wolf, T., Ahrens, B., *et al* (1996) Mortality of patients who dropped out from regular lithium prophylaxis. *Acta Psychiatrica Scandinavica*, **94**, 344–347.

Myers, D. H., Carter, R. A., Burns, B. H., *et al* (1985) A prospective study of the effect of lithium on thyroid function and on the prevalence of antithyroid antibodies. *Psychological Medicine*, **15**, 55–61.

Peet, M. & Pratt, J. P. (1993) Lithium. Current status in psychiatric disorder. *Drugs*, **46**, 7–17.

Perry, P. J., Alexander, B., Prince, R. A., *et al* (1986) The utility of a single-point dosing protocol for predicting steady-state lithium levels. *British Journal of Psychiatry*, **148**, 401–405.

Post, R. M. (1993) Issues in the long-term management of bipolar affective illness. *Psychiatric Annals*, **23**, 86–93.

Price, L. H., Chamey, D. S. & Henninger, G. R. (1986) Variability of response to lithium augmentation in refractory depression. *American Journal of Psychiatry*, **143**, 1387–1392.

Prien, R. F., Caffey, E. M. & Klett, C. J. (1972) Relationship between serum lithium level and clinical response in acute mania treated with lithium. *British Journal of Psychiatry*, **120**, 189–192.

Schou, M. (1984) Long lasting neurological sequelae after lithium intoxication. *Acta Psychiatrica Scandinavica*, **70**, 594–602.

—— (1988) Effects of long-term lithium treatment on kidney function; an overview. *Journal of Psychiatric Research*, **22**, 287– 296.

—— (1997) Forty years of lithium treatment. *Archives of General Psychiatry*, **54**, 9–13.

Sheean, G. L. (1993) Lithium neurotoxicity. *Clinical and Experimental Neurology*, **14**, 112–127.

Small, J. G & Millstein, V. (1990) Lithium interactions; lithium and electroconvulsive therapy. *Journal of Clinical Psychopharmacology*, **10**, 346–350.

Swann, A. C., Bowden, C. L., Morris, D., *et al* (1997) Depression during mania. Treatment response to lithium or divalproex. *Archives of General Psychiatry*, **54**, 37-42.

Swartz, C. M. & Jones, P. (1994) Hyperlithemia correction and persistent delirium. *Journal of Clinical Pharmacology*, **34**, 865–870.

Tondo, L., Baldessarini, R. J., Floris, G., *et al* (1997) Effectiveness of re-starting lithium treatment after its discontinuation in bipolar I and bipolar II disorders. *American Journal of Psychiatry*, **154**, 548–550.

Tyrer, S. P. (1987) Maintenance lithium. *Lancet, i*, 866–867.

—— (1994) Lithium and treatment of aggressive behaviour. *European Neuropsychopharmacology*, **4**, 234–236.

—— (1996) Lithium intoxication; appropriate treatment. *CNS Drugs*, **6**, 426–439.

——, Shopsin, B. & Aronson, M. (1983) Dangers of reducing lithium. *British Journal of Psychiatry*, **142**, 427.

Verdoux, H. & Bourgeois, M. L. (1990) A case of lithium neurotoxicity with irreversible cerebellar syndrome. *Journal of Nervous and Mental Diseases*, **178**, 761–762.

Vestergaard, P., Poulstrup, I., Schou, M. (1988) Studies on a lithium cohort, 3; tremor, weight gain, diarrhoea, psychological complaints. *Acta Psychiatrica Scandinavica*, **78**, 434–441.

——, Licht, R. W., Brodersen, A., *et al* (1998) Outcome of lithium prophylaxis: A prospective follow up of affective disorder patients assigned to high and low serum lithium levels. *Acta Psychiatrica Scandinavica*, **98**, 310–315.

Wilson, R., McKillop, J. H., Crocket, G. I, *et al* (1991) The effect of lithium therapy on parameters thought to be involved in the development of auto-immune thyroid disease. *Clinical Endocrinology*, **34**, 357–361.

Wright, B. A. & Jarrett, D. B. (1991) Lithium and calcium channel blockers: possible neurotoxicity. *Biological Psychiatry*, **30**, 635–636.

Brief dynamic psychotherapy

Jeremy Holmes

The notion of brief dynamic psychotherapy (BDP) may seem at first sight to be a contradiction in terms. 'Dynamic' is a Freudian psychoanalytic term implying conflictual psychological forces – an opposition between the conscious and unconscious mind, and the use of defence mechanisms to arrive at a compromise between them. The rigidity of a person with an obsessional disorder whose self-expression is traded for security, the self-reproaches of a person with depression reflecting inhibited aggression, the clinging of the phobic individual who lacks an inner sense of a secure base – these would be examples of the relationship between dynamic conflict and psychiatric symptoms. But the image of psychoanalysis conjures up a picture of prolonged and intensive couch-based therapy. How can this be brief?

There are several answers to this. Freud's original conception of psychoanalysis was, by modern psychoanalytic standards, extremely short – a therapy lasting six months would have been considered long, and occasionally consisted of no more than a brisk walk with the master round the Vienna woods.

As analyses became more and more prolonged, some early analysts, notably Ferenczi and Rank, saw the need for more circumscribed, time-limited treatments, and began to discuss techniques to make these effective, such as reducing therapist passivity and focusing on the here-and-now rather than on the reconstruction of past trauma.

Freud himself addressed the problem of the 'interminability' of some analyses (Freud, 1937) and experimented with setting a definite date for ending.

Research suggests a negative logarithmic 'dose–effect' curve in psychotherapy (Howard *et al*, 1986), such that more than two-thirds of the total therapeutic benefit is achieved within the first 25 sessions.

There is evidence that quality rather than quantity of good attachment experience in childhood is linked with security and self-confidence and, by analogy, the same may be true in psychotherapy (Holmes, 1993).

Finally, it has been found that psychotherapy based in community mental health centres in the USA has a median length of treatment of 13 sessions

Box 1. Pioneers of BDP

Active therapist – Rank and Ferenczi
Setting a date for termination – Freud
Corrective emotional experience – Alexander and French
Focal therapy – Michael and Enid Balint
Brief dynamic psychotherapy – Malan
Short-term anxiety-provoking therapy – Sifneos and Davanloo
Core conflictual relationship theme – Luborsky
Time-limited psychotherapy – Mann
Cognitive analytical therapy – Ryle

(Howard *et al*, 1989): BDP can be conceptualised as an organised form of what otherwise would be a premature closure of therapy.

BDP can be defined as a time-limited form of psychoanalytically-based therapy, usually lasting between 6 and 40 sessions, characterised by high levels of therapist activity, and the attempt to work with a psychodynamic 'focus' which links the presenting problem, past conflict or trauma, and the relationship with the therapist (Delaselva, 1996; McCullough-Valiant, 1997). Although there are distinct schools of BDP (see Box 1), this chapter synthesises the main clinical features common to all of them, and highlights important differences where relevant.

Assessment: indications and contraindications

Most authors emphasise the need for careful assessment before embarking upon BDP, but there is little systematic research on the specific indications for it, as opposed to dynamic therapy generally. An exception was Horowitz *et al* (1984), who found in brief therapy following bereavement that more disturbed patients did better with behavioural supportive therapy, while those with greater ego strength improved more with BDP. This is consistent with the usually cited indications for BDP, which include high motivation for change, a circumscribed problem, evidence of at least one good relationship in the past, and the capacity for self-reflection or 'psychological mindedness' (see Box 2).

Malan (1963, 1976*a,b*, 1979), a pioneer of BDP, indicates contraindications such as:

(a) chronic addiction;

(b) serious suicide attempts;

(c) chronically incapacitating phobic or obsessional symptoms;

(d) evidence of gross destructive or self-destructive 'acting out' behaviours.

However, there is clinical evidence (Malan, 1979; Ryle, 1990) that quite disturbed patients with long-standing difficulties can, if sufficiently motivated, be helped with BDP. Since Malan's list contains qualifying terms such as 'gross' and 'serious', which are matters of judgement, in the end the 'feel' of the assessment interview remains a critical determinant of whether BDP is likely to be helpful. This is consistent with research indicating that a positive therapeutic alliance and the capacity to show affect in the early sessions of therapy are the best predictors of good outcomes in therapy generally (Orlinsky & Howard, 1986). This finding can be linked with Malan's picture of therapeutic 'leap-frogging' in BDP, in which the therapist responds to the patient's material with a brief comment or interpretation, leading to deepening of rapport, and further elaboration by the patient, perhaps with an affective response – usually sadness or anger –

followed by another intervention by the therapist, and so on.

Therapeutic contract

If the decision is to proceed with BDP, the patient should be informed at the outset what the terms of the therapeutic contract are:

(a) how many sessions are being offered;

(b) how long they will last, what the arrangements are in case of missed sessions;

(c) where 'homework' is part of the therapy, as in cognitive analytical therapy (Ryle, 1990), what is expected.

Most BDP includes a follow-up session after treatment has ended, and this too should be mentioned at the outset. Sometimes BDP is defined by time rather than number of sessions (e.g. six months, or 'from now until Easter'). This may seem less draconian than defining a number of sessions, and leaves room for transferential reactions as to whether six months, say, is a 'long' or 'short' time, but has the disadvantage of promising rather more than is often delivered because of holidays and other avoidable or unavoidable 'breaks'.

Finding a focus

Balint & Balint (1961) introduced the notion of a 'focus' in dynamic therapy, and indeed 'focal therapy' is often used interchangeably with BDP, although the phrase could equally be applied to cognitive therapies. A focus brings together:

(a) the patient's presenting problem;

(b) past difficulty – usually a 'hidden impulse' or affect related to loss or trauma;

(c) the current transferential relationship with the therapist.

The focus thus is a crystallisation of the patient's core or nuclear problem, based in the past, but permeating present difficulties and conflicts. The idea of focus operates at several levels in the course of dynamic therapy. It provides an overall conceptualisation or formulation of the problem; it ensures that patient and therapist do not becomes distracted by interesting but irrelevant side issues; and it acts as a guide to the therapist's interventions.

The man who beat his wife

John was a 30-year-old panel beater, whose marriage was in tatters when he presented for help with his

---

Box 2.   Factors predicting good outcomes in BDP

Circumscribed problem
Strong motivation
Able to express feeling at assessment
Psychological-mindedness
At least one good relationship
Evidence of achievement
Not actively suicidal
Not chronically obsessional or phobic
Not grossly destructive or self-destructive
Not actively misusing illicit drugs

intense jealousy (bordering on morbidity) of his wife. She responded to his jealous outbursts with provocative flirtation, and so a vicious circle built up. Both had been married before, but they had two children together and were desperate for the marriage to succeed. John was clearly depressed, with a score of 28 on the Beck Depression Inventory. The final straw had come when, rather than just shouting at his wife, he had physically assaulted her.

Although not particularly psychologically minded, and with no educational qualifications, he was strongly motivated for change, made a good rapport with the therapist, and was taken into a project specifically offering BDP to men with problems of violence.

He came from a family of four; when he was seven years old his sister developed cancer and eventually died; at the same time he and his brother were sent to a children's home about 150 km from his home town for a year. His parents visited once a fortnight.

The therapist made a focal link between his feelings of abandonment as a child and the emotions which were aroused in him when he imagined his wife was attracted to other men. John then recalled his feelings of fury and incomprehension when his parents left after visiting the home, and how he would invariably get into a fight with one of the other boys at that moment, for which he would be severely punished (just as he now was by his wife's withdrawal from him, and, sometimes, by the law), further fuelling his feelings of rage and injustice. In the sessions he was generally friendly, punctual and positive, and relations with his wife seemed to improve. The therapist often felt rather overwhelmed and importuned by John's rapid-fire delivery, which made it hard for him to get a word in, and it was often a relief when the session came to an end. This countertransferential reaction provided a view into how stifled John's wife might feel, perhaps based on John's feeling that any space or distance in a relationship was equivalent to abandonment. This was highlighted when the therapist mentioned he would be unavoidably away in two sessions' time. John became despondent, and referred at the next session to the therapist "going away on your holidays". The therapist pointed out that he had not said he would be on holiday, but simply 'away' (in fact his absence was work-related). John conceded that this was true, and revealed that he thought the therapist had had enough of him, needed a break, and was "flying off for a bit of sun". Once more he felt abandoned, and this led to discussion of how he imagined his parents having a good time away from him as a child, when in fact they were struggling with his sister's death, which was never openly discussed in the family. When he returned from the childrens' home she was simply not there. This in turn led onto his misery at the thought of losing his children if the marriage broke up. He missed the next session after the break, but returned for the following one, saying that things had been very bad with his wife, confirming Malan's view that the patient's worst problem will manifest itself at some point during therapy. This was once more taken up around the focal notion of abandonment and his furious reaction to it. Thereafter he continued to improve. At follow-up there had been no more serious outbreaks of violence, and he was still using his 'mood diary' when he felt bad, a device which had been suggested in the course of therapy.

The capacity to find and work with a focus is central to BDP, and several authors have developed conceptual tools to help therapists think focally. Malan (1979) extended Menninger's idea of a psychodynamic 'triangle of insight' into his 'triangle of person' and 'triangle of defence' (see Fig. 1). The former links the relationship with the 'significant other' (in John's case his wife), the therapist and the parent; the latter connects a hidden impulse or forbidden feeling, a defence, and a resulting anxiety. John's hidden feeling was abandonment; his defence was to attack and fight and so punish in the hope of preventing his 'object' from leaving him; and his anxiety manifested itself in his jealousy.

Molnos (1984) combined these into her four triangles in which the triangle of defence is experienced at different times in relation to other, therapist and parent.

Ryle (1990) similarly uses pictorial means to crystallise a focus, in his 'sequential diagrammatic reformulation' (SDR) (see Fig. 2), which emphasises the self-perpetuating nature of neurotic difficulty – John's violent 'defence' against abandonment producing the very result it aimed to prevent.

Like Ryle, Luborsky (1984) uses for research purposes a set of standard foci, or 'core conflictual relationship themes' (CCRT). These comprise:

(a) a wish;
(b) an imagined response by the other;
(c) the reaction of the self to that response.

For John this would be the wish not to be abandoned, the abandonment, and his consequent violent retaliations, his behaviour as a child and his reaction to the therapist's absence.

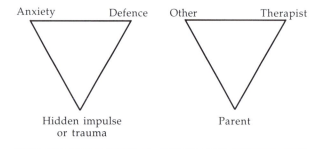

Fig. 1.   Malan's triangles

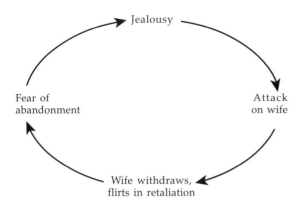

Exits
Count to 10 (*behavioural*).
Awareness of fear of abandonment from childhood (*dynamic*).
Perhaps wife is just friendly, not unfaithful (*cognitive*).

Fig. 2.   Sequential diagrammatic reformulation

The corrective emotional experience

Alexander & French (1946), who pioneered BDP in the USA in the 1940s, popularised Strachey's (1934) idea that cure in dynamic therapy comes about not, as Freud originally suggested, through intellectual insight alone, but by a reworking of relationship patterns with the therapist in a way that disconfirms previous neurotic expectations – the 'corrective emotional experience'. John's riposte to the therapist's missed session was to fail to turn up next time himself, but the therapist reacted to this with understanding, not punishment, a response which John was perhaps able to internalise and use when he next felt let down by his wife.

Managing resistance

Entering therapy is risky – patients are invited to abandon defences which may have served them reasonably well for many years. BDP offers two contradictory strategies for overcoming resistance – the cautious and the confrontative. Malan originally counselled caution, arguing that it is best to proceed from interpretations directed against anxiety and defence before going to the underlying feeling that is being defended. In John's case the therapist suggested that his jealousy was not some inherently evil part of his character, but could be understood

dynamically to arise from his fear of abandonment. The sequence was from his fear of splitting up with his wife (anxiety) to his jealousy (defence). Only later were the underlying feelings of rage and murderousness towards those who threatened to leave him (parents, wife, therapist) tackled.

Later, Malan became strongly influenced by the work of Davanloo (1980, 1990), a pupil of Sifneos (1979) who developed the method of 'short-term, anxiety-provoking psychotherapy' (STAPP). Davanloo, a powerful and charismatic figure, went further than Sifneos and advocated the relentless confrontation of resistance, in which patients are held in the here-and-now by a therapist who will not let them go until they have faced their negative feelings and destructiveness. A patient with depression is confronted with his or her anger for example, and if he or she denies it, the therapist will interpret the denial until the patient actually becomes angry in the session with the therapist. Expressing such 'healing anger' is a great relief to the patient, who at this point usually begins to let go of other feelings, especially sadness (Ashurst, 1991).

This cathartic approach can, in the right hands, be highly potent, but is not a necessary part of routine BDP practice. Ryle, for example, in his cognitive analytic therapy, which combines the techniques of BDP and cognitive therapy much more gently, urges the patient to consider possible 'exits' from his or her self-perpetuating vicious circles of neurosis. John used a variety of these, including the folk-wisdom of 'counting to 10' when he felt enraged, identifying the fear of abandonment that underlay his violence, and discussing with himself the possibility that his wife was simply being civil when talking to other men, rather than planning to go to bed with them.

Active therapist

Implicit in the above is the requirement of an active therapist, intervening frequently, holding the patient to the focus, attending to the here-and-now interactions. This is very different to the caricature of the passive analytic or Rogerian therapist who says little and suggests not at all. Whether such therapists exist in reality, even in full psychoanalysis, is debatable, but BDP undoubtedly implies active collaboration between therapist and patient, a relationship based as much on learning as holding and interpreting.

Malan studied the types of interventions made by therapists and claimed that good outcomes were particularly associated with high frequency of transference interpretations ('therapist–parent links') – for those committed to psychoanalysis, a particularly satisfying result. However, this finding has not been replicated, and may well be an artefact (Marziali, 1984), quality rather than quantity of interpretation being the more likely candidate for therapeutic efficacy. This view is supported by Piper *et al*'s (1991) study showing that high frequencies of transference interpretations were related to poor outcomes, although whether this was a causal relationship, or merely a desperate attempt by therapists to salvage an already rocky therapeutic alliance, was unclear.

Termination

Perhaps the defining feature of BDP is that it is time-limited, attempting to turn to advantage what, from a traditional psychoanalytic viewpoint, might seem a major drawback (Rosen, 1986). The limit to the contract, it is claimed, as well as being cost-effective, concentrates the mind of both patient and therapist, intensifies feelings, and enables a working through of themes of loss which are so central to many neurotic difficulties.

Mann's (1973) time-limited psychotherapy (TLP) particularly stresses termination, and the patient is informed at each session how many are left. This aspect of brief therapy can be stressful for therapists when first embarking on BDP, especially if from a psychoanalytic background. It is often clear towards the end of therapy that much psychological work has been left undone, but this is balanced by an affirmation of the patient's autonomy and capacity to cope, and for the therapist of a feeling of a job begun and completed. Ryle's cognitive analytic therapy includes a 'goodbye' letter, given to the patient at the penultimate session, and, as mentioned, most BDP schemata include a three-month follow-up. While most patients are satisfied with BDP, there will be some who require either a further course of BDP or a move into another mode of therapy, perhaps marital therapy or a long-term analytical group therapy.

Outcome

The evaluation of controlled studies of psychotherapy remains controversial. Two meta-analyses of outcome in BDP compared with waiting-list controls (Crits-Cristoph, 1992; Svartberg & Styles, 1992) confirmed impressive effect sizes (0.8–1.1) in target symptoms, general psychiatric symptoms and social adjustment, with treated patients being better off than 90% of those awaiting treatment. However, the improvements were less impressive when compared with non-specific treatments such as 'clinical mangement' and self-help groups, although on target symptoms BDP patients were still better off than 60% of controls.

Crits-Cristoph (1992) found that the effect size for 11 studies when compared with alternative treatments was on average only 0.32. But in two studies from highly reputable centres the effect sizes were much higher: Luborsky's group (Woody *et al*, 1990) compared BDP with routine drug counselling (effect size 0.74), and Weissman's group (DiMascio *et al*, 1979) contrasted interpersonal therapy (IPT) with 'low contact therapy' (effect size 0.67). Winston *et al* (1994) compared two different BDP models, 'brief adaptive therapy' and 'short-term dynamic psychotherapy' in the treatment of personality disorders. As in most psychotherapy outcome studies, no consistently significant differences emerged between the different BDP models, although both were superior to waiting-list controls on all measures.

In general, depression, especially as measured with the Beck Depression Inventory (BDI; Beck *et al*, 1961; Elkin *et al*, 1989), seems to respond well to psychological treatments such as BDP, and, in the follow-up studies performed, such interventions can be as effective as antidepressant medication in preventing relapse.

Conclusions

BDP is a successful, logical, cost-effective, teachable and appropriate form of therapy for a wide range of patients with neurotic disorders and moderately severe personality disorders (Stevenson & Meares, 1992; Winston *et al*, 1994). It is relevant to the work of NHS psychiatric departments, and should be part of the repertoire of most psychiatrists.

Interesting convergences are beginning to emerge between BDP and cognitive therapy, as the former acknowledges the cognitive component of much analytical work, while the latter recognises the importance of resistance and transference (Teasdale, 1993). To be effective, therapists should learn and stick within a particular model of therapy: Frank *et al* (1991) have shown that for IPT good outcomes can be linked to the extent to which therapists remain faithful to the method they purport to practise.

Training manuals are available for a number of forms of BDP (e.g. Luborsky, 1984; Ryle, 1990), and most psychotherapy departments provide relevant

---

Box 3.　Requirements for successful practice of brief dynamic psychotherapy

Appropriate setting – regular time, quiet place

Commitment

Focal thinking

Positive therapeutic alliance

Sticking to a particular model

Good supervision

Experience of personal therapy (desirable but not essential)

---

training and supervision (see Box 3). An essential prerequisite of practising BDP, as indeed with all forms of psychotherapy, is regular supervision, which, in the current political climate, can be characterised as continuing professional development or quality control.

References

Alexander, F. & French, T. M. (1946) Psychoanalytic Psychotherapy. Lincoln, Nebraska: University of Nebraska Press.

Ashurst, P. (1991) Brief psychotherapy. In *Textbook of Psychotherapy in Psychiatric Practice* (ed. J. Holmes), pp. 187–212. Edinburgh: Churchill Livingstone.

Balint, M. & Balint, E. (1961) *Psychotherapeutic Techniques in Medicine*. London: Tavistock.

Beck, A. T., Ward, C. H., Mendelson, M., *et al* (1961) An inventory for measuring depression. *Archives of General Psychiatry*, **4**, 561–571.

Crits-Cristoph, P. (1992) The efficacy of brief dynamic psychotherapy: a meta-analysis. *American Journal of Psychiatry*, **149**, 151–158.

Davanloo, H. (ed.) (1980) *Short Term Dynamic Psychotherapy*. New York: Aronson.

—— (1990) *Unlocking the Unconcious*. Chichester: Wiley.

Delaselva, P. (1996) *Intensive Short-Term Dynamic Psychotherapy*. Chichester: Wiley.

DiMascio, A., Weissman, M., Prusoff, B., *et al* (1979) Differental symptom reduction by drugs and psychotherapy in acute depression. *Archives of General Psychiatry*, **36**, 1450–1456.

Elkin, I., Shea, M., Watkins, J., *et al* (1989) NIMH treatment of depression collaborative research program: general effectiveness of treatments. *Archives of General Psychiatry*, **46**, 971–982.

Frank, E., Kupfer, D., Wagner, E., *et al* (1991) Efficacy of interpersonal psychotherapy as a maintenance treatment for recurrent depression. *Archives of General Psychiatry*, **48**, 1053–1059.

Freud, S. (1937) *Analysis, Terminable and Interminable. Standard Edition, Vol. 23*. London: Hogarth.

Holmes, J. (1993) *John Bowlby and Attachment Theory*. London: Routledge.

Horowitz, M., Marmar, C., Weiss, D., *et al* (1984) Brief psychotherapy of bereavement reactions: the relationship of process to outcome. *Archives of General Psychiatry*, **41**, 438–448.

Howard, K., Kopta, S., Krause, M., *et al* (1986) The dose–effect relationship in psychotherapy. *American Psychologist*, **41**, 159–164.

——, Davidson, C., O'Mahoney, M., *et al* (1989) Patterns of psychotherapy utilisation. *American Journal of Psychiatry*, **146**, 775–778.

Luborsky, L. (1984) *Principles of Psychoanalytic Psychotherapy: A Manual for Supportive-Expressive Treatment*. New York: Basic Books.

McCullough-Valiant, L. (1997) *Changing Character*. New York: Basic Books.

Malan, D. (1963) *A Study of Brief Psychotherapy*. London: Tavistock.

—— (1976a) *Frontier of Brief Psychotherapy*. New York: Plenum.

—— (1976b) *Towards the Validation of Dynamic Psychotherapy: A Replication*. New York: Plenum.

—— (1979) *Individual Psychotherapy and the Science of Psychodynamics*. London: Butterworths.

Mann, J. (1973) *Time Limited Psychotherapy*. Cambridge: Harvard University Press.

Marziali, E. (1984) Three viewpoints on the therapeutic alliance. *Journal of Nervous and Mental Disease*, **7**, 417–423.

Molnos, A. (1984) The two triangles are four: a diagram to teach the process of dynamic brief psychotherapy. *British Journal of Psychotherapy*, **1**, 112-125.

Orlinsky, D. & Howard, K. (1986) Process and outcome in psychotherapy. In *Handbook of Psychotherapy and Behaviour Change* (eds S. Garfield & A. Bergin), pp. 56–102. Chichester: Wiley.

Piper, W., Hassan, F., Joyce, A., *et al* (1991) Transference interpretations, therapeutic alliance, and outcome in short-term individual psychotherapy. *Archives of General Psychiatry*, **48**, 946–953.

Rosen, B. (1986) Brief focal psychotherapy. In *An Introduction to the Psychotherapies* (ed. S. Bloch), pp. 55-79. Oxford: Oxford University Press.

Ryle, A. (1990) *Cognitive Analytic Therapy: Active Participation in Change*. Chichester: Wiley.

Sifneos, P. (1979) *Short-Term Psychotherapy and Emotional Crisis*. Cambridge, MA: Harvard University Press.

Stevenson, J. & Meares, R. (1992) An outcome study of psychotherapy for patients with borderline personality disorder. *American Journal of Psychiatry*, **149**, 358–362.

Strachey, J. (1934) The nature of the therapeutic action of psychoanalysis. *International Journal of Psychoanalysis*, **15**, 127–159.

Svartberg, M. & Styles, T. (1992) Comparative effects of short-term psycho-dynamic psychotherapy: a meta analysis. *Journal of Consulting and Clinical Psychology*, **59**, 704–714.

Teasdale, J. (1993) Emotion and two kinds of meaning: cognitive therapy and applied cognitive science. *Behaviour Therapy Research*, **31**, 339–354.

Winston, A., Laikin, M., Pollack, J., *et al* (1994) Short-term psychotherapy of personality disorders. *American Journal of Psychiatry*, **151**, 190–194.

Woody, G., Luborsky, L., McLellan, A., *et al* (1990) Corrections and revised analysis for psychotherapy in methadone maintenance patients. *Archives of General Psychiatry*, **47**, 788–789.

Cognitive–behavioural therapy for whom?

Stirling Moorey

In many ways cognitive and behavioural therapies represent the acceptable face of psychotherapy for the general psychiatrist. They are brief, focused, problem-oriented treatments, which take symptoms seriously. They show an affinity for the medical model in their acceptance of diagnostic categories and their commitment to effective evaluation of treatments through randomised controlled trials. The wide applicability of these therapies is also attractive to the general psychiatrist. Cognitive and behavioural techniques are of major importance in the treatment of anxiety disorders, depression, eating disorders and sexual dysfunctions, and beyond this core group the methods can be applied to enhance coping and change unwanted behaviours in conditions as diverse as cancer, chronic pain, substance misuse, anger control, schizophrenia, and challenging behaviours in people with learning disabilities.

Despite these attractions, relatively few psychiatrists are trained in cognitive–behavioural techniques, and there is uncertainty about who should be referred. This article describes the conditions which cognitive–behavioural therapy (CBT) can treat, and the characteristics of the patients who are most likely to benefit. It also suggests some ways in which the process of referral can itself be used to increase the chances that the patient will engage in therapy.

Cognitive and behavioural psychotherapies

Behaviour therapy has its roots in learning theory: classical (Pavlovian) conditioning or operant (Skinnerian) conditioning. The behaviourist is primarily interested in observable behaviour and the way in which environmental events increase or decrease behavioural responses. In its most radical

form behaviourism sees internal mental processes, such as thoughts and beliefs, as epiphenomena. Even now some behaviour therapists still consider that behaviour change always precedes cognitive change, and so cognitive techniques can add nothing to behavioural interventions.

By contrast, cognitive therapy (based on the work of pioneers like Ellis (1962) and Beck (1976)) asserts that understanding thoughts, images and beliefs is the most important component of therapy. A cognitive therapist would consider behavioural techniques to work by producing cognitive change. For instance, in the treatment of a phobia the behaviour therapist believes that exposure has a direct effect on the conditioned fear responses, independent of cognitions. The cognitive therapist, however, sees exposure in humans as a form of behavioural experiment which demonstrates that a feared consequence does not occur: change comes from disproving the patient's erroneous belief. The impact of the 'cognitive revolution' on behaviour therapy has been profound, and in practice most behaviour therapists use cognitive techniques alongside conventional behavioural ones, hence the term CBT.

Cognitive and behavioural therapies are characterised by a focus on the patient's current life problems. The therapist is active and collaborates with the patient in identifying problems and finding solutions; the problems are defined in a way that allows their severity and frequency of occurrence to be measured to assess change. There is an emphasis on participation in the therapy through the use of self-help assignments between sessions. Within this framework the therapist uses a variety of techniques to produce change. Self-monitoring of thoughts, beliefs, emotions and behaviours can give information about the problem and also help the patient to begin to gain some control over it.

Behavioural techniques include: graded exposure to feared situations (phobias/obsessive–compulsive disorder (OCD)); graded tasks and activity scheduling (depression); removing the reinforcing consequences of maladaptive behaviour; and rewarding adaptive behaviour (challenging behaviours).

Cognitive techniques include: daily diaries to identify dysfunctional thoughts and beliefs; labelling types of distortion in negative thoughts; reality testing by questioning the evidence for negative interpretations; setting up experiments to test erroneous beliefs; and cognitive rehearsal of coping with difficult situations.

Length of treatment varies depending on the problem treated. For a simple phobia a few hours of therapist time with self-exposure between sessions is sufficient to produce complete cure, cognitive therapy for depression is traditionally one hour of therapy once a week for 10–20 sessions, while cognitive therapy for personality disorders or psychosis may require a year or more of therapy.

Applications of CBT

Exposure for phobias and OCD

Graded exposure is a simple and effective treatment for specific anxiety disorders. The patient and therapist construct a hierarchy of feared situations, and the patient is encouraged to confront them in a graded way. Exposure is more effective if it is in real life rather than imagination (Emmelkamp & Wessels, 1975), prolonged rather than brief (Stern & Marks, 1973) and practised regularly with self-exposure tasks (McDonald et al, 1978). Exposure is most effective with simple phobias such as animal phobias, where the phobic stimulus is clear. About two-thirds of the people who suffer from agoraphobia are successfully treated with exposure alone, and these gains are maintained at two-year follow-up (Munby & Johnston, 1980). Social phobia has also been effectively treated with exposure (Butler et al, 1984). Despite these successes a significant percentage of patients do not improve with exposure alone, and adding anxiety management or cognitive procedures may enhance the effects of exposure (Butler et al, 1984).

Exposure has also proved successful in the treatment of OCD. Obsessional patients try to neutralise fears by rituals, such as checking, handwashing, etc. Therapy consists of graded and prolonged exposure to the feared stimuli (e.g. contamination) with the additional component of preventing any neutralising rituals (response prevention). A combination of exposure and response prevention seems to be most effective,

producing a median success rate of 75% improvement in patients who complete treatment. However, because of treatment refusal, drop-out or failure, only 50% of all patients with OCD are actually helped (Salkovskis, 1989).

Obsessional ruminations without overt rituals are more difficult to treat. Exposing the patient to the ruminations by using a loop tape played on a personal stereo is sometimes effective. There is evidence for the efficacy of serotonin reuptake inhibitors in treating OCD, but the long-term outcome has not been satisfactorily evaluated: there is a high relapse rate when drug therapy is discontinued (Pato et al, 1988). With behaviour therapy, on the other hand, gains in people with phobias (Fava et al, 1995) and obsessions can be maintained at four-year follow-up.

Exposure with or without the addition of cognitive restructuring should therefore be considered the treatment of choice for phobias and OCD. In uncomplicated cases a referral for CBT should be made directly. Patients with OCD who are clinically depressed, whose obsessional symptoms are so severe they could not immediately use therapy, or who are unwilling to take part in treatment, should be treated with clomipramine or a selective serotonin reuptake inhibitor; but one of the main aims of treatment should be to prepare the patient for a course of CBT.

Generalised anxiety, panic disorder without agoraphobia and hypochondriasis

These conditions differ from phobias and OCD in that there is not a readily identifiable external stimulus to which the patient can be exposed. Behaviour therapy attempts to identify internal stimuli such as physiological cues for panic, and to expose the patient to them. The cognitive model of anxiety stresses the overestimation of the risk of catastrophe, misperception of danger and underestimation of coping abilities. Cognitive therapy challenges unrealistic thoughts and sets up experiments to test the negative predictions associated with anxiety.

The cognitive model of panic stresses the specific interpretations that the patient makes about the physical symptoms of anxiety. According to this model, catastrophic misattributions are made about symptoms such as palpitations, dizziness, faintness and breathlessness, which are really due to autonomic manifestations of anxiety, but are seen as signs of impending death, madness or loss of control. A vicious circle develops in which the automatic thoughts produce more anxiety and therefore more symptoms. Therapy consists of helping the patient to test their attributions through logical discussion and setting up behavioural experiments. Clark *et al* (1994) compared cognitive therapy, imipramine, applied relaxation and a waiting list control in patients with panic disorder and mild to moderate agoraphobia. The active treatments were all more effective than the waiting list, and cognitive therapy was the most effective treatment after completion and at follow-up.

The cognitive approach to hypochondriasis is similar to panic: patients misinterpret bodily symptoms as signs of physical illness, but do not believe they are about to die immediately. Reassurance seeking and avoidance act to maintain the hypochondriacal beliefs. Cognitive therapy develops an alternative explanation for the patient's symptoms, while behaviour therapy stresses overcoming avoidance and a ban on reassurance seeking. Preliminary studies show that both treatments may be helpful for these difficult patients (Salkovskis & Warwick, 1986). Whereas brief CBT can be effective in hypochondriacal conditions which have strong obsessional and anxious features, with other forms of somatisation (e.g. somatisation disorder) interpersonal and personality factors may predominate, making it difficult to engage in collaborative problem-solving. These patients may require longer term CBT. Patients with somatic conditions are increasingly being treated with CBT, and there are promising preliminary results with chronic fatigue syndrome.

Many patients with anxiety disorders will respond to a combination of education about their symptoms, support and drug therapy. Patients experiencing problems with long-term prescribing of benzodiazepines often want to learn anxiety management strategies which they can apply themselves. Therefore, if symptoms do not resolve within a few weeks a CBT referral should be considered.

Cognitive therapy for depression

Beck's cognitive model of depression states that the depressed person has a negative view of the self, the world and the future (Beck *et al*, 1979), which leads to the distortion of information to fit this negative set. Cognitive therapy is now widely accepted as an effective treatment for non-psychotic, unipolar, out-patients with depression. Behavioural techniques such as graded task assignment and activity scheduling are used to distract the patient from negative thoughts and provide experiences of success and pleasure. Patients are then taught to identify and challenge their distorted thinking.

Finally the dysfunctional assumptions which underlie the depressive thinking and make the patient vulnerable to depression are challenged. In numerous studies of out-patients with depression cognitive therapy has proved as effective or more effective than antidepressant medication (Dobson, 1989). Several follow-up studies have reported a relapse prevention effect for cognitive therapy. A review of these studies by DeRubeis & Crits-Cristoph (1998) found that if cognitive therapy and anti-depressants are withdrawn shortly after remission the relapse rate in the patients treated with cognitive therapy alone is 24% compared with 64% in those treated with medication alone. One large multi-centre trial found that cognitive therapy did less well than tricyclic antidepressants and interpersonal therapy with patients with more severe depression (Elkin *et al*, 1989). However, Stuart & Bowers (1995) reviewed studies of in-patients (*n*=203) and found combined treatment with medication and cognitive therapy superior to medication.

Most patients with depression will respond well to antidepressant medication, and it is also not practical for all to receive cognitive therapy. A number of factors might be considered when deciding which depressed patient should be referred. First, not all patients are able or willing to take antidepressants: some refuse medication, others cannot tolerate side-effects, and a small number have medical conditions which preclude drug treatment. Cognitive therapy may be the best first line of treatment in these cases. Second, not all patients make a complete recovery with pharmacotherapy. This sort of chronic low-grade depression can be very disabling, and may respond to cognitive therapy (Fava *et al*, 1994). Finally, there is now strong evidence that depression is a relapsing condition. Maintenance antidepressants prevent relapse, but their protective effect is lost when treatment is ended. If a patient experiences two or more depressive episodes a referral for cognitive therapy should be considered seriously.

Eating disorders

Fairburn *et al* (1986) suggest that people with bulimia have a tendency to judge self-worth in terms of shape and weight. Strict dietary control and perfectionistic attitudes mean that any lapse from the diet is seen as catastrophic and leads to a temporary abandonment of all control over eating. Therapy consists of monitoring binges and food intake, adopting a more normal dietary pattern and challenging maladaptive beliefs. Fairburn *et al* (1991) compared CBT, behaviour therapy and interpersonal therapy. All treatments produced improvements, but cognitive therapy was more effective than the other treatments in modifying disturbed attitudes to shape and weight and reducing extreme dieting. CBT has been found to be more effective than imipramine (Mitchell *et al*, 1990). Compas *et al* (1998) reviewed 33 studies and concluded that CBT produces an 80% reduction in binge–purge episodes, and 50–60% of patients are in remission at one-year follow-up. CBT for anorexia nervosa is less well established. This evidence suggests that CBT should be the primary intervention in patients with bulimia nervosa. The acute stage of anorexia nervosa often requires hospital treatment to induce weight gain. There may be a place for CBT in challenging maladaptive attitudes about food, shape and weight once the patient is out of the life threatening stage of the illness.

Other conditions

In general adult psychiatry, promising results have been obtained with patients with borderline (Linehan *et al*, 1993) and other personality disorders (Beck & Freeman, 1990). Behavioural techniques have had a place in the rehabilitation of patients with long-term mental illness for many years. Recent developments in work with schizophrenia have used cognitive–behavioural family interventions to teach problem solving skills (Falloon, 1988), reduce high expressed emotion (Leff *et al*, 1982) and to teach patients and families to recognise early signs of relapse. Another exciting development is the application of cognitive–behavioural principles to coping with psychotic symptoms and even challenging delusional ideas (Garety *et al*, 1994; Kuipers *et al*, 1997).

Box 1 lists the conditions for which CBT should be considered the psychological therapy of choice. A good summary of the evidence base for CBT and other therapies for a variety of disorders can be found in Roth & Fonagy (1996).

Factors influencing outcome in CBT

Coexisting diagnoses

Because both cognitive and behavioural techniques require the commitment and active participation of the patient, coexisting diagnoses such as depression and substance misuse can interfere with treatment. Secondary depression and anxiety, and also poor work, social or marital adjustment are associated with a poorer response to behaviour therapy for

phobias and OCD (Marks, 1987). These conditions respond to exposure if clinical depression is first treated with drugs (Baer *et al*, 1985).

People with social phobias and to a lesser extent those with agoraphobia may resort to alcohol and drug use as a way of dampening down anxiety. Alcohol misuse and excessive use of benzodiazepines can interfere with the effectiveness of exposure, and it may be necessary to treat these conditions before CBT is commenced.

Chronicity and severity

In general the more severe and chronic a disorder the poorer will be the outcome with any form of therapy. Marks (1987) claims that for phobias and OCD, chronicity does not augur poorer outcome with exposure.

In out-patient cognitive therapy for depression, chronicity and severity are associated with a poor outcome. Modification of standard CBT may be needed when treating severely depressed inpatients. The finding that chronicity and severity predict poor outcome is not specific to cognitive therapy: these variables also predict poor response

---

> **Box 1. Which diagnostic groups benefit from cognitive–behavioural therapies?**
>
> *Strongest evidence for efficacy* (large number of randomised controlled trials (RCTs))
> **Depression**
> **Agoraphobia**
> **Panic disorder**
> **Social phobia**
> **Specific phobia**
> **Obsessive–compulsive disorder**
> **Bulimia nervosa**
> **Sexual dysfunction**
>
> *Good evidence for efficacy* (several RCTs)
> **Hypochondriasis**
> **Chronic fatigue syndrome**
> **Post-traumatic stress disorder**
> **Schizophrenia**
>
> *Some evidence for efficacy* (more trials needed)
> **Borderline, antisocial and avoidant personality disorders**
> **Self-harm behaviours**
> **Bipolar affective disorder**
> **Substance misuse**

to antidepressants. Some studies have found a combination of cognitive therapy and antidepressants to be superior to either alone, while others have not found any advantage of combined treatment. In clinical practice it is rare for a patient with moderate to severe depression to be referred for cognitive therapy without also receiving drug therapy. The National Institute of Mental Health (Elkin *et al*, 1989) study suggests that cognitive therapy alone may not be the most effective treatment for severe depression.

Psychosocial factors

The association of depression with psychosocial factors might suggest that CBT will be less effective in socially disadvantaged groups and in people facing major life stress. In fact, both CBT and tricyclic antidepressants seem to be equally effective in patients experiencing high social stressors (Garvey *et al*, 1994).

Personality and interpersonal relationships

There is some evidence that the presence of a comorbid personality disorder predicts poor outcome in generalised anxiety (Noyes *et al*, 1990), agoraphobia (Fava *et al*, 1995) and bulimia nervosa (Rossiter *et al*, 1993). Sanderson *et al* (1994) found that patients with personality disorders with generalised anxiety disorder did not do less well, but were more likely to drop out.

Interpersonal and relationship difficulties are often felt to be clinically important in agoraphobia: the quality of a marriage does not predict short-term outcome (Cobb *et al*, 1984) but may be associated with long-term follow-up. A high proportion of women with agoraphobia report marital difficulties, but this is not a contraindication to behaviour therapy, since marital satisfaction improves following successful treatment with exposure .

Personality disorder should not be considered an absolute contraindication to referral, but treatment may take longer than with more straightforward patients (Beck & Freeman, 1990). Tarrier *et al* (1998) describe the clinical application of CBT to complex cases.

Cognitive factors

Patients are often referred for CBT because they display conspicuously negative thinking patterns, with the assumption that they are therefore ideal candidates. In fact, cognitive variables such as

---

> **Box 2.　Making a referral**
>
> **Is CBT a proven treatment for this diagnostic group?**
> **Are there any contraindications, e.g. severe depression, substance misuse**
> **Is the patient motivated to work psychologically?**
> **Can the patient identify problems and goals to work on?**
> **Does the patient accept the therapeutic model?**
> **Is the patient prepared to carry out self-help assignments?**

---

hopelessness, frequency of negative thoughts, cognitive distortions and maladaptive assumptions are highly correlated with mood and are not predictive of response to therapy in their own right. Patients who do better with cognitive therapy actually have lower scores on dysfunctional attitudes (see Moorey, 1989 for a review of patient factors associated with outcome in CBT for depression). Patients with more cognitive distortions often have life-long, fixed negative beliefs about themselves which are not amenable to standard cognitive interventions, but may need longer, schema-focused therapy (Beck & Freeman, 1990).

These findings would suggest that there are not any clear cognitive predictors of outcome with CBT, and that the degree of negative thinking should not be a factor in deciding whether or not to make a referral.

It is also sometimes assumed that patients need to be of a certain intellectual standard to engage in CBT or that they need to have a high degree of education. In fact , education and IQ have no effect on the outcome of cognitive therapy for depression.

Motivation for change

Clinically, the patient's desire to find relief from symptoms and to solve personal problems is considered important in assessing suitability for therapy. From a research perspective, attempts to predict outcome by measuring a unitary variable of 'desire to change' have not been successful. Even if it seems obvious that a symptom is disabling, it does not mean that the patient wishes to deal with it. The therapists' time can be saved if the referrer checks that the patient actually does want to give up the particular symptom.

Box 3.   Self-help material for patients

General cognitive therapy
Beck, A. T. (1976) *Cognitive Therapy and the Emotional Disorders.* New York: Penguin.
Greenberger, D. & Padesky, C. (1995) *Mind Over Mood.* New York: Guildford.
Butler, G. & Hope, T. (1995) *Manage Your Mind.* Oxford: Oxford University Press.

Anxiety disorders
Marks, I. (1980) *Living with Fear.* New York: McGraw Hill.
Kennerley, H. (1997) *Overcoming Anxiety.* London: Robinson.

Depression
Gilbert, P. (1997) Overcoming Depression. London: Robinson.
Burns, D. D. (1989) *The Feeling Good Handbook.* New York: Morrow.

Eating disorders
Schmidt, U. & Treasure, J. (1993) *Getting Better Bit(e) by Bit(e).* Hove: Laurence Erlbaum Associates.

Personality problems
Klosko, J. S. & Young, J. E. (1994) *Reinventing Your Life.* New York: Penguin.

Goals for therapy

In general, CBT is more applicable if patients have clear ideas of the problems they wish to work on and clear goals for therapy. 'Understanding myself better' does not augur well as a goal, whereas 'being able to drive more than 10 miles on my own without anxiety' does. CBT is a problem-solving therapy and works best when patients have problems in the here and now. Patients who wish to gain insight, to explore their past or resolve conflicts are more suitable for dynamic psychotherapy. Again it is helpful for the clinician to discuss this explicitly with the patient before referring for therapy.

Acceptance of the therapeutic model

Frank (1973) has argued that therapy is most effective if the patient feels confident in the therapist and accepts the therapist's explanation of the cause and cure of their problems. In CBT this applies not

only to what goes on within the session, but also to the patient's compliance with self-help assignments outside the session. There is some evidence that patients who already think in a problem-solving way are more likely to respond to CBT. Simons *et al* (1985) found that a measure of 'learned resourcefulness' (a tendency to use problem-solving and self-control skills) predicted good response to cognitive therapy and poor response to drug treatment. While some studies have replicated this finding, others have not. Fennell & Teasdale (1987) found that patients who had a positive response to a booklet describing cognitive therapy and went on to have a successful first homework assignment recovered more rapidly. The effectiveness of exposure for phobias and OCD depends to a large extent on the patient's willingness to engage in self-directed exposure homework (Marks, 1987). In cognitive therapy for depression, homework compliance is associated with better outcome. Burns & Holen-Hoeksema (1991) found that expectations about the value of coping strategies did not correlate with outcome, but willingness to carry out self-help assignments and homework adherence did.

Taken together these findings suggest that individuals who tend to think in a problem-focused way may find it easier to accept the rationale for CBT and so do better in therapy. Both the behavioural and more cognitive forms of CBT work better if the patient is prepared to engage in self-help assignments. An important part of assessment for CBT must therefore involve assessing the patients' acceptance of the therapeutic model. It is worth describing the rationale for therapy (principles of exposure for phobias and obsessions, and the cognitive model for depression, anxiety, eating disorders) to the patient before a referral is made, while emphasising the importance of homework assignments. If a patient resolutely refuses to consider that the psychological model has merit, or indicates that they will not be able to do homework, a referral is probably not worthwhile. Some general psychiatrists take this one stage further and give the patient reading material about CBT. This is in effect a behavioural experiment. If the patient responds negatively to the information in the literature, or does not often carry out the assignment, this may be a contraindication.

Referral considerations

The increasing evidence for the wide range of applications of CBT in psychiatry means that many of the patients a psychiatrist encounters in out-patients could potentially benefit from this approach. Availability of CBT is still limited. There are increasing numbers of trained nurse behaviour therapists but they are not all trained in cognitive therapy. Most clinical psychology departments will provide CBT, but in psychiatry there are still only a handful of consultant psychotherapy posts which are CBT-based rather than psychoanalytically-based. Given the need to be selective in which patients are referred, these guidelines may be helpful in choosing the patients most likely to benefit from CBT. But in the long run they are no substitute for providing adequate resources, and training psychiatrists themselves in the application of CBT.

Acknowledgement

I am grateful to Mrs Ruth Williams who made helpful comments on an earlier draft of this paper.

References

Baer, B. L., Minichiello, W. E. & Jenike, M. A. (1985) Behavioural treatment in two cases of OCD with concomitant bipolar affective disorder. *American Journal of Psychiatry*, **142**, 358–360.

Beck, A. T. (1976) *Cognitive Therapy and the Emotional Disorders*. New York: International Universities Press.

——, Rush, A. J., Shaw, B. F., *et al* (1979) *Cognitive Therapy of Depression*. New York: Guilford.

—— & Freeman, A. (1990) *Cognitive Therapy of Personality Disorders*. New York: Guilford.

Burns, D. D. & Holen-Hoeksema, S. (1991) Coping styles, homework compliance, and the effectiveness of cognitive-behavioral therapy. *Journal of Consulting and Clinical Psychology*, **59**, 305–311.

Butler, G., Cullington, A., Munby, M., *et al* (1984) Exposure and anxiety management in the treatment of social phobia. *Journal of Consulting and Clinical Psychology*, **52**, 642–650.

Clark, D. M., Salkovskis, P. M., Hackmann, A., *et al* (1994) A comparison of cognitive therapy, applied relaxation and imipramine in the treatment of panic disorder. *British Journal of Psychiatry*, **164**, 759–769.

Cobb, J. P., Mathews, A. M., Childs-Clark, A., *et al* (1984) The spouse as co-therapist in the treatment of agoraphobia. *British Journal of Psychiatry*, **144**, 282–287.

Dobson, K. S. (1989) A meta-analysis of the efficacy of cognitive therapy for depression. *Journal of Consulting and Clinical Psychology*, **57**, 414–419.

DeRubeis, R. J. & Crits-Cristoph, P. (1998) Empirically supported individual and group psychological treatments for adult mental disorders. *Journal of Consulting and Clinical Psychology*, **66**, 37–52.

Elkin, I., Shea, T., Watkins, J. T., *et al* (1989) NIMH Treatment of depression collaborative research program. I. General effectiveness of treatments. *Archives of General Psychiatry*, **46**, 971–982.

Ellis, A. (1962) *Reason and Emotion in Psychotherapy*. New York: Lyle Stuart.

Emmelkamp, P. M. G. & Wessels, H. (1975) Flooding in imagination versus flooding *in vivo* for agoraphobics. *Behaviour Research and Therapy*, **13**, 7–15.

Fairburn, C. G., Cooper, Z. & Cooper, P. J. (1986) The clinical features and maintenance of anorexia nervosa. In *Handbook of Eating Disorders: Physiology, Psychology and Treatment of Obesity, Anorexia and Bulimia*, (eds K. D. Brownell & J. P. Foreyt). New York: Basic Books.

Fairburn, C. G., Jones, R., Peveler, R. C., *et al* (1991) Three psychological treatments for bulimia nervosa. *Archives of General Psychiatry*, **48**, 453–469.

Falloon, I. R. H. (1988) *Handbook of Behavioural Family Therapy*. London: Unwin Hyman.

Fava, G. A., Grandi, S., Zielezny, M., *et al* (1994) Cognitive–behavioral treatment of residual symptoms in primary major depressive disorder. *American Journal of Psychiatry*, **151**,1295–1299.

——, Zielezny, M., Savron, G., *et al* (1995) Long-term effects for behavioural treatment of panic disorder with agoraphobia. *British Journal of Psychiatry*, **166**, 87–92.

Fennell, M. J. V. & Teasdale, J. D. (1987) Cognitive therapy for depression: individual differences and the process of change. *Cognitive Therapy and Research*, **11**, 253–271.

Frank, J. (1973) *Persuasion and Healing: A Comparative Study of Psychotherapy* (2nd edn). Baltimore, MD: Johns Hopkins University Press.

Garety, P. A., Kuipers, l., Fowler, D., *et al* (1994) Cognitive–behavioural therapy for drug-resistant psychosis. *British Journal of Psychiatry*, **167**, 259–271.

Garvey, M. J., Hollon, S. D. & DeRubeis, R. J. (1994) Do depressed patients with higher pre-treatment stress levels respond better to cognitive therapy than imipramine? *Journal of Affective Disorders*, **32**, 45–50.

Kuipers, E., Garety, P., Fowler, D., *et al* (1997) London–East Anglia randomised-controlled trial of cognitive–behavioural therapy for psychosis. *British Journal of Psychiatry*, **171**, 319–327.

Leff, J., Kuipers, L., Berkowitz, R., *et al* (1982) A controlled trial of intervention in the families of schizophrenic patients. *British Journal of Psychiatry*, **141**, 121–134.

Linehan, M. M. (1993) *Cognitive-Behavioral Treatment of Borderline Personality Disorder*. New York: Guilford Press.

McDonald, R., Sartory, G., Grey, S. J., *et al* (1978) Effects of self-exposure instructions on agoraphobic out-patients. *Behaviour Research and Therapy*, **17**, 83–85.

Marks, I. M. (1987) *Fears, Phobias and Rituals: Panic, Anxiety, and their Disorders*. New York: Oxford University Press.

Mitchell, J. E., Pyle, R. L., Eckert, E. D., *et al* (1990) A comparison study of antidepressants and structured group therapy in the treatment of bulimia nervosa. *Archives of General Psychiatry*, **47**, 149–157.

Munby, M. & Johnston, G. W. (1980) Agoraphobia: the long-term follow-up of behavioural treatment. *British Journal of Psychiatry*, **137**, 418–427.

Moorey, S. (1989) Cognitive therapy of depression: patient factors related to outcome. In *Cognitive Psychotherapy: Stasis and Change* (eds W. Dryden & P. Tower) London: Cassell.

Noyes, R. J., Reich, J., Christiansen, J., *et al* (1990) Outcome of panic disorder. *Archives of General Psychiatry*, **47**, 809–818.

Pato, M. T., Zoka-Kadouch, R., Zohar, J., *et al* (1988) Return of symptoms after desensitization of clomipramine in patients with obsessive–compulsive disorder. *American Journal of Psychiatry*, **145**, 1521–1525.

Rossiter, E. M., Agras, W. S., Telch, C. F., *et al* (1993) Cluster B personality disorder characteristics predict outcome in the treatment of bulimia nervosa. *International Journal of Eating Disorders*, **13**, 349–357.

Roth, A. & Fonagy, P. (1996) *What Works for Whom? A Critical Review of Psychotherapy Research*. London: Guilford.

Salkovskis, P. M. (1989) Somatic disorders. In *Cognitive Behaviour Therapy for Psychiatric Problems: A Practical Guide*. (eds K. Hawton, P. M. Salkovskis, J. W. Kirk, *et al*). Oxford: Oxford University Press.

—— & Warwick, H. M. (1986) Morbid preoccupations, health anxiety and reassurance: a cognitive behavioural approach to hypochondriasis. *Behaviour Research and Therapy*, **24**, 597–602.

Sanderson, W. C., Beck, A. T. & McGinn, L. K. (1994) Cognitive therapy for generalised anxiety disorder: significance of co-morbid personality disorders. *Journal of Cognitive Psycho-therapy: An International Quarterly*, **8**, 13–18.

Simons, A. D., Lustman, P. J., Wetzel, R. D., *et al* (1985) Predicting response to cognitive therapy of depression: The role of learned resourcefulness. *Cognitive Therapy and Research*, **9**, 79–89.

Stern, R. & Marks, I. M. (1973) Brief and prolonged flooding: a comparison in agoraphobic patients. *Archives of General Psychiatry*, **28**, 270–276.

Stuart, S. & Bowers, W. A. (1995) Cognitive therapy with in-patients – review and meta-analysis. *Journal of Cognitive Psychotherapy*, **9**, 85–92.

Tarrier, N., Wells, A. & Haddock, G. (1998) *Treating Complex Cases: the Cognitive–Behavioural Approach*. Chichester: Wiley.

Behavioural therapy and drug treatments for obsessive–compulsive disorder

C. Duggan

Three recent advances have increased the importance of obsessive–compulsive disorder (OCD) for the general psychiatrist. It is a more common disorder than previously realised, there are effective treatments, and the basic neurobiological substrate for the condition is being identified. This chapter will consider these advances but focus mainly on the practical aspects of assessing the condition and planning treatment.

Diagnostic criteria

OCD is an anxiety disorder, with the anxiety arising from certain cues which have to be neutralised either by a behavioural or mental ritual. Anxiogenic cues may be either thoughts or behaviours which the OCD sufferer has to undo with anxiolytic responses which, again, may be either thoughts or behaviours. Failure to carry out the 'undoing' ritual results in an increase in anxiety.

Obsessions are defined as recurrent and persistent ideas, thoughts or impulses which are experienced, at least initially, as intrusive and senseless. They commonly focus on thoughts of contamination, violence, doubting and worries about sexual or religious prohibitions. These are invariably distressing so an attempt is made to resist, suppress or neutralise them with some other thought or action. The individual recognises that these are the product of his or her own mind and not imposed from outside.

Compulsions are repetitive, purposeful and intentional behaviours which are performed in response to an obsession, or according to certain rules or in a stereotyped fashion. They frequently involve checking, washing and counting. The behaviour is designed to neutralise or to prevent discomfort from some dreaded event or situation.

The person recognises the behaviour as excessive or unreasonable.

In addition to these phenomenological criteria, recent definitions also include the requirement that the obsessions or compulsions should cause distress, take up more than an hour a day and interfere with occupational or social functioning. Obsessional slowness refers to abnormal length of time spent in performing everyday tasks. This is usually secondary either to ruminating on whether a particular act has been carried out properly or to being abnormally indecisive.

Associated features

Secondary avoidance is common, with idiosyncratic thinking and the belief that the slightest infringement of the rules will spell catastrophe. This is often extensive and may result in the core anxiety feature of the disorder not being evident.

Family members are often forced to offer repeated reassurance and go to extraordinary lengths to comply with the avoidant behaviour. Thus, the impact of the disorder often extends far beyond the affected individual. Relatives often make useful allies in a treatment intervention.

Comorbidity often occurs with OCD; the most frequently found disorders are depression (30%), other anxiety states and drug misuse (frequently iatrogenic).

Epidemiology

OCD was regarded as an uncommon disorder with a lifetime prevalence rate of 0.1% before the recent epidemiological surveys. The ECA survey, for instance, showed rates of 2–3%, making OCD the fourth most common psychiatric disorder (Myers *et al*, 1984). The discrepancy between estimated and true rates suggests a hidden morbidity in the community. This perception is supported by the experience of specialised referral centres where there is often a delay of many years between the onset of the disorder and presentation.

Other epidemiological aspects of OCD include an equal gender ratio, although compulsive washing and obsessional slowness are more common among females and males respectively (Marks, 1987). The age of onset is in early adolescence or early adulthood although there is an interesting additional increase among females over 60 years of age. OCD has a variable course with exacerbations often being precipitated by adverse life events (Rasmussen & Eisen, 1988).

Aetiology

Current theories involve an interaction between biological vulnerability and social learning. Attention has focused on the orbito-frontal cortex, cingulate cortex and caudate nucleus and it is suggested that these form a hyperactive circuit in OCD (Insel, 1992). Of particular interest is Baxter *et al*'s (1992) positron emission tomography scan finding that caudate nucleus activity decreased in OCD subjects treated with either fluoxetine or 10 weeks of behavioural therapy. These advances need to be integrated with the psychological models of how the avoidance and neutralising rituals prevent the extinction of conditioned anxiety.

Assessment strategies

In the assessment of OCD, a behavioural analysis provides a comprehensive examination of the disorder. This involves identification of the anxiogenic stimulus (usually the obsession), the resultant anxiety state and then the anxiolytic response. The anxiogenic stimulus may occur spontaneously or be cued by a number of stimuli which that individual will avoid to prevent its occurrence. The undoing ritual may be overt, in the form of a behaviour which is excessive, or covert, in the form of a mental ritual. As the ritual reduces anxiety, it has an important maintaining, reinforcing or even a pre-emptive function.

One should also establish the impact on the individual's relationships, and occupational functioning. The recruiting of an informant, such as a close family member, is often very useful in that the OCD sufferer may minimise his or her level of disability or omit crucial avoidances, and family members may need guidance in avoiding offering reassurance. This often involves explicit coaching, for example, encouraging the relative to respond to requests for reassurance with the same neutral and monotonous response – 'the hospital has instructed me to say no answer' (Marks, 1986).

One should enquire about previous treatments, their appropriateness, and the nature of the response. One also needs to assess the daily drug and alcohol intake of the patient. No more than 5 mg of diazepam or two units of alcohol should be taken while participating in the exposure therapy as this will affect habituation. Finally it is important to assess the mental state to decide if there is any depression or evidence of psychosis.

It is essential to check out continually that the formulation is in accord with the individual's own perception as, apart from the need to obtain accuracy, this will help cement the therapeutic alliance. Focusing on the presenting problem in considerable depth has therapeutic properties as well as being helpful in the assessment.

The therapist and patient together should also determine a list of specific targets which the patient wishes to achieve. These should be quantified and form a baseline whereby the impact of the therapy may be judged. There are several instruments which give a quantitative assessment of OCD symptoms. As a routine package in the assessment of OCD, I would advise using the Self-Report Obsessive Compulsive Checklist, (Marks, 1986), the Fear Questionnaire (Marks & Matthews, 1979), and the Beck Depression Inventory (Beck *et al*, 1961).

Differential diagnoses

Obsessive–compulsive personality disorder

Conventionally, obsessive–compulsive personality disorder (OCPD) traits are considered egosyntonic (i.e. not distressing or alien) whereas OCD symptoms are egodystonic. This separation becomes difficult when the phenomena of OCD become embedded with such a degree of secondary avoidance that subjective distress becomes minimal and resistance to the intrusion disappears (Tallis *et al*, 1988). Research has shown that many personality disorders other than OCPD co-occur with OCD and this hampers the treatment of OCD with medication, behavioural treatment and with self-help methods in general.

Depression

This is the most important and common co-occurrent condition with a lifetime prevalence of 70% in those with OCD; 25–30% of these are depressed at presentation (Rasmussen & Eisen, 1988). Comorbid depression may cause an individual with long-standing OCD to present for treatment, may increase the severity of OCD and may reduce the response of OCD to treatment.

Other anxiety states

It may be difficult to distinguish an individual with a phobia from one with OCD (Marks, 1987). In addition, the co-occurrence of OCD with other anxiety states is common, with one study showing that other phobias and panic disorder occurred in 40% and 10%, respectively, of those with OCD (Mulder *et al*, 1991).

OCD as a prelude to psychosis

It may sometimes be difficult to distinguish OCD from an overvalued idea, especially if the belief has been held for some time and resistance has disappeared. An overvalued idea is considered to be reasonable (versus futile), natural (versus intrusive) and not resisted (McKenna, 1984). One needs also to consider whether the OCD sympto-matology represents a defence against either an acute psychotic breakdown or a more gradual deterioration of personality.

Treatment

OCD is a chronic condition; if the symptoms have been established for more than a year spontaneous recovery is unusual. Given that it takes most individuals many years to present for treatment, there is much untreated morbidity from OCD in the community. One of the challenges for the mental health professional is to make sufferers aware that effective treatments are available and how these might be accessed. Controlled research has identified two treatments as being effective for OCD – behavioural therapy and pharmacotherapy.

Behavioural therapy

Successful behavioural treatment of OCD was first developed in the mid 1960s by Victor Meyer (1966). Initially, it was both lengthy and expensive as it involved therapist-assisted exposure. This has now been shown to be unnecessary and treatment time has been reduced to 10–15 sessions, making it potentially available to many more individuals (Marks, 1991).

The principles of this treatment are extremely simple. The patient has to expose himself or herself to the anxiogenic cue and thereafter resist the undoing ritual. Thus, someone who is fearful of contamination would, as part of their treatment, deliberately contaminate themselves (exposure) and then resist the compulsion to wash (response prevention). Someone who is compulsively neat would be expected to leave their possessions in disarray and then resist the compulsion to tidy them and so on. The essential manoeuvre of the treatment is that the behaviour should generate anxiety which must then be tolerated in the absence of the undoing ritual.

Controlled research has shown that if the therapy is practised in a systematic manner, then it is successful in most cases. These gains are maintained for many years of follow-up (O'Sullivan & Marks, 1990). Foa *et al* (1985) reviewed studies of patients treated with behavioural therapy and concluded that half of the patients achieved a 70% reduction in symptoms.

Relapse prevention

Since we know that adverse life events are often associated with a recrudescence of the OCD, the patient can predict the times of future relapse so that appropriate self-exposure and response prevention can be commenced. Short booster courses of therapy, for example one or two sessions, may be necessary to re-establish the previous programme.

Pure obsessional ruminations

This subset of OCD involves thoughts which intrude into the mind despite, as Henry Maudsley described, 'the most earnest wish to turn and keep them out'. In the past, obsessional ruminations had a particularly poor response to behavioural techniques of thought stopping and distraction (Rachman, 1983). More sophisticated conceptualisations of this disturbance have improved treatment response. These view obsessional ruminations as comprising anxiogenic thoughts together with anxiolytic or cognitive neutralising rituals – which have the same maintaining effect on the rumination as overt compulsive behaviour (Salkovskis & Westbrook, 1989). Treatment consists of the patient (again as a part of a homework task) recording their anxiogenic thoughts on a looped cassette tape and then playing these thoughts continually until habituation occurs, while at the same time omitting anxiolytic or cognitive neutralising thoughts.

In-patient units

In the past OCD was thought to be such a serious and refractory disorder that intensive in-patient work was required to effect change. The recent emphasis on self-exposure means that in-patient treatment is rarely necessary. Indications for in-patient treatment have now been refined to include: those who do not have access to behavioural therapy locally; those who have severe OCD or co-occurrent depression; and where members of the family need to rehearse not giving reassurance (Thornicroft *et al*, 1991). In the main, however, hospitalisation is not necessary and it is likely that gains made in hospital may well be lost after discharge.

Cognitive therapy

The need for cognitive restructuring in addition to behavioural therapy is not entirely established (Emmelkamp & Beens, 1991). Certainly, the unwary or inexperienced practitioner should avoid debating the validity of a particular thought or behaviour with an OCD sufferer, as this may offer a subtle form of reassurance. Cognitive therapy may be of advantage in persuading an individual to take the risk of engaging in a behavioural experiment, or in making the thought more egodystonic so that it can be challenged. This especially applies when the obsession has the quality of overvalued ideation (Salkovskis & Warwick, 1985). Cognitive therapy may also be used to improve adherence, which is a major problem with behavioural therapy.

Treatment failures in behavioural therapy

Treatment failure in OCD may arise from:

(a) Treatment refusal (5–25%).
(b) Treatment drop-outs (10%).
(c) True treatment failures (10%).
(d) Treatment relapse (20%).

Thus, of the patients with OCD referred for treatment and believed to be suitable for behavioural therapy, some 30–50% will make little progress (Duggan *et al*, 1993). Foa *et al* (1985) have investigated some of the predictors of failure in OCD. They identified initial severe depression, late age of symptom onset, pre-treatment anxiety and over-valued ideation as having had a negative effect on outcome. Depression prevented habituation taking place at all whereas with overvalued ideation, habituation took place within but not outside the session. Neither duration nor severity of symptoms affected outcome.

Problems in carrying out behavioural interventions

To a non-believer in behavioural therapy, it may seem extraordinary that an activity which has been the kernel of the pathology for so many years can suddenly be confronted in such a bare-faced way and that this approach can be so successful. How does the therapist convince and coax someone to take on an activity which had hitherto been avoided so stringently? At the point of assessment, it is essential that the patient recognises that only he or she can alter his condition and that it is his or her responsibility to do so. Although many individuals will recognise the validity of the behavioural analysis, this intellectual acquiescence does not mean that they are willing to take a risk with the treatment. To encourage the patient to take this risky step, one can point to the following: although anxiety is uncomfortable, it may well not be as uncomfortable as the patient anticipates; the amplitude and duration of anxiety will diminish over time, and the prediction that something catastrophic will happen may be disconfirmed by the behavioural experiment.

Failures to habituate

Since habituation is the most crucial aspect of successful treatment it may be helpful to list the reasons for a failure to habituate (see Box 1). By far the most common is that homework between sessions is not carried out satisfactorily. Patients generally underestimate the amount of homework involvement necessary to overcome their OCD. Patients need to spend at least one hour every day practising homework tasks. Records should be made of the homework in a simple diary. Taking homework seriously is as important for the therapist as for the patient. A large proportion of every session should be given over to an examination of the homework diary. This will help identify many potential pitfalls in treatment. These include: (a) not doing homework at all – which unfortunately is quite common; (b) doing homework, but not systematically or regularly enough to be effective (e.g. only two days out of seven); (c) carrying out an inadequate exposure exercise – shown by a low

---

Box 1. Behavioural therapy for OCD

Failure to habituate may be caused by:

Inadequate homework or covert neutralising

Co-occurrent major depression

Covert consumption of anxiolytic drugs or alcohol

Physiological non-habituation

anxiety score, either because the task was not sufficiently anxiety provoking, it was ended prematurely, or some mode of distraction was used.

Review of the homework exercises will focus on: examining the previous tasks since the last session; discussing any difficulties which may have arisen in carrying out the homework exercises and setting homework exercises for the next session. The patient should set more and more of the homework tasks themselves in a successful treatment, so that the length of a session can be shortened to the order of 15–20 minutes.

Co-occurrent depression appears to increase the severity of OCD, and to decrease learning and motivation and so must be treated urgently. The therapist also needs to enquire repeatedly into the illicit use of anxiolytic substances. There remains a small group of patients who, despite carrying out homework assignments, do not habituate. Unfortunately, they are a group who can only be discovered by default and cannot be predicted in advance.

Pharmacotherapy

There have been individual case reports of successful treatment with a diverse series of drugs, but the only medications with consistent anti-obsessional effects are those which act on the serotonergic system. Controlled evaluation points to the efficacy of clomipramine and, more recently, several of the specific serotonergic reuptake inhibitors (SSRIs). These drugs achieve a significant symptom reduction in 30–60% of cases (White & Cole, 1990). Even in cases where there is residual symptomatology, the individual usually regards the reduction as a major benefit (Jenike, 1990).

Clomipramine has been the most extensively studied drug prescribed for OCD. Placebo-controlled trials have shown that it is effective, for example the Clomipramine Collaborative Study showed a significant reduction in an OCD group compared with a placebo control group (Clomipramine Collaborative Study Group, 1991).

Several of the modern SSRI drugs (fluoxetine, fluvoxamine and sertraline) have been shown to be efficacious in treating OCD (Chouinard *et al*, 1990; Goodman *et al*, 1992). For instance, double-blind placebo-controlled studies of fluvoxamine have shown an effect independent of the baseline depressive ratings (Jenike *et al*, 1990). There have also been encouraging reports of the efficacy of fluoxetine in OCD where, as with clomipramine, high doses are necessary (Jenike, 1990). Although the side-effect profile of these drugs is less than that of clomipramine, they can cause gastrointestinal upsets, nausea, diarrhoea and motor restlessness. A comparison between clomipramine and fluoxetine

by means of meta-analysis showed the former to have the greater effect size but also to have more side-effects (Jenike, 1990). Although the chances of obtaining symptomatic relief are high, relapse is common on discontinuing medication (Pato *et al*, 1988). The important practice points when using pharmacotherapy for OCD are listed in Box 2.

Treatment resistance

When the patient fails with a mainline drug, the first step is to switch to an alternative SSRI. After this, the standard medication could be augmented by a range of drugs including lithium (10% respond), an MAOI, buspirone, tryptophan or neuroleptics, although there are no clear data to support the effectiveness of most of these.

Selecting optimal treatment strategies

The advantage of behavioural therapy over drugs is that it produces greater overall improvement which, once established, tends to persist (unlike treatment with medication) and, is cheaper in the long term. The disadvantages are the need for trained therapists to supervise the treatment, a significant involvement at the initial stages to get the therapy underway and the greater drop-out rate. Since there is no research to inform us on the indications for either of these treatments, selection must depend on patient preference and the availability of trained behavioural therapists.

Assessment of comorbid depression is important as this will require treatment in its own right if behavioural therapy is offered as the front-line treatment. Augmentation of behavioural therapy

---

Box 2. Drug treatment for OCD – practice points

Only drugs affecting the serotonergic system are effective

Dosage needs to be high (e.g. 250–300 mg clomipramine, 60 mg fluoxetine)

Response is slow and may not occur for several weeks

Response to OCD is independent of baseline depressive symptomatology

Relapse is the norm on stopping medication

with cognitive therapy would appear to be indicated for an overvalued idea. As other diagnoses are documented in addition to OCD, then it may be possible to develop a rational policy of management for the overall treatment of the patient. Thus, although certain authors argue that there is no role for anxiety management (e.g. Marks, 1991), there may be a role for the same in a subgroup of patients where the anxiety level is so high it either prevents the patient engaging in the task, or prevents habituation. Similarly, individuals with personality disorder and OCD may well require extensive treatment for their personality disorder in order to improve their adherence with a behaviour programme.

Combining drugs with behavioural therapy

Since neither pharmacotherapy or behavioural therapy for the treatment of OCD is entirely satisfactory when prescribed singly, is there an advantage in combining these two approaches? Marks and colleagues compared clomipramine and exposure with exposure alone. They found that although clomipramine initially enhanced the effect of exposure, this drug effect had disappeared at two years' follow-up (Marks *et al*, 1988).

Another combination study by Foa *et al* (1992) tested the hypothesis that treating patients with OCD with an antidepressant before treatment with behavioural therapy would enhance the response to the latter in patients with OCD and severe depression. Contrary to their hypothesis, they found: pre-treatment with antidepressants did not enhance the effects of behavioural therapy for OCD (as compared with placebo); the antidepressant reduced the depressive but not the OCD symptoms and behavioural therapy reduced the OCD symptoms. Present evidence suggests, therefore, that a behavioural approach used as the primary intervention is a sufficient treatment in itself and does not require adjunctive medication. However, when medication is used as the primary intervention, it is useful to complement it with behavioural therapy to prevent relapse once the medication is stopped.

Psychosurgery

For those who remain severely disabled with OCD and who have not responded to either medication or behavioural therapy, psychosurgical techniques such as cingulotomy, anterior capsulotomy or modified leucotomy have been shown to have some effect. Jenike *et al* (1991) recently reviewed the long-term outcome of 33 patients with OCD after cingulotomy. They concluded that 25–30% had benefited substantially from the procedure. The main side-effects were seizures (9%) and transient mania (6%). They also suggested that improvement occurs over weeks or months and that conventional treatments which might have failed pre-surgery are well worth trying post-operatively as the response may then be significantly improved.

Summary

OCD is a common psychiatric condition with a lifetime prevalence of 2.5%. The basic neuropathology, centring on the orbito-frontal cortex, is gradually being clarified. Behavioural therapy or drugs have been shown to be effective in controlled research.

Behavioural therapy is successful in up to 70% of cases treated and these gains have been shown to persist in several long-term follow-up studies. Obsessional ruminations can now be treated successfully with a behavioural approach. Drugs which act to increase serotonin also produce substantial symptom reductions in between 30–60% of patients, however, relapse is common once the medication has been stopped. Future research needs to focus on unmet need in the community, on those who refuse treatment and the role of anxiety management training.

References

Baxter, L. T. Jr., Schwartz, J. M., Bergman, K. S., *et al* (1992) Caudate glucose metabolic rate changes with both drug and behavioural therapy for obsessive compulsive disorder. *Archives of General Psychiatry*, **49**, 681–689.

Beck, A. T., Ward, C. H., Mendelson, M., *et al* (1961) An inventory for measuring depression. *Archives of General Psychiatry*, **4**, 561–571.

Chouinard, G., Goodman, W. & Griest, J. (1990) Obsessive–compulsive disorder – treatment with sertraline: a multicenter study. *Psychopharmacological Bulletin*, **26**, 279–284.

Clomipramine Collaborative Study Group (1991) Clomipramine in the treatment of patients with obsessive–compulsive disorder. *Archives of General Psychiatry*, **48**, 730–738.

Thiggen, C. E., Marks, I. & Richards, D. (1993) Clinical audit of behaviour therapy training of nurses. *Health Trends*, **25**, 25–30.

Emmelkamp, P. M. G. & Beens, H. (1991) Cognitive therapy with obsessive–compulsive disorder: a comparative evaluation. *Behaviour Research Therapy*, **29**, 293–300.

Foa, E. B., Steketee, G. S. & Ozarow, B. J. (1985) Behaviour therapy with OCD. In *Obsessive Compulsive Disorder* (ed M. Mavissakalian), pp. 49–129. New York: Plenum.

——, Kozak, M. J., Steketee, G. S., *et al* (1992) Treatment of depressive and obsessive–compulsive symptoms in OCD by imipramine and behaviour therapy. *British Journal of Clinical Psychology*, **31**, 279–292.

Goodman, W. K., McDougle, C. J. & Price, L. H. (1992) Pharmacotherapy of obsessive compulsive disorder. *Journal of Clinical Psychiatry*, **53**, 29–37.

Insel, T. R. (1992) Toward a neuroanatomy of obsessive–compulsive disorder. *Archives of General Psychiatry*, **49**, 739–744.

Jenike, M. A. (1990) The pharmacological treatment of obsessive–compulsive disorders. *International Review of Psychiatry*, **2**, 411–425.

––– , Baer, L. & Greist, J. H. (1990) Clomipramine vs fluoxetine in obsessive–compulsive disorder: a retrospective comparison of side-effects and efficacy. *Journal of Clinical Psychopharmacology*, **10**, 122–124.

––– , ––– , Ballantine, M. D., *et al* (1991) Cingulotomy for refractory obsessive compulsive disorder. *Archives of General Psychiatry*, **48**, 548–550.

Lelliott, P. T., Noshirvani, H. F., Basaglu, M., *et al* (1988) Obsessive–compulsive beliefs and treatment outcome. *Psychological Medicine*, **18**, 697–707.

Marks, I. M. (1986) *Behavioural Psychotherapy: The Maudsley Pocketbook of Clinical Management*. Bristol: Wright.

––– (1987) *Fears, Phobias and Rituals*. Oxford: Oxford University Press.

–– (1991) Self-administered behavioral treatment. *Behavioral Psychotherapy*, **19**, 42–46.

–– & Matthews, A. M. (1979) Brief standard self-rating for phobic patients. *Behaviour Research and Therapy*, **17**, 263–267.

–––, Lelliot, P., Basoglu, M., *et al* (1988) Clomipramine, self-exposure and therapist-aided exposure for obsessive–compulsive rituals. *British Journal of Psychiatry*, **152**, 522–534.

McKenna, P. J. (1984) Disorders with overvalued ideas. *British Journal of Psychiatry*, **145**, 579–585.

Meyer, V. (1966) Modification of expectations in cases with obsessional rituals. *Behaviour Research and Therapy*, **4**, 273–280.

Mulder, R. T., Sellman, D. & Joyce, P. R. (1991) The comorbidity of anxiety disorders with personality, depressive, alcohol and drug disorders. *International Review of Psychiatry*, **3**, 253–263.

Myers, J. K., Weissman, M. M., Tischler, G. L., *et al* (1984) Six month prevalence of psychiatric disorders in three communities. *Archives of General Psychiatry*, **41**, 959–967.

O'Sullivan, G. & Marks, I. M. (1990) The treatment of anxiety. In *Handbook of Anxiety* (ed M. Roth). New York: Elsevier.

Pato, M. T., Zohar-Kadouch, R. & Zohar, J. (1988) Return of symptoms after discontinuation of clomipramine in patients with obsessive compulsive disorder. *American Journal of Psychiatry*, **144**, 1543–1548.

Rachman, S. J. (1983) Obstacles to the successful treatment of obsessions. In *Failures in Behaviour Therapy* (eds E. B. Foa & P. Emmelkamp), pp. 35–57. New York: John Wiley & Sons.

Rasmussen, S. A. & Eisen, J. L. (1988) Clinical and epidemiological findings of significance to neuro-pharmacological trials in obsessive–compulsive disorder. *Psychopharmacological Bulletin*, **24**, 466–470.

Salkovskis, P. M. & Warwick, H. M. C. (1985) Cognitive therapy of obsessive–compulsive disorder: Treating treatment failures. *Behavioural Psychotherapy*, **13**, 243–255.

––– & Westbrook, D. (1989) Behaviour therapy and obsessional ruminations: Can failure be turned into success? *Behavioural Research and Therapy*, **27**, 149–160.

Thornicroft, G., Colson, L. & Marks, I. (1991) An in-patient behavioral psychotherapy unit: Description and audit. *British Journal of Psychiatry*, **158**, 362–367.

White, K. & Cole, J. (1990) Pharmacotherapy. In *Handbook of Comparative Treatments* (eds A. S. Bellack & M. Hersen), pp. 266–284. New York: John Wiley & Sons.

Management of somatisation

Graeme C. Smith

Somatisation remains a matter of bewilderment in medicine. Medical students have trouble defining it, psychiatry trainees wilt in its presence, and all doctors are prone to become entangled in it. The current spate of reviews on the topic is appropriate (Mayou *et al*, 1995*a*; Gill & Bass, 1997; Kisely *et al*, 1997; Barsky, 1998). There is a great need for those required to manage patients with 'medically unexplained symptoms' to be informed sufficiently to take a stance on the theoretical issues involved and develop appropriate management plans.

Faced with a display of physical symptoms for which neither lesion nor pathophysiological cause can be substantiated, the practitioner has the choice of admitting ignorance, suspecting fraud or evoking the concept of psychogenesis, mind-made disorder, as an explanatory model. How well is the modern doctor, let alone the patient, prepared to deal with models of uncertainty, fraudulence and mind? Feelings of impotence are invoked on the part of the doctor, and feelings of responsibility, even blame, on the part of the patient. The doctor–patient relationship, on which resolution will depend, is under grave threat in the presence of medically unexplained physical symptoms, of which somatisation is an example.

Just as Freud, in offering a model for the understanding of symptom formation and a psychological mode of treatment, liberated both patient and doctor from the tyranny of unexplained symptoms in this century, so too are a new generation of empirical studies providing rational treatment models that are re-empowering practitioners to deal with such problems as they now present (Smith *et al*, 1995). This chapter aims to trace this evolution and identify guidelines that will facilitate practice.

Definition

A widely quoted definition of somatisation is that of Lipowski (1988):

"The tendency to experience and communicate somatic distress and somatic symptoms unaccounted for by relevant pathological findings, to attribute them to physical illness, and to seek medical help for them."

Most doctors will be familiar with extreme examples of somatisation. Typically such patients present frequently and to many types of doctor, always communicating their complaints in the language of the body. They induce many investigations and treatments, and often develop iatrogenic illnesses as complications of invasive procedures. They are prescribed multiple drugs, and develop adverse reactions and 'allergies'. They develop skills of gaining medical attention and admission. They often become victims of abnormal doctor behaviour by inducing markedly ambivalent feelings in all health care personnel involved. Such cases illustrate the three components of Lipowski's definition quoted above; the experiential, the cognitive and the behavioural.

The wider perspective

Lipowski's definition, and the case illustration, are extremes. A broader perspective is required to avoid marginalising somatisation as something bizarre and unusual. It is essential to grasp the point that somatisation as a phenomenon is not equivalent to, nor confined to, the more severe cases defined by the ICD–10 category 'somatisation disorder' (World Health Organization, 1992) or its DSM–IV equivalent (American Psychiatric Association, 1994). Rather, somatisation is a ubiquitous tendency present in many cultures (Kirmayer *et al*, 1994), and more likely than not to be a comorbid feature of other psychiatric disorders and physical disorders (Bass, 1994).

Somatisation is not confined to communication with health care professionals. It forms part of everyday communication. It is how humans think about themselves, and is reflected in their cultural productions:

"He first deceased; she for a little tried
To live without him, liked it not and died."
Wotton (1642)

Is somatisation a medical matter at all? Or is it a sociological phenomenon best understood as playing out the sick role, which draws on somatic and mental models but which does not necessarily imply disorder of either? This post-modern reading commands attention. Nevertheless, in Western culture people who somatise often present to doctors, and some are referred to psychiatrists, who must deal with them rationally.

When patients come to psychiatrists we expect to hear mental symptoms; what we get with somatisers are symptoms of the body. Value judgements appear; we regard the somatiser as having opted for a lower order metaphor. The derogatory use of the term hysteric epitomises this. Why is the body so important to patients in general and somatisers in particular? Why are bodily symptoms chosen as the vehicle for expression rather than externally directed behaviour or mental anguish?

History gives some clues. Scholarly accounts of the history of psychiatry remind us that Western psychiatry embraced psychological thinking only a century ago (Berrios & Porter, 1995). Psychiatry invented its psychological language at that time. It borrowed the physical term 'depression' to name the affective component of its newly conceived mood disorder, and it purloined the terms and concepts of 'neurosis' and 'anxiety' from physicians, transforming their clinical meaning from a physical to a psychological one. While lay people may long have had an inherent sense of how intimately social and physical events are related, they have not necessarily adopted the psychogenic model; that is, they find it hard to share the view that mind processes can cause physical symptoms in a way that does not have disease process as an intermediary. Those from other cultures may never have had the chance to be exposed to such notions.

Somatisation is, therefore, likely to be part of the phenomenology of all illness. It occasionally (dramatically) presents as a pure and acute psychosocial metaphor, as in hysterical conversion, but most often it is part of a complex biopsychosocial web which health professionals must unravel (Hiller *et al*, 1995; Mayou, 1996; Robbins & Kirmayer, 1996; Rogers *et al*, 1996). This is captured in the concept of Bass & Murphy (1995) that chronic somatisation is like a personality disorder. This has important implications for management.

Origins of the term

Changes in the way that somatisation has been conceptualised and defined add to the bewilderment. The word somatisation dates from the height of the psychosomatic movement in North America

in the 1940s, when Stekel and Menninger used it as a name for an unconscious defence (Menninger, 1947). But it was inherent in Freud's revolutionary concept of the psychogenesis of neurotic symptoms through a direct physiological reaction or a symbolic conversion. In this vein, Lipowski (1968) originally postulated a continuum of somatisation reactions from the "conversion and hypochondriacal disorders" to the "psychophysiological disorders". The somatic components of anxiety disorders and depression, and disorders of sleep, eating and sexual function all came within his concept of somatisation, as did factitious disorders. While all of these latter examples of expression of psychogenic symptoms in physical terms are excluded from Lipowski's later definition of somatisation, their mention serves to remind us how ubiquitous such expression is, as illustrated by the following theoretical scenario. An elderly, recently widowed lady from an ethnic minority group who has recently entered a nursing home develops chest pain after hearing the news that her only son is returning to his homeland. She has had a myocardial infarct previously, and her family practitioner has been treating her for a depressive illness.

Are we dealing with myocardial infarction, angina, a psychophysiological reaction, an anxiety attack, worsening depression, hysterical conversion, hypochondriasis or factitious disorder? Whichever one or combination of these it is, the setting is that of abnormal bereavement which has transcultural undertones. In assessing the case, the clinician would also have in mind the concepts of abnormal illness behaviour and alexithymia. Another way of putting it is to say that the clinician will have to decide to what extent physical disease is present, how ill the patient feels, and how all this is being played out as sickness. These concepts represent recent attempts to deconstruct the phenomenon of somatisation and reframe it in cultural terms.

Thus the current trend in thinking about somatisation, which focuses only on the circumscribed issue of patients who frequently complain of physical symptoms that either lack demonstrable organic bases or are judged to be grossly in excess of what one would expect to find on the grounds of objective medical findings, promotes an artificial demarcation. It promotes the mind/body split in situations where an integrated biopsychosocial approach is required.

The ICD and DSM classifications

Changing terminology in the official classifications adds to the difficulty in comprehending somatisation. The term 'somatoform disorder' was coined by the authors of DSM–III as part of their strategy to remove the term 'neurosis'. In DSM–IV it refers to "the presence of physical symptoms which suggest a general medical condition", and covers acute and chronic conversion conditions. ICD–10 has adopted the term, but limits it to the chronic forms of conversion, using the term 'dissociative' (conversion) to cover the acute forms. It has re-introduced the term 'neurasthenia' to describe chronic fatigue phenomena. This division into acute and chronic presentations is widely supported (Mayou *et al*, 1995*b*). Thus those with somatoform disorders somatise in a particular way, but not all those who somatise have somatoform disorder.

Alternative terminology

Other doctors use a different language. The term 'medically unexplained symptoms' is in common use. It seems less pejorative; it does not imply cause, and it acknowledges that a problem exists for which further assessment is appropriate. The term 'functional' has been in use for two centuries. It seems to have arisen as a synonym for physiological in the first half of the 19th century. It was used by Charcot in this way at the end of the 19th century, but as ideogenic notions took hold in the 20th century it embraced these as well. It is, thus, broader than the term somatoform, and covers both dissociative (conversion) and psychophysiological phenomena, for which ICD–10 uses the awkward term "psychological and behavioural factors associated with disorders or diseases classified elsewhere".

A term used by doctors for much of this century and now part of common language is 'psycho-somatic'. Its modern use became consolidated in the 1930s, when Alexander developed Freud's concept of organ neuroses into that of psychosomatic disorders, later to become psychophysiological disorders. The term came to be used to describe the field of medicine concerned with the relationship of biological and psychological factors in general. It entered popular language, and remains in use in a pejorative way. For that reason psychiatrists specialising in this field now call themselves consultation/liaison psychiatrists rather than psychosomaticists.

Related concepts

Persisting disagreement between patient and doctor about diagnosis or treatment, such as tends to occur

in cases of somatisation, has been conceptualised by Pilowsky as abnormal illness behaviour (Pilow-sky, 1997). This has proved to be an extremely useful concept in helping us to come to grips with the systems issues involved, and the multifactorial determinants. Its pejorative connotation with respect to the patient has been leavened by Singh's concept of abnormal treatment behaviour (Singh *et al*, 1981).

The term 'alexithymia' is a neologism which refers to difficulty in feeling or expressing emotions, and in experiencing or expressing fantasies (Taylor, 1987). Like somatisation, it is a popular and seemingly well understood descriptive term and explanatory concept in the field, but it has proved difficult to operationalise and research. Taylor admits these difficulties while holding to the inherent, conventional wisdom of the concept (Taylor, 1987). He claims for it the value of a risk factor both for susceptibility to disease and for response to psychotherapy. The presence of alexithymia in doctors would presumably make collusion with somatisation easier.

Conditions embraced by somatisation

Despite the history of frequent changes in terminology and the fact that there are three overlapping categorisations of somatisation – ICD–10, DSM–IV and the 'folk-loric' language which doctors use in their communication with each other – the clinician is likely to have in mind three enduring terms and concepts when faced with somatisation. These are hysteria, hypochondriasis and neurasthenia, and it is important that their history be understood.

The phenomena embraced by the term 'hysteria' have been regarded as a distinct syndrome for millennia, and the syndrome, its name and its theoretical constructs have provided in the last 100 years the arena in which patients and doctors alike played out the debate about somatisation. Hysteria, like its parent term 'neurosis', has now been largely excluded from the international classifications, but not from doctors' and patients' everyday language. Such a disjunction has major implications.

Although there had been some implications of psychogenicity since the 17th century, it was not until Freud proposed that conversion of psychic conflict into physical and mental symptoms by means of mental dissociation was at work in neurosis that psychogenetic thinking became fashionable. Early classifiers split hysteria into dissociative disorders (of memory, consciousness and personality) and conversion disorders (of somatic function), but this division is now blurred. For instance, ICD–10 gives priority to dissociation over conversion, and uses that term to replace hysteria.

The term 'hypochondriasis' fell out of use in the last half of the 19th century, its components being dispersed to other psychiatric diagnoses. Now it has returned, though not yet clearly distinguished from depression and anxiety, nor indeed from the other somatoform disorders. It is defined as belief or attitude; ICD–10 describes it as a persistent preoccupation with the possibility of having one or more serious and progressive physical disorders. It thus represents a particular cognitive set which has certain behavioural consequences, but it often involves a somatic experience of some sort. There is often an element of hypochondriasis in other somatoform disorders. A useful distinction between acute and chronic types can be made (Robbins & Kirmayer, 1996).

'Neurasthenia' was an important 19th century term which the American, Beard (1869), used to draw together different types of neurosis, particularly those in which the patient had an aggregate of physical and psychological symptoms. It is a term still used in many non-Western countries and appears in ICD–10 where it is defined as either a complaint of increased fatigue after mental effort, or of feelings of bodily or physical weakness and exhaustion after only minimal effort. Recent studies suggest that it is not a distinct entity, but rather a continuum, and that it has a high degree of association with other psychiatric illnesses, especially anxiety and depression. It describes chronic fatigue syndrome which, although difficult to define, has become the test case to prove or disprove psychogenicity of a physical disorder, replacing repetitive strain injury as the arena for public positioning of polarised views about medically unexplained symptoms.

respect to alternative medicine. These are tricky matters to handle. People who somatise often demand practical answers, but the psychiatrist needs to be alert to what others have missed, and to do this needs to listen to the patient's narrative. Premature closure of this may destroy the chance to detect that one slip of the tongue, that particular construct, or those many other sorts of subtle clues which allow the psychiatrist into areas from which others have been excluded. A useful strategy is to ask the patient, "When were you last really well?" They will often say, "Do you mean mentally or physically?" This provides the chance to remind the patient that you are interested in their construct, and in exploring their attitudes. They have raised the issue of the mind/body split, and reminding them of this gives them a chance to educate the psychiatrist about their own mind-set and culture, their belief system and practices, and the way in which illness is constructed within that environment (see Box 2).

In any event, such matters should be dealt with in a way that will encourage the patient to see that you have respect for their construct of the illness, that you acknowledge that you are dealing with unexplained symptoms, and that you are interested in working toward a joint understanding of the meaning and significance of the sickness rather than dismissing them as having nothing wrong, as others have done. The attitude displayed during these negotiations will reveal the cognitive set of the patient and help determine which type of somatisation predominates, and will guide the rest of the assessment. Is there any sign at all of psychological mindedness that will permit a joint exploration of the possibility of mind-caused factors being relevant?

Assessment

Biopsychosocial assessment

An individual who somatises is fixated on the biological. To widen the agenda takes time, patience and educational skills. Referral to the psychiatrist will usually have been made with difficulty and against resistance, perhaps sold as being to a psychiatrist who is 'different' (see Box 1 for some relevant questions). The patient may be unclear as to whether or not the psychiatrist is a doctor, and if so, what expectations they can expect to have about familiarity with the physical aspects of their presentation. Models encompassed by the psychiatrist may be questioned, especially with

---

Box 1.   Questions for use in assessment of somatisers

What is your understanding of why you were referred?

How did you feel about that?

What do you expect from this referral?

When were you last really well?

Of all the things that worry you, what worries you most?

What is your understanding of how you came to be the way you are?

Box 2. Some golden rules for assessing somatisation

Know where you stand on the theoretical issues involved

Find common ground for completing the assessment

Instil hope but not the promise of cure

Find out all possible treatable primary and secondary psychiatric and physical conditions

Listen with the psychiatrist's ear to the patient's narrative

Negotiate a formulation with all concerned, including the patient

Educate all concerned, including the patient, about the mechanisms involved

---

It is more likely than not that the psychiatrist will perform a physical examination, at least of the relevant parts, if this seems natural in the situation; such examination often throws light on the cognitive set and will act as a reminder to consider drug and alcohol misuse.

An interview with family members will usually be required; they may or may not be somatisers, and they may be compulsive carers. In complex cases data will have to be gathered from a number of sources. It is useful to test hypotheses with these other sources, sharing with them the uncertainty. A multi-disciplinary assessment involving all relevant doctors is common, and indeed often it is this process that brings to light the gap which clinches the psychodynamic formulation. For example:

> Mrs H has ulcerative colitis. She infuriates the medical and nursing staff with her excessive vigilance over her treatment. The psychiatrist has acted as a broker for years. Only when she developed breast cancer and accepted treatment of that with

equanimity was it possible to understand that she had a differential perception of her illnesses based on the concept described by Freud in his writing on the death instinct, wherein he argued that each person has an unconsciously determined preferred way of dying, and opposes every other way. It now became possible to work with the patient on the meaning of her ulcerative colitis, and achieve a more harmonious relationship with staff.

At some point the patient will expect education about how the psychiatrist views the problem. People who somatise do not handle uncertainty well, and the formulation and its delivery must allow for this.

Formulation

Formulation, or the answer to the question, "Why is this patient ill in this way at this time?", requires negotiation with the patient, the family, and the other clinicians involved. The biopsychosocial model is the basis, but it needs spelling out in a multi-causal, interactive aetiological model such as that espoused by Mayou *et al* (1995*b*) and illustrated in Table 1.

Key aetiological mechanisms should be spelt out in detail, and an explanation of how this will provide a rational basis for management should be given. This is a critical point, and if not negotiated well, the patient is likely to withdraw. In particular, the distinction between dissociative (conversion) and psychophysiological mechanisms needs to be made. Demonstration of the effects of hyperventilation may be a useful strategy. Likening the tendency to somatise to the holding of other personality traits and cultural beliefs is a way of helping the patient conceptualise the process. Of course, the language must be appropriate to the situation, and the lesson is unlikely to be learned in one sitting. If a positive diagnosis such as conversion disorder has been made, emphasise that it is not simply a diagnosis of exclusion, but rather that it has been made positively on the basis of the whole range of evidence available.

Table 1. A grid for recording and classifying the multi-causal factors of the interactive aetiological model, with examples (after Sharpe *et al*, 1995)

	Biological	Psychological	Social
Predisposing	Genetic	Somatising personality	Cultural attitudes
Precipitating	Physical illness	Stress	Job loss
Perpetuating	Psychotropic drug side-effects	Depressive illness	Sick role rewards

Management

A positive attitude to management is necessary and justifiable. Improvement in functional outcome and decrease in health care utilisation and costs can be expected even with simple interventions (see Box 3).

Acknowledgement

Acknowledging to oneself that somatisation is a cultural norm likely to be directing the doctor's thinking as much as the patient's is the first step required. Some doctors are more prone to that way of thinking than others. Goldberg *et al* (1989) have shown that it is possible to re-train doctors to treat somatisation, but not all doctors are so educable (Cohen-Cole *et al*, 1991). Acknowledgement to the patient that both parties are confronting a highly valued way of thinking with roots largely inaccessible to patient and doctor alike is also required.

Case management

Once the formulation is agreed to by all parties including the patient, interventions and their coordinated management should be negotiated. Someone must be the case manager (Barsky, 1998). It is difficult for the psychiatrist to play this role; somatisation is a powerful process which can push the psychiatrist's comfort with physical medicine to the limits. The case manager needs to be someone who feels comfortable with uncertainty and is prepared to take the risk of non-investigation. The psychiatrist has a major role to play in supporting such a case manager and counselling the patient about how to handle their various doctors. A single letter from a psychiatrist to a primary care physician, explaining the diagnosis and suggesting a rational management plan, can have an extraordinary impact (Smith *et al*, 1995). The use of a patient-held case record can help minimise confusion and conflict.

Specific interventions

If somatisation is an episodic component of a reactive disorder, resolution can be expected. Treatment of underlying depression or anxiety will be required, with explanation to all concerned that the somatisation is largely reactive but requires firm but supportive handling. A major role for the psychiatrist in such cases is to help prevent the condition becoming chronic, and to help prevent iatrogenic physical complications.

If somatising traits dominate the picture, it will be important to dissect out primary and secondary effects (Robbins & Kirmayer, 1996). Medication will be needed for severe anxiety and depression, and is of proven value in chronic pain. Although antidepressants are often used for the treatment of the depressive component of neurasthenia, their efficacy is not proven (Vercoulen *et al*, 1996). Since chronic somatising patients are more likely than not to have comorbid physical disorder, iatrogenic or otherwise, and certainly likely to be on multiple and diverse drugs including analgesics, the psychiatrist is often operating beyond the boundaries of evidence-based medicine in prescribing psychotropic drugs in such situations. Addition of psychotropic medication to that pot is a potentially hazardous exercise requiring close monitoring and coordination (Jachna *et al*, 1996). Involving the pharmacist helps. The tendency of the patient to experience side-effects at low threshold levels and to incorporate them into their somatising mind set is a further challenge.

Physical treatments

Patients may already be undertaking physiotherapy, relaxation therapy, or similar but more

---

Box 3. Some golden rules for managing somatisation

Negotiate a management plan with all involved, including the patient

Agree about who will be the case manager, and offer support to that person

Give the patient a role in case management by use of diaries and patient-held case records

Base treatment on evidence-based recommendations: treatment of comorbid physical and psychiatric conditions; use of Smith *et al*'s (1995) management plan for primary physicians; cognitive–behavioural psychotherapy individually or in groups; modified psychodynamic and interpersonal therapy for selected conditions; involve families and ethnic health workers

Use a multi-disciplinary approach, and recognise that an allied health professional may be the most acceptable key therapist

marginal therapies. These may be specifically indicated, as in the presence of anxiety symptoms, or their use may be a non-specific correlate of the fact that the patient somatises and finds physical attention appropriate. Used wisely, the physical therapists can become major allies in the management plan, acceptable therapists who are able to contain the situation.

Psychotherapeutic interventions

Psychotherapeutic intervention for a psychological problem seems to have such face validity that one might expect there to be considerable evidence-based guidelines available. In the case of those patients likely to be seen by psychiatrists, this has not been so until recently. People who somatise tend to be so chronic and complex that it is difficult to design appropriate studies and recruit satisfactorily. Nevertheless, we have clues about what therapies are worth trying in certain groups of patients. They include cognitive–behavioural and psychodynamic therapies.

Barsky (1998) has reviewed the cognitive–educational techniques which seem useful in the management of chronic hypochondriasis. Group therapy involves didactic presentation, experiential learning and discussion. A similar programme for patients with somatisation disorder yielded significant improvement in physical and mental health and a decrease in health care costs (Kashner *et al*, 1995).

There are recent evidence-based demonstrations of the efficacy of a cognitive–behavioural approach in a number of conditions, including pain, irritable bowel syndrome and dyspepsia, reviewed by Guthrie (1996), and for chronic fatigue syndrome (Sharpe *et al*, 1996; Deale *et al*, 1997). Psychodynamic therapy appears to be effective in the treatment of irritable bowel syndrome (Guthrie *et al*, 1991) and hypochondriasis (Warwick *et al*, 1996).

Replication has been a problem, and this raises the possibility that what really works is a confident team, dedicated to helping patients make some sort of sense of why something that seems so naturally physical to them responds best to psychosocial interventions that seem so unnatural to them. Many of these issues have been discussed extensively in Mayou *et al* (1995a).

References

American Psychiatric Association (1994) *Diagnostic and Statistical Manual Of Mental Disorders Fourth Edition DSM–IV.* Washington, DC: American Psychiatric Association.

Barsky, A. (1998) A comprehensive approach to the chronically somatizing patient. *Journal of Psychosomatic Research*, **45**, 301–306.

Bass, C. (1994) Somatisation disorder: the need for effective intervention studies. *General Hospital Psychiatry*, **16**, 379–380.

—— & Murphy, M. (1995) Somatoform and personality disorders: syndromal comorbidity and overlapping developmental pathways. *Journal of Psychosomatic Research*, **39**, 403–427.

Beard, G. (1869) Neurasthenia or nervous exhaustion. *Boston Medical and Surgical Journal*, **80**, 217–221.

Berrios, G. & Porter, R. (eds) (1995) *A History of Clinical Psychiatry.* London: Athlone.

Cohen-Cole, S. A., Howell, E. F., Barrett, J. E., *et al* (1991) Consultation–liaison research: four selected topics. In *Handbook of Studies on General Hospital Psychiatry* (eds F. K. Judd, G. B. Burrows & D. R. Lipsitt), pp. 79–98. Amsterdam: Elsevier.

Deale, A., Chalder, T., Marks, I., *et al* (1997) Cognitive behaviour therapy for chronic fatigue syndrome: a randomised controlled trial. *American Journal of Psychiatry*, **154**, 408–414.

Gill, D. & Bass, C. (1997) Somatoform and dissociative disorders: assessment and treatment. *Advances in Psychiatric Treatment*, **3**, 9–16.

Goldberg, D., Gask, L. & O'Dowd, T. (1989) The treatment of somatisation: teaching techniques of reattribution. *Journal of Psychosomatic Research*, **33**, 689–695.

Guthrie, E. (1996) Emotional disorder in chronic illness: psychotherapeutic interventions. *British Journal of Psychiatry*, **168**, 265–273.

——, Creed, F. H., Dawson, D., *et al* (1991) A controlled study of psychological treatment of the irritable bowel syndrome. *Gastroenterology*, **100**, 450–457.

Hiller, W., Rief, W. & Fichter, M. M. (1995) Further evidence for a broader concept of somatisation disorder using the somatic symptom index. *Psychosomatics*, **36**, 285–294.

Jachna, J. S., Lane R. D. & Gelenberg, A. J. (1996) Psychopharmacology. In *Textbook of Consultation–Liaison Psychiatry* (eds J. R. Rundell & M. G. Wise), pp. 958–1005. Washington: American Psychiatric Press.

Kashner, T. M., Rost, K., Cohern, B., *et al* (1995) Enhancing the health of somatisation disorder patients. Effectiveness of short-term group therapy. *Psychosomatics*, **36**, 462–470.

Kirmayer, L. J., Robbins, J. M. & Paris, J. (1994) Somatoform disorders: personality and the social matrix. *Journal of Abnormal Psychology*, **103**, 125–136.

Kisely, S., Goldberg, D. & Simon, G. (1997) A comparison between somatic symptoms with and without clear organic cause: results of an international study. *Psychological Medicine*, **27**, 1011–1019.

Lipowski, Z. J. (1968) Review of consultation psychiatry and psychosomatic medicine: III. Theoretical issues. *Psychosomatic Medicine*, **30**, 394–422.

—— (1988) Somatisation: the concept and its clinical application. *American Journal of Psychiatry*, **145**, 1358–1368.

Mayou, R. (1996) Accident neurosis revisited. *British Journal of Psychiatry*, **168**, 399–403.

——, Bass, C. & Sharpe, M. (eds) (1995a) *Treatment of Functional Somatic Symptoms.* Oxford: Oxford University Press.

——, —— & —— (1995b) Overview of epidemiology, classification, and aetiology. In *Treatment of Functional Somatic Symptoms* (eds R. Mayou, C. Bass & M. Sharpe), pp. 42–65. Oxford: Oxford University Press.

Menninger, W. C. (1947) Psychosomatic medicine: somatization reactions. *Psychosomatic Medicine*, **9**, 92–97.

Pilowsky, I. (1997) *Abnormal Illness Behaviour.* Chichester: John Wiley and Sons.

Robbins, J. M. & Kirmayer, L. J. (1996) Transient and persistent hypochondriacal worry in primary care. *Psychological Medicine*, **26**, 575–589.

Rogers, M. P., Weishenker, N. J., Warshaw, M.G., *et al* (1996) Prevalence of somatoform disorders in a large sample of patients with anxiety disorders. *Psychosomatics*, **37**, 17–22.

Sharpe, M., Bass, C. & Mayou, R. (1995) An overview of the treatment of somatic symptoms. In *Treatment of Functional Somatic Symptoms* (eds R. Mayou, C. Bass & M. Sharpe), pp. 66–86. Oxford: Oxford University Press.

——, Hawton, K., Simkin, S. S., *et al* (1996) Cognitive–behaviour therapy for the chronic fatigue syndrome: a randomised controlled trial. *British Medical Journal*, **312**, 22–26.

Singh, B., Nunn, K., Martin, J., *et al* (1981) Abnormal treatment behaviour. *British Journal of Medical Psychology*, **54**, 131–137.

Smith, G. R., Rost, K. & Kashner, T. M. (1995) A trial of the effect of a standardised psychiatric consultation on health outcomes and costs in somatising patients. *Archives of General Psychiatry*, **52**, 238–243.

Taylor, G. J. (1987) Psychosomatic medicine and contemporary psychoanalysis. *International Universities Press Stress and Health Series Monograph 3* (ed. G. Goldberger). Madison: International Universities Press.

Vercoulen, J. H., Swanik, C. M., Zitman, F. G., *et al* (1996) Randomised, double-blind, placebo-controlled study of fluoxetine in chronic fatigue syndrome. *Lancet*, **347**, 858–861.

Warwick, H. M. C., Clark, D. M., Cobb, A.M., *et al* (1996) A controlled trial of cognitive-behavioural treatment of hypochondriasis. *British Journal of Psychiatry*, **169**, 189–195.

World Health Organization (1992) *The ICD–10 Classification of Mental and Behavioural Disorders*. Geneva: World Health Organization.

Wotton, H. (1642) Upon the death of Sir Albert Morton's wife. In *Familiar Quotations by John Bartlett, 14th edn* (1968) (ed. E. M. Beck), p. 300. London: MacMillan.

Management of patients with personality disorder

Kingsley Norton

"...therapy often becomes part of the problem rather than vice versa." (Lockwood, 1992)

Ten per cent of the general adult population have a diagnosable personality disorder (Zimmerman & Coryell, 1990) and in 4% this is severe (Tyrer, 1988). The clinical management of such patients may be difficult. However, much clinical difficulty is generated by interpersonal aspects deriving from the particular interaction of the patient and psychiatrist involved and the respective roles they take.

It is important, therefore, to distinguish between the clinical problem proper and those aspects of the personal interaction of patient and psychiatrist which may unhelpfully (including via stigmatic labelling) contribute to the complexity of the case, further complicating the clinical management of it (Norton & Smith, 1994). This is because interpersonal issues often become so prominent, in clinical transactions with personality disordered patients, that they make it impossible to achieve or maintain an ordinary clinical focus which could identify relevant and achievable treatment goals (Norton & McGauley, 1997).

The psychiatrist can be side-tracked by such interpersonal aspects but recognising this may be problematic, since the distraction from a proper clinical focus may be subtle and is not necessarily negative in quality. Thus, there may be an inappropriately positive interpersonal influence, at least initially (Yeomans, 1993). Whether the distraction is positive or negative, what is missing is an appropriate level of mutual respect and trust, so vital for carrying out the professional level clinical tasks. Too often the psychiatrist mistakenly takes its existence for granted.

The aim of this chapter is to identify some of the common pitfalls in the engagement and clinical management of patients with personality disorder, indicating how these can be avoided or otherwise dealt with, so making treatment less arduous.

Diagnosis and engagement

An unreliable or invalid diagnosis of personality disorder often reflects poor diagnostic technique, as much as it reflects inadequate definitions or inaccurate measures of personality disorder. Thus, sometimes there appears to be ignorance of the need to engage the personality disordered individual, as a patient, rather than to take for granted their ability to perform the role of patient successfully. Without adequate engagement, it is not possible to elicit an accurate history or mental state examination and so on, hence no diagnosis is reliable.

Diagnostic subcategories

The validity of subcategories of personality disorder is uncertain (Oldham, 1991) and some prefer to view personality disorder as a unitary syndrome (Coid, 1989), a view given support by the presence of more than one personality disorder subtype diagnosis in individual patients (Zimmerman et al, 1991). The number of personality disorder subtype diagnoses, per patient with personality disorder, is associated with the particular psychiatric setting (see Dolan et al, 1995), the highest numbers being recorded in the most secure in-patient settings, wherein are experienced some of the greatest clinical management problems. In such settings it may be the exception, rather than the rule, to find single subcategory personality disorder diagnosis. The number of personality disorder subtype diagnoses in an individual patient therefore may be a marker of the severity of the overall personality disorder (Dolan et al, 1995; Tyrer & Johnson, 1996).

In view of the presence of more than one personality disorder subtype in so many personality disordered psychiatric patients, especially in those

> **Box 1.   Clinical difficulty and patients with personality disorder**
>
> Personality disorder is not in itself inherently untreatable
>
> Patients with personality disorder can be difficult to manage because of:
>
> (a)   difficulties in diagnosing personality disorder or a missed diagnosis of personality disorder
>
> (b)   the coexistence of symptom disorder which complicates the treatment of personality disorder
>
> Some patients with personality disorder cannot or will not play their complementary role as patients
>
> Interpersonal problems between the psychiatrist and patient with personality disorder, arising from the problems mentioned above, become the focus of the clinical encounter, thereby supplanting relevant clinical tasks and complicating treatment

who present extreme difficulty in their clinical management, personality disorder will be considered here as a unitary syndrome.

The patient's role

Initially, many people with personality disorder who come into contact with psychiatrists are not meaningfully 'patients', in the sense of having a capacity to present a complaint or symptom with the expectation that appropriate professional treatment or help will be forthcoming. Their non-verbal, and sometimes their verbal, behaviour says: "Here I am! I've done my bit by turning up. Now it's over to you. What are you going to do about it (me)?"

> Mr A was smoking a cigarette as he entered the consulting room. The consultant psychiatrist had initially interviewed him the previous week, making a diagnosis of generalised anxiety disorder and personality disorder. He now indicated the discreet 'No Smoking' sign situated on the desk. Apparently not heeding this non-verbal request to extinguish the cigarette, Mr A continued to inhale. Indeed, he put the cigarette up to his lips and then removed it in an ostentatious manner. All the time he kept his eyes fixed on the consultant. The latter, attempting to meet Mr A's steady gaze, silently fumed! After a short while, and no longer able to contain his impatience

with what he perceived to be Mr A's contemptuous and provocative silence, he blurted out, "Really, Mr A, I must ask you to show more consideration for other people and to refrain from smoking". He then added, with a hint of remorse, "In any case, it's a very bad habit".

> The consultant later confided to a colleague that he had regretted this outburst, albeit controlled, not least because Mr A had, in response, silently stood up and left the room, quietly closing the door behind him. He subsequently failed further appointments which were sent to him.

The first clinical task is thus to ensure that the patient is engaged as a patient. Engagement entails the successful establishment of a collaborative clinical enterprise between psychiatrist and personality disordered individual, resulting in the negotiating of more or less clear and relevant treatment goals. In the above example, the consultant had thought he had successfully engaged Mr A at their first interview and he believed there was sufficient trust and respect to permit him his non-verbal request to the patient. He was not aware that he would again have to prove his trustworthiness and could not take this for granted at the second interview.

Obstacles to engagement

There are many obstacles to engagement (see Box 1), yet the development of a therapeutic alliance with the patient is essential as a vehicle of change (Horwitz, 1974; Frank, 1991). Some personality disordered individuals have totally unrealistic expectations of professionals (too high, too low or constantly oscillating between the two extremes) and so will make inappropriate or unrealistic demands. Disabusing them of their misapprehension or educating them about what is realistically available is crucial, but it is often experienced as patronising or humiliating and the professional relationship may break down under the burden of the resulting disagreement, anger or disappointment (Gunderson *et al*, 1989). Failure to engage and maintain a therapeutic alliance (as with Mr A) only serves to reinforce the patient's basic mistrust of professionals and the psychiatrist's notion of the difficulty and untreatability of the patient.

Some individuals with personality disorder, by virtue of their style of presentation, impel or seduce professionals into attempting to offer more than is realistically available. Such a temptation for the psychiatrist to be 'too good' or 'too powerful', often a reaction to the patient's unrealistically high expectations and the former's unwillingness to state limits which might disappoint or frustrate the patient, needs to be avoided (Yeomans, 1993).

Insecure and disorganised attachments

The past

Patients with personality disorder have basic and pervasive mistrust of others which stems from being neglected and/or abused during childhood by parents (or their substitute adults) who misused their authority, avoided their parental responsibilities or were highly inconsistent in attitude or behaviour towards their children, many parents having personality disorder themselves (Zanarini *et al*, 1990; Norton & Dolan, 1995*b*). The patients' formative years are thus scarred by insecure and disorganised attachments. As a result, their internal working models, influencing their later expectations of others and their styles of relating to them, reflect this (Bowlby, 1973; West *et al*, 1993).

Many personality disordered patients thus expect professionals to fail them (as did their parents) even though, usually secretly, they crave an individual who could meet their every need. In the face of this, psychiatrists often feel as if they cannot succeed. If psychiatrists only reinforce part of the patient's view – that no reliable help is available – then they fail the secret view (against all odds and previous experience) that there exists someone who will help responsibly and not abuse their authority. However, any help which is provided is often perceived as

insufficient. Falling so far short of the idealised 'perfect help', it can cause further pain and disappointment. As a consequence, the psychiatrist may feel 'damned if he does and damned if he does not' treat.

Patients' lack of familiarity with secure attachments and their ambivalence towards the psychiatrist and treatment therefore need to be assumed and addressed directly, as part of the (ongoing) task of engagement and the forging of a therapeutic alliance (see Box 2).

The present

In-patient staff, particularly, experience difficulties in providing care of consistently high quality in the face of the patient's ambivalent wish for it and their consequent lack of engagement. Inconsistency in the delivery of planned treatment increases with the number of staff or number of different agencies involved with it. This occurs for two main reasons: covert inter-staff disagreements with the treatment approach, which are either unspoken and/or unresolved; and breakdowns in inter-staff communication or the communication of partial or inaccurate information between staff or between agencies (Stanton & Schwartz, 1954; Main, 1957).

For many patients, the combined thrill and terror of the in-patient chase and capture, followed by enforced sedation and/or seclusion or 'specialling', represents familiar (albeit insecure) emotional territory. Paradoxically, they are reassured by many, though not all, aspects of it. This frantic mutual activity, however, disallows a novel experience which might impel the patients to question their habitual maladaptive attitudes and behaviour – its cognitive and emotional origins, antecedents, and its consequences. The patients' ingrained behaviour patterns and inflexible responses thus endure (Norton & Dolan, 1995*c*).

Where physical containment (for example, locked wards, enforced medication) predominates, patients with personality disorder survive and function. This is because their current 'inflexible responses' (part of the definition of personality disorder, World Health Organization, 1992) have been shaped by issues of domination and control in the abusive and/or neglecting interpersonal experiences received during their childhood and adolescence. In such an in-patient environment, just as in the past, apparent care and respect readily transform, either to punishment or else to a remote professional neutrality perceived by the patient as indifference or neglect. Professional care is then viewed as counterfeit and simply as a manipulative or seductive camouflage.

Box 2. Engaging an individual with personality disorder as a patient

The patient's capacity to engage in treatment should not be assumed

Engagement is the result of an active and collaborative endeavour between psychiatrist and patient

Without adequate engagement the quality and reliability of assessment information is impaired leading to diagnostic and treatment difficulties

Commonly encountered obstacles to engagement include the patient's:

(a) unrealistic expectations of treatment

(b) basic mistrust in professionals

(c) ambivalence about seeking and receiving help

Box 3. Correctable reasons for treatment failure

Inadequate engagement in treatment

Unrealistic treatment expectations

Inconsistent delivery of treatment due to the involvement of more than one agent or agency, leading to:

    (i)   covert staff disagreements which are unresolved

    (ii) breakdown or other inadequacy in inter-staff communication

Undue delay in response to deterioration or improvement in the patient's clinical status

---

Although simple physical containment can afford personality disordered patients temporary and familiar relief, in the longer term they are left feeling misunderstood, righteously indignant and victimised (Gunderson *et al*, 1989). Indeed, they can appear to be enveloped by such feelings as if in a welcomed embrace. In the absence of anxiety evoked by an environmental response which is felt by them to be empathic, hence novel, patients do not experience distress sufficiently within themselves – there is a relative absence of a conflictual internal dialogue. They tend to remain more in conflict with others, mainly staff. Thereby a potentially creative internal conflict is instead enacted interpersonally. Internal energy, which would be derived from an experience of conflict, is expended through maintaining the interpersonal discord.

The future

If patients are to change their mistrustful attitudes to staff, and to begin to work with them collaboratively, they need to give up their oppositional stance (Norton, 1997). However, this is only achievable if the staff's response is other than to reinforce such a stance. To facilitate this requires of the staff a capacity to consistently apply a treatment approach (withstanding the destructive aspects of staff disagreements and communication problems), and provide a response to the patients' testing behaviour (often violent and manipulative but sometimes involving seductive or erotic behaviour) which does not simply condemn or condone (Norton & Dolan, 1995*a*). Thus, staff are required to strive to

remain balanced, not taking sides simply for or against, and to examine the particular situation and its relevance to the patient. This approach may include reiterating that certain aspects of the patient's behaviour are not acceptable and will not be tolerated but it requires, in addition, a questioning attitude and a quest to understand the antecedents and consequences of the behaviour (Main, 1983; Norton, 1992).

In this way, the patient's behaviour may be both condemned and understood. This is a more complex construction than simply condemning or condoning and it can be communicated to the patient. Through this process, patients can learn to understand that they are perceived by others as more than just their 'behaviour' and that the condemnation of their behaviour is not a damning personal attack. The aim is to help the patients, in spite of their ambivalence about receiving help and their basic mistrust, to become 'talkers' and 'feelers' rather than simply the 'actors' of maladaptive behaviour (Masterson, 1972).

Using a treatment contract

Even with patients with personality disorder who have not been particularly dangerous or disturbed, clinical transactions may be complicated rather than straightforward. Thus the ordinary collaborative goal-directed activity of the clinical encounter (out-patient or in-patient) may require buttressing by the establishment of a treatment contract.

A treatment contract involves formalising the usually implicit agreement which exists between patient and psychiatrist in a straightforward clinical transaction. If it is established early, before basic mistrust and prior insecure or disorganised attachment patterns are reinforced by the current relationship and interaction, it can serve to anchor an agreement to achieve relevant goals by minimising the influence of destructive or distracting personality 'clashes' between patient and doctor. As a beneficial by-product, the patient may derive enhanced self-esteem, through being enabled to perform the role of patient more successfully, and the psychiatrist may gain professional satisfaction.

The treatment contract may usefully involve people from the patient's wider social network, especially where they are likely to be directly affected by the meeting of contractual conditions. It can help to have the patient, staff and, in some cases, family and/or friends, as literal co-signatories to the contract (Miller, 1989). The more staff or agencies who are involved the more urgent is the need to have regular meetings of all concerned, lest inconsistencies in the treatment approach develop and remain undetected and unremedied.

Establishing a treatment contract is easier said than done. It often entails: exploring and changing the patient's basic mistrust; ambivalence about seeking help; low self-esteem; ways of dealing with impulses to injure (self or others); and idiosyncratic obstacles to giving up an immature chemical dependence (on drugs or alcohol) in favour of a more mature dependence on people.

Pitfalls

The most common pitfall is for the treatment contract to be introduced at a time when either or both the psychiatrist and the patient are feeling hostile to one another. Under such circumstances it is not likely to succeed in its stated aims. Hostility, especially where this may have formed part of the psychiatrist's motivation to implement the contract in the first place, must have begun to subside before a treatment contract can be successfully negotiated.

Negotiating the contract may require considerable time, tact and diplomacy just when such attributes are in short supply. The patient may experience the psychiatrist as authoritarian or patronising, especially if there is, or has been in the past, compulsory treatment or if contractual conditions are set which the patient cannot meet. If this is the case, the contract is likely to break down even if there has been an apparent initial agreement to it.

> Ms B, an in-patient for more than six months, had been compulsorily admitted. The diagnosis was of anorexia nervosa with features of a coexisting affective disorder (including serious suicidal ideation and parasuicidal activity) and an underlying dysocial personality disorder. She made little progress initially and, with staff's mounting anxiety about the unlikelihood of her survival, a treatment contract was established out of desperation and frustration, with little staff confidence that it might help.
>
> The contract stated that Ms B would accept a high calorie diet with the aim of achieving a weight increase to a mutually agreed level. Staff agreed to stop their cajoling and coaxing of Ms B to eat in return for her agreement to attend and speak in her individual sessions. (She had often found reasons not to attend and had avoided talking in depth.)

To the surprise of the team, Ms B began to accept her diet and achieved her contracted target weight. However, she did this without divulging any personal difficulties or other information about herself. The staff treating her were grateful that compliance with re-feeding had resulted and that the immediate threat of suicide and death had receded. The treatment contract was regarded to have 'worked' in spite of the fact that she had not complied fully with the contractual agreement. Consequently,

discharge from hospital was arranged. At this point Ms B broke a mirror in the unit and used the shards to repeatedly cut her forearms. Feeling frustrated and defeated, the staff felt compelled to shelve the discharge plans.

Treatment contracts require monitoring and if specified goals are not achieved these need discarding, re-negotiating or else discussion to establish why. If the contractual conditions pertaining to the patient with personality disorder are too restrictive or require them to give up the only defences they have against intolerable feelings, and if no viable alternative outlet or coping strategy is provided or available to them, the contract will not succeed. Therefore it is important that any conditions attached to the contract are realistically achievable. With Ms B, it was eventually decided to reinstate and update the treatment contract and to reiterate the need for her to speak in her individual sessions in order to address the maladaptive self-harming behaviour. With regard to the latter, nursing staff's time was made available to her whenever she recognised the impulse to self-mutilate, regardless of the time of day or night. It was important to ensure that the treatment contract did not become a substitute for support and active psychotherapy (Miller, 1989).

Prescribing medication

Symptom disorder and personality disorder comorbidity is common (Du Fort *et al*, 1993), therefore a substantial proportion of patients with personality disorder have a coexisting symptom disorder which may require treatment in its own right, including relevant pharmacotherapy. While psychological treatments of the personality disorder itself form the mainstay, there is a limited role for drug treatment (see Stein, 1992 for review).

A constructive approach to pharmacotherapy is to engage a patient with personality disorder as an ally who will study, along with the prescribing psychiatrist, responses to the various drugs (Gunderson & Sabo, 1993). This helps to curb patients' unrealistic expectations of the drug effect, encourages them to step back and identify their own behaviour and symptom patterns and fosters collaboration rather than an adversarial inter-personal relationship with the psychiatrist. Its symptomatic focus facilitates a closer tailoring of treatment to patients' needs than does an approach which links drugs to a specific personality disorder sub-category or sub-categories (see Stein, 1992).

Symptoms of personality disorder such as depersonalisation, de-realisation, illusions, ideas of reference and brief paranoid states may respond to low-dose neuroleptics (Goldberg *et al*, 1986; Soloff *et al*, 1986). The characteristic 'depression' of many patients with personality disorder (associated with chronic emptiness, boredom and discomfort in being alone) may be responsive to monoamine oxidase inhibition. Where intense anger and hostility are prominent, low-dose neuroleptics are probably the drugs of choice (Soloff *et al*, 1989) since benzodiazepines may disinhibit the patient and thereby increase hostility, self-destructiveness and assaultiveness (Gardner & Cowdry, 1985).

Some favourable results in the management of impulsiveness have been reported with serotonergic reuptake inhibition (Norden, 1989) but so has suicide and self-mutilation (Teicher *et al*, 1990). Therefore, neuroleptics are probably still the drugs of choice for impulsiveness in both the short-term (Soloff *et al*, 1989) and long-term management (Montgomery & Montgomery, 1982). There may be a role for carbamazepine (Cowdry & Gardner, 1988) or lithium, however, a controlled study of the latter found it to be only slightly superior to placebo (Links *et al*, 1990).

Drug treatment may be used in combination with many psychological interventions (Layden *et al*, 1993), including in-patient admission. The possibility of the patient's self-destructive use of medication, however, should be entertained. Prescribing and dispensing relatively small quantities of drugs, especially to those with a history of parasuicide or addiction, should thus form part of any treatment regime. 'Cocktails' of drugs should be avoided. Failure to achieve the desired effect or the presence of side-effects that are too great should lead to a cessation of a given medication and to a discussion of the potential benefits of commencing another drug.

Psychological treatments

If patients with personality disorder receive any treatment, it is most likely to be individual supportive psychotherapy. The aim is to improve the patient's adaptation through diminishing self-destructive responses to expectable interpersonal frustrations (Rockland, 1989). The aim is not to change the patient's personality, but there is some evidence of personality change resulting (Wallerstein, 1986). Patients who drop out of ambitious long-term psychotherapy may also benefit from supportive approaches. However, starting with a supportive approach may prepare some for more intensive therapies.

Dynamic psychotherapy aims at personality re-organisation through the resolution of intra-psychic structural conflicts and/or deficits thought to lie at the heart of the disorder, via interpretation of the transference–countertransference relationship, as part of a modified, more active, psychoanalytic technique (Kernberg, 1984). Cognitive psychotherapy focuses on the identification of the patient's important cognitive distortions or schemas and examines the way in which these are reiterated and maintained in everyday life. Discussion of such self-defeating and maladaptive manoeuvres is aimed at atrophying their use and replacing them with more self-affirming and adaptive cognitive strategies linked with appropriate affect (Linehan, 1987; Young, 1990; Ryle & Marlowe, 1995).

A review of treatment outcome and related issues is beyond the scope of this chapter and is available elsewhere (Higgitt & Fonagy, 1992; Stein, 1992; Dolan & Coid, 1993; Shearer & Linehan, 1994; Norton & Dolan, 1995*c*; Reugg & Frances, 1995).

Non-individual therapies

For a disorder which is known to have such prominent environmental aetiological factors, it is surprising that family therapy is under-represented in the personality disorder literature and perhaps under-utilised as a therapy in clinical practice. This may reflect the absence of an intact family and/or the presence of acrimonious or ambivalent relationships with those family members with whom the patient is still in contact. Sometimes, however, it

---

Box 4. Managing the destructive effect of inter-staff 'splits'

Education of staff regarding the phenomenon of 'splitting' and its inevitable presence in treatment involving more than one staff member and/or agency

The use of treatment contracts which specify what staff are able and prepared to provide and/or tolerate

Regular meetings of all relevant staff to identify and resolve differing attitudes to treatment which affect the consistency and speed of its delivery

Staff support systems for those involved in significant face-to-face contact with patients with personality disorder in residential settings

is not entertained as a treatment because the psychiatrist feels unskilled and/or it is not otherwise available. Family therapy, where family members and treatment resources permit, may have a therapeutic contribution to make, especially in patients' families which are separation-sensitive or enmeshed. However it is best considered as an adjunct to individual therapy, especially where this is threatened by an adverse family network (Gunderson & Sabo, 1993).

Reports of the use of group therapy are also under-represented in the literature (Dolan & Coid, 1993), given that many patients with personality disorder find their way into psychotherapy and clinical psychology departments where they are treated by group dynamic psychotherapeutic methods. The beneficial effect of peer group influences in challenging and shaping personality disordered patients' aberrant or maladaptive attitudes and behaviour, however, is well-established (Bion, 1961; Foulkes, 1964; Tschuschke & Dies, 1994). Controversy remains over the advisability of having more than one patient with personality disorder in an out-patient group and whether concurrent individual therapy is superior to group therapy alone (Gunderson & Sabo, 1993).

Specialist in-patient units

Referral to a specialist in-patient unit may be indicated where there is: a history of failed out-patient and general psychiatric in-patient treatment; an accumulating number of failed relationships; a poor occupational record; and evidence that hopelessness and destructive living styles have become incorporated into the patient's personality (Greben, 1983). Basic educational achievement, a period of stable employment, maintenance of interpersonal stability in an intimate relationship for longer than six months and a recall of a positive enduring relationship during childhood may be good prognostic indicators of a successful outcome with specialist treatment (Whiteley, 1970; Healy & Kennedy, 1993). Any referral and/or transfer, however, needs to be carefully discussed with the patient with personality disorder if it is not to be experienced by them as a rejection or as a confirmation of their inherent badness, paradoxically, as confirmation of their untreatability.

One of the advantages of the specialist in-patient unit lies in its power to select its patients and to deploy a coherent and coordinated treatment strategy via staff who have become expert in the particular method. The usual therapeutic emphasis is psychodynamic and in some units no psychotropic medication is prescribed (Norton, 1992).

Units vary in the extent to which they utilise the therapeutic influence of the personality disordered patient's peer group (Hinshelwood, 1988; Norton & Dolan, 1995a; Reiss et al, 1996). Most require motivated and voluntary participation in treatment and some capacity to experience subjective distress. Treatment lasts between six and 18 months and there is accumulating evidence of the success of such units in terms of change in behaviour (Copas et al, 1986; Cullen, 1994), psychological improvement (Dolan et al, 1992; Stone, 1993) and cost offset following treatment (Dolan et al, 1996).

In spite of such intensive and expert treatment, after-care is often required in many cases of severe personality disorder and treatment may need to be long term, lasting for a number of years. Information regarding this can be shared with the patient to facilitate engagement in treatment, not least because of introduction of a realistic time-frame in which treatment goals can be negotiated and tackled. Failure to convey this information early on can contribute to unrealistic expectations and treatment failure, however, such information needs to be imparted sensitively so as not to extinguish all hope or optimism that the patient has in the treatment.

Conclusions

Many of the clinical needs of patients with personality disorder do not differ fundamentally from those of other non-psychotic patients. However, the experience of most psychiatrists is that some of these patients are numbered among the most problematic clinical management problems which they encounter. Characteristically, difficulties arise because the patient is relatively or absolutely unable to perform the role of patient and because clinical issues are supplanted by interpersonal problems. Knowing this can save the psychiatrist some disappointment and frustration since it can lead to education of the patient about the expected role of patients, thus keeping expectations of help and treatment within reasonable bounds.

The therapeutic endeavour can be supported by the careful and judicious introduction of a treatment contract. The latter serves to bolster the legitimate professional activity by describing the actual limits of the professional input, including the proscription of some of the interpersonal aspects whose distracting presence only undermines the professional level activity. However, there are many pitfalls in the use of treatment contracts which need to be avoided.

In the management of any case where more than one professional or more than one agency are involved, there is a potential for unhelpful 'splitting'. The most regular destructive effect of this is the production of an inconsistent delivery of treatment, regardless of type or model. To avoid this, all relevant staff must meet regularly and, if necessary, frequently, to iron out disagreements or other inconsistencies. Only in this way can the patient experience treatment which is simultaneously emotionally containing and appropriately confronting and challenging.

The marshalling of professional resources, and in some cases those of other patients (as in group, milieu or therapeutic community treatment) or members of the personality disordered patient's wider social network (as in marital and family work), need to be carefully coordinated. Only if this is so can the predictable (external) organisational structure be assimilated by the patient for later internalisation. Well organised and coordinated treatment plans can convey a predictable and responsive experience of the world to patients for whom this was previously lacking. Maintaining such a concerted stance, however, may require specialised in-patient psychotherapeutic management as part of a long-term treatment plan.

Acknowledgement

I thank Dr Bridget Dolan for her helpful editorial comments and suggested improvements to an earlier draft of this paper.

References

Bion, W. R. (1961) *Experience in Groups*. London: Tavistock.

Bowlby, J. (1973) *Attachment and Loss, Vol. 2. Separation: Anxiety and Anger*. New York: Basic Books.

Coid, J. W. (1989) Psychopathic disorders. *Current Opinion in Psychiatry*, **2**, 750–756.

Copas, J. B., O'Brien, M., Roberts, J.C., *et al* (1986) Treatment outcome in personality disorder: the effect of social, psychological and behavioural variables. *Personality and Individual Differences*, **5**, 565–573.

Cowdry, R. & Gardner, D. (1988) Pharmacotherapy of borderline personality disorder: alprazolam, carbamazepine, trifluoperazine and tranylcypromine. *Archives of General Psychiatry*, **45**, 111–119.

Cullen, E. (1994) Grendon: The therapeutic prison that works. *Therapeutic Communities*, **15**, 301–311.

Dolan, B., Evans, C. & Wilson, J. (1992) Therapeutic community treatment for personality disordered adults: changes in neurotic symptomatology on follow-up. *International Journal of Social Psychiatry*, **38**, 242–250.

—— & Coid, J. (1993) *Psychopathic and Antisocial Personality Disorders: Treatment and Research Issues*. London: Gaskell.

——, Evans, C. & Norton, K. (1995) Multiple Axis II diagnosis of personality disorder. *British Journal of Psychiatry*, **166**, 107–112.

——, Warren, F., Menzies, D., *et al* (1996) Cost-offset following specialist treatment of severe personality disorders. *Psychiatric Bulletin*, **20**, 413–417.

Du Fort , G. G., Newman, S. C. & Bland, R. C. (1993) Psychiatric comorbidity and treatment seeking: sources of selection bias in the study of clinical populations. *Journal of Nervous and Mental Diseases*, **18**, 467–474.

Foulkes, S. (1964) *Therapeutic Group Analysis*. London: George Allen & Unwin.

Frank, A. F. (1991) The therapeutic alliances of borderline patients. In *Borderline Personality Disorder: Clinical and Empirical Perspectives* (eds J. Clarkin, E. Marziali & H. Munroe-Blum). New York: Guilford.

Gardner, D. L. & Cowdry, R. W. (1985) Alprazolam induced dyscontrol in borderline personality disorder. *American Journal of Psychiatry*, **143**, 519–522.

Goldberg, S. C., Schulz, S. C., Schulz, P. M., *et al* (1986) Borderline and schizotypical personality disorders treated with low-dose thiothixene vs placebo. *Archives of General Psychiatry*, **43**, 680–686.

Greben, S. (1983) The multi-dimensional inpatient treatment of severe character disorders. *Canadian Journal of Psychiatry*, **28**, 97–101.

Gunderson, J. G., Frank, A. F., Ronningstam, E. F., *et al* (1989) Early discontinuance of borderline patients from psychotherapy. *Journal of Nervous and Mental Disorders*, **177**, 38–42.

—— & Sabo, A. N. (1993) Treatment of borderline personality disorder: a critical review. In *Borderline Personality Disorder: Aetiology and Treatment* (ed. J. Paris), pp. 385–406. Washington, DC: American Psychiatric Press.

Healey, K. & Kennedy, R. (1993) Which families benefit from in-patient psychotherapeutic work at the Cassel Hospital? *British Journal of Psychotherapy*, **9**, 394–404.

Higgitt, A. & Fonagy, P. (1992) Psychotherapy in borderline and narcissistic personality disorder. *British Journal of Psychiatry*, **161**, 23–43.

Hinshelwood, R. (1988) Psychotherapy in an in-patient setting. *Current Opinion in Psychiatry*, **1**, 304–308.

Horwitz, L. (1974) *Clinical Prediction in Psychotherapy*. New York: Jason Aronson.

Kernberg, O. F. (1984) *Severe Personality Disorders: Psychotherapeutic Strategies*. New Haven and London: Yale University Press.

Layden, M. A., Newman, C. F., Freeman, A., *et al* (1993) *Cognitive Therapy of Borderline Personality Disorder*. Massachusetts: Allyn and Bacon.

Linehan, M. M. (1987) Dialectical behaviour therapy: a cognitive–behavioural approach to parasuicide. *Journal of Personality Disorders*, **4**, 328–333.

Links, P. S., Steiner, M., Boiago, I., *et al* (1990) Lithium therapy for borderline patients: preliminary findings. *Journal of Personality Disorders*, **4**, 173–181.

Lockwood, G. (1992) Psychoanalysis and the cognitive therapy of personality disorders. *Journal of Cognitive Psychotherapy*, **6**, 25–42.

Main, T. (1957) The ailment. *British Journal of Medical Psychology*, **30**, 129–145. Reprinted in T. Main (1989) *The Ailment and other Psycho-Analytic Essays*. London: Free Association Books.

—— (1983) The concept of the therapeutic community: its variations and vicissitudes. In *The Evolution of Group Analysis* (ed. M. Pines), pp. 197–217. London: Routledge and Kegan Paul.

Masterson, J. F. (1972) *Treatment of the Borderline Adolescent: A Development Approach*. New York: Wiley.

Miller, L. J. (1989) Inpatient management of borderline personality disorder: a review and update. *Journal of Personality Disorders*, **3**, 122–134.

Montgomery, S. A. & Montgomery, D. (1982) Pharmacological prevention of suicidal behaviour. *Journal of Affective Disorders*, **4**, 291–298.

Norden, M. J. (1989) Fluoxetine in borderline personality disorder. *Progress in Neurophyschopharmacology and Biological Psychiatry*, **13**, 885–893.

Norton, K. R. W. (1992) Personality disordered individuals: the Henderson Hospital model of treatment. *Criminal Behaviour and Mental Health*, **2**, 80–191.

––– (1997) In-patient psychotherapy: integrating the other 23 hours. *Current Medical Literature – Psychiatry*, **8**, 31–71.

–– & Smith, S. (1994) *Problems with Patients: Managing Complicated Clinical Transactions*. Cambridge: Cambridge University Press.

–– & Dolan, B. (1995a) Acting out and the institutional response. *Journal of Forensic Psychiatry*, **6**, 317–332.

–– & –– (1995b) Personality disorders and parenting. In *Parental Psychiatric Disorders* (eds M. Gopfert, J. Webster & M. Seeman), pp. 219–232. Cambridge: Cambridge University Press.

–– & –– (1995c) Personality disorder: assessing change. *Current Opinions in Psychiatry*, **8**, 371–375.

––– & McGauley, G. (1997) *Counselling Difficult Clients*. London: Sage.

Oldham, J. M. (1991) *Personality Disorders: New Perspectives on Diagnostic Validity*. Washington, DC: American Psychiatric Press.

Reiss, D., Grubin, D. & Meux, C. (1996) Young 'psychopaths' in special hospitals: treatment and outcome. *British Journal of Psychiatry*, **168**, 99–104.

Reugg, R. & Frances, A. (1995) New research in personality disorders. *Journal of Personality Disorders*, **9**, 1–48.

Rockland, L. H. (1989) *Supportive Therapy: A Psychodynamic Approach*. New York: Basic Books.

Ryle, A. & Marlowe, M. (1995) Cognitive–analytical therapy of borderline personality disorder: theory, practice and the clinical and research uses of the self-states sequential diagram. *International Journal of Short-Term Psychotherapy*, **10**, 21–34.

Shearer, E. N. & Linehan, M. (1994) Dialectical behaviour therapy for borderline personality disorder: theoretical and empirical foundations. *Acta Psychiatrica Scandinavica*, **89** (suppl. 379), 61–68.

Soloff, P. H. , George, A. & Nathan, R. S. (1986) Progress in pharmacotherapy of borderline personality disorders. *Archives of General Psychiatry*, **43**, 691–697.

–––, ––– & Northam, R. L. (1989) Amitriptyline versus halopcridol in borderlines: final outcomes and predictors of response. *Journal of Clinical Psychopharmacology*, **9**, 238–246.

Stanton, A. H. & Schwartz, M. S. (1954) *The Mental Hospital*. New York: Basic Books.

Stein, G. (1992) Drug treatment of the personality disorders. *British Journal of Psychiatry*, **161**, 167–184.

Stone, M. H. (1993) Long-term outcome in personality disorder. *British Journal of Psychiatry*, **162**, 299–313.

Teicher, M. H., Glod, C. & Cole, J. O. (1990) Emergence of intense suicidal preoccupation during fluoxetine treatment. *American Journal of Psychiatry*, **147**, 207–210.

Tschuschke, V. & Dies, R. R. (1994) Intensive analysis of therapeutic factors and outcome in long-term in-patient groups. *International Journal of Group Psychotherapy*, **44**, 185–208.

Tyrer, P. (1988) *Personality Disorder, Diagnosis, Management and Care*. London: Wright.

–– & Johnson, T. (1996) Establishing the severity of personality disorder. *American Journal of Psychiatry*, **153**, 1593–1597.

Wallerstein, R. (1986) *Forty-Two Lives in Treatment: A Study of Psychoanalysis and Psychotherapy*. New York: Guilford.

West, M. , Keller, A., Links, P., *et al* (1993) Borderline disorder and attachment pathology. *Canadian Journal of Psychiatry*, **38**, 1–6.

Whiteley, S. (1970) The response of psychopaths to a therapeutic community. *British Journal of Psychiatry*, **116**, 517–529.

World Health Organization (1992) *The Tenth Revision of the International Classification of Mental and Behavioural Disorders* (ICD–10). Geneva: WHO.

Yeomans, F. (1993) When a therapist over-indulges a demanding borderline patient. *Hospital and Community Psychiatry*, **44**, 334–336.

Young, J. (1990) *Cognitive Therapy for Personality Disorders: A Schema Focused Approach*. Sarasota, FL: Professional Resources Exchange.

Zanarini, M. C., Gunderson, J. G., Marino, M. F., *et al* (1990) Psychiatric disorders in the families of borderline outpatients. In *Family Environment and Borderline Personality Disorder* (ed. P. S. Links), pp. 67–84. Washington, DC: American Psychiatric Press.

Zimmerman, M. & Coryell, W. H. (1990) Diagnosing personality disorder in the community. *Archives of General Psychiatry*, **47**, 527–531.

––, Pfohl, B. & Coryell, W. H. (1991) Major depression and personality disorder. *Journal of Affective Disorders*, **22**, 199–210.

Management of alcohol misuse within the context of general psychiatry

Duncan Raistrick

The general psychiatrist and the addiction specialist have a shared agenda of concerns and interests about the misuse of alcohol. The task of this chapter is to highlight and develop thoughts on items for inclusion on the shared agenda, rather than to define, or limit in any other way, how the generalist role might unfold in a particular place at a particular time. It is certain that the general psychiatrist will see a role that is more than just signposting their own specialist colleagues, local counselling services or self-help groups such as Alcoholics Anonymous, but opinion on just how broad that role could or should be will vary considerably. One difference may be a mismatch of views as to where patients with alcohol misuse problems are best treated – the general psychiatrist seeing alcohol misuse, or even dependence, as having little to do with general psychiatry and belonging within a specialist service, and the specialist seeing alcohol misuse as very much part of the everyday work of the general psychiatrist.

Alcohol misuse is everyone's business: the politician, the publican, the parent, the tax payer, the doctor; the list could go on. A shared agenda, possibly informing the content of journal clubs or case conferences, needs to invoke some passion and to promise benefits for psychiatry. The agenda might include:

(a) Raising awareness of alcohol misuse within the profession.
(b) Achieving *Health of the Nation* targets.
(c) Understanding brief interventions for alcohol misuse.
(d) Managing dual diagnosis patients.

Whether they are aware of the fact or not, general psychiatrists see many patients whose problems include alcohol misuse. In the most recent survey of drinking patterns in the general population, the Office for National Statistics (1999) found 27% of men and 14% of women drinking above low-risk levels (21 units per week for men and 14 units per week for women),

with 6% of men and 2% of women drinking at high-risk levels (51+ units and 36+ units). In a health district of 300 000 this would equate to between 9000 and 61 000 people misusing alcohol, depending upon the cut-off point which is selected. Even if only 10% of these people seek help or find themselves in hospital or out-patient services for reasons other than alcohol misuse at any given time, it would be ludicrous to think that such numbers could be handled by the resources of an addiction team, even if this were considered a good idea. Some 20% of patients in general medical wards, and rather greater numbers in psychiatric wards, have alcohol-related problems (although these are not necessarily the cause of admission), but 20% of doctors are not addiction specialists, and no-one would think it sensible to create such numbers. So, the inescapable implication of these figures is that people who misuse alcohol will be a challenge to all doctors in their day to day practice.

Raising awareness

The medical profession has steadily reduced its own *per capita* intake of alcohol over the last 10–20 years and come to see drinking as incompatible with the workplace. Medical students and doctors now have similar consumption levels, when matched by age and gender, to the general population, having in the past had much higher levels. This should not be taken as a reason for complacency as the reduction in alcohol-related problems among doctors is only down to the levels of alcohol-related harm in the general population, which remain high. It is to be expected that social trends will be reflected in the behaviour of medical students and young doctors. In a study comparing lifestyles of Newcastle medical students in 1983–84 with 1993–94, Ashton & Kamali (1995) found a modest increase in alcohol consumption between the two periods, with 32% of men and 21% of women drinking above low-risk levels: 94% gave 'pleasure', and 9% 'exam pressures' as reasons for drinking. There was an increase in those who had 'ever used' cannabis from 26% to 54% for men and from 15% to 46% for women, and an increase for both groups from 3% to 22% for having 'ever used' other illicit drugs. These findings are not confined to Newcastle, nor to medical students, indeed medical students compare favourably to other students.

Clearly progress has been made on raising awareness of alcohol misuse within the profession. Nonetheless, situations involving alcohol or other drugs still contributed 31 of 55 cases entering the General Medical Council health procedures in 1994, and only three doctors in that year were successfully returned to practice. General Medical Council procedures have since been subject to reform. In a retrospective casenote study of 144 doctors with substance misuse problems, Brooke (1995) identified stress of work or of life events coupled with a vulnerable personality, usually characterised by traits such as anxiety, introversion or obsessionality, to be frequent companions of substance misuse. Other risk factors are isolation and collusion by family, friends and colleagues with the net result that intervention often comes too late. On the positive side, doctors have the potential to mobilise powerful protective mechanisms through their knowledge base, peer support and formal professional support.

From the point of view of self-awareness and patient care, the effects of alcohol and other psychoactive drugs on health need to be discussed throughout medical training. Psychiatrists as a group have traditionally led the call for alcohol education in the medical curriculum (Ritson, 1990). A failure to permeate alcohol education into the new medical curricula will be to neglect a responsibility of the profession to trainee doctors and their patients. It is equally important that awareness is maintained as part of continuing education. Consultants can set the clinical standard by rigorously accounting for the contribution of alcohol to physical and mental illness in their routine practice. Practices that partition alcohol misuse and mental health are unhelpful, even damaging. In addition, consultants in psychiatry share a special role within the health care community, namely to engender good mental health. Alcohol misuse will be one of the more common barriers to achieving this goal.

Understanding dependence

Tober (1992) theorises on the meaning of dependence and concludes that dependence is important because it is the essence of addiction. The arguments underpinning this deceptively obvious conclusion are more complex than might at first be assumed and are not universally accepted. The concept of a dependence syndrome was first described in provisional form by Edwards & Gross (1976) and was incorporated into ICD–9 after approval by the World Health Organization in 1979. The dependence syndrome departed from the notion of 'alcoholism', a disease concept, in two important ways: first, dependence was seen as existing along a continuum of severity, implying the need for different treatments and different outcome goals; second, alcohol-related disabilities in the physical, psychological and social spheres were to be seen as belonging to a separate domain. Dependence was described as a biopsychosocial syndrome consisting of seven markers:

(a) Narrowing of drinking repertoire.
(b) Salience of drink-related behaviour.
(c) Increased tolerance to alcohol.
(d) Repeated withdrawal symptoms.
(e) Relief or avoidance of withdrawal symptoms by further drinking.
(f) A subjective awareness of a compulsion to drink.
(g) Rapid reinstatement after a period of abstinence.

A number of criticisms followed, the most damaging of which was the contention that the dependence syndrome had little predictive validity, limited clinical utility, and that estimates of alcohol intake and patterns of consumption are more helpful (Robertson, 1986). It is true that the largest proportion of outcome variance is accounted for by social stability factors, however, it does not follow that dependence is of limited utility. Rather, it follows that social treatments are effective at extinguishing learned behaviour such as dependence. This point is illustrated by Azrin *et al* (1982) who described favourable outcomes using a Community Reinforcement Approach – a comprehensive package of social interventions – to treat alcohol misuse problems. When making treatment decisions, the clinician needs to assess the extent to which dependence is driving continued excessive drinking in order to determine 'how much' treatment will be needed. As dependence becomes more severe the social cues for drinking diminish and pharmacological cues come to dominate (see Fig. 1). This does not mean that social therapy is necessarily less effective than cognitive–behavioural or spiritual interventions for more severely dependent patients. The effectiveness of any therapy depends on the extent to which it is able to optimise benefits of cue avoidance, or cue exposure and reinforce behaviours incompatible with drinking.

The biopsychosocial description of dependence has been further criticised for placing unwarranted emphasis on withdrawal symptoms. While the anticipation or experience of withdrawal may indeed be a potent source of negative reinforcement for drinking it is not the only source of reinforcement, and it may be that the positive reinforcement of a pharmacological (alcohol) effect is more important whether or not an individual also experiences withdrawal.

Room (1989) succinctly captures the political dimension of the debate submitting that "the de-emphasis of cognitive and experiential dimensions in medical definitions and operationalisations of dependence reflects a strong pull towards reductionist and psychological conceptions in medical thought". A consequence has been confusion over the meaning of dependence – some authors continue to distinguish between physical dependence, which seems to be code for medical territory, and psychological dependence, code for psychological territory. In other words, the clinical understanding of tolerance and withdrawal has been lost in a contest for medical or for psychological hegemony. The important end point of this debate is that the terms 'psychological' and 'physical' dependence should be considered obsolete; physical dependence refers to withdrawal symptoms and to tolerance which are best seen as separate phenomena to dependence and referred to collectively as neuroadaptation.

Raistrick *et al* (1994) have proposed a modified description of the dependence syndrome and developed the idea of substance dependence as a purely psychological phenomenon where tolerance and withdrawal are understood as consequences of regular drinking, rather than being a part of dependence. The withdrawal symptoms themselves are one step removed from the cognitive response to the symptoms, which may or may not include thoughts about drinking. If withdrawal symptoms were themselves a defining element of dependence

then different drugs would be associated with different kinds of dependence, but this is not a widely held view, rather it is believed that dependence can readily shift from one substance to another (Kosten *et al*, 1987). The markers of substance dependence translate the neuroadaptive elements of the biopsychosocial description of dependence into cues which condition cognitions and behaviours and are therefore of more universal application. There are 10 markers of substance dependence:

(a) Preoccupation with drinking or taking drugs.
(b) Salience of substance use behaviour.
(c) Compulsion to start using drink or drugs.
(d) Planning drink- or drug-related behaviours.
(e) Maximising the substance effect.
(f) Narrowing of substance use repertoire.
(g) Compulsion to continue using drink or drugs.
(h) Primacy of psychoactive effect.
(i) Maintaining a constant state (of intoxication).
(j) Expectations of need for substance use.

Substance dependence also departs from the broader psychological view of dependence proposed by Orford (1985) which embraces such objects of dependence as people and activities. In many ways this ubiquitous dependence is a restatement of learning theory. What distinguishes substance dependence from other behavioural dependencies, like gambling or exercise, is the way in which addictive drugs alter the physiological substrate upon which they act thereby increasing reinforcement potential. The distinction is imperfect but serves to define boundaries which have found clinical relevance.

The Leeds Dependence Questionnaire (LDQ; Raistrick *et al*, 1994) was derived from the idea of substance dependence and was designed to measure dependence on any psychoactive drug; to date the questionnaire has been validated for use with alcohol and heroin users. The dominant view in the addiction field is that dependence is a learned phenomenon where expectations play a central part: in other words beliefs about, for example, what will happen on taking a drink after a period of abstinence have a greater effect on outcome than alcohol does itself. How these learned cognitions and behaviours change is not yet understood. Is it the case that dependent behaviour, drinking, can be extinguished, or is it that the behaviour changes as a result of cognitive control resulting in avoidance? Most likely both of these mechanisms can operate. This distinction is an important one in that social drinking, controlled drinking or abstinence from drinking are possible drinking goals, but the appropriate goal will depend upon the degree of cue extinction that can be achieved.

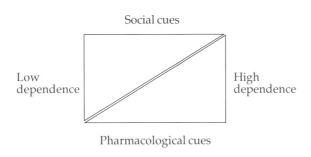

Social cues

Low dependence   High dependence

Pharmacological cues

Fig. 1.   Relationship between dependence and drinking cues

In summary, dependence is conceptualised in psychological terms and can be assessed by questionnaire or by clinical interview. At lower levels of dependence social cues will be more important than pharmacological cues for drinking, but as dependence increases so this relationship is reversed and dependence becomes more fixed indicating that social or controlled drinking goals are unlikely to be successful (Fig. 1). It follows from this that at low levels of dependence a brief alcohol-focused intervention or a social intervention, suitable for use in general psychiatry, is likely to be effective. Brief interventions may be no more than an information leaflet, a drinking diary, or five minutes' advice and information which is sensitive to a patient's particular problem but, importantly, includes a follow-up session.

Dual diagnosis

The most frequent problem for the general psychiatrist is not the straightforward case of alcohol dependence or misuse but the patient with a dual diagnosis. Penick *et al* (1988) administered a DSM–III compatible diagnostic interview to 241 male 'alcoholics' during an in-patient admission and again at 1 year: 30% were deemed to have one additional psychiatric syndrome, 18% two, and 9% three or more additional syndromes. Depression and antisocial personality were the most common diagnoses. There was some fluidity of diagnostic category between intake and follow-up interview: only 62% of men diagnosed with antisocial personality, 53% with depression and 38% with panic attacks had the same diagnosis at both interviews. Rounsaville *et al* (1987) found alcohol dependence complicating psychopathology to be an unfavourable and robust predictor of outcome. However, the authors suggested that, while a dimensional measure of psychopathology is an independent predictor of outcome, categorical diagnosis brings additional predictive power, for example, alcohol misuse secondary to affective disorder carries a relatively favourable prognosis. Chappel (1993) has recommended that treatment of dual diagnosis patients should be conducted by one clinical team in one setting; this approach has benefits in terms of simplifying communication between clinical staff and ensuring that the links between substance use and psychiatric disorder are fully investigated and dealt with.

Anxiety

The relationship between alcohol and anxiety is complex and each case requires careful clinical assessment. At a pharmacological level, alcohol has an initial, but short-lived, stimulant effect which is superseded by an anxiolytic effect. The use of alcohol to self-medicate anxiety symptoms has long been recognised. It is less appreciated, especially by patients, that more alcohol does not mean more anxiety relief, but rather chronic alcohol use can itself become a stressor and increase anxiety. In proposing a revised tension reduction hypothesis, Young *et al* (1990) illustrate the interaction of expectations and pharmacology. Their preliminary conclusions, with specific caveats that the effects of gender and high versus low dose alcohol need further elucidation, stress the possible difference between 'normal' and 'patient' populations. 'Socially impaired' individuals are more likely to take on positive expectations of the effects of alcohol but actually perform worse under the influence of alcohol, compared with placebo, while continuing to believe their performance to be enhanced. On the other hand, 'normal' subjects with positive expectations for alcohol in socially stressful situations perform better, subjectively and objectively, but only with the enabling effect of alcohol not placebo.

Estimates of the prevalence of anxiety disorder among patients with an alcohol dependence diagnosis typically fall between 10 and 30%, while of in-patients who have a primary diagnosis of phobic anxiety only 10% have the secondary diagnosis of alcohol dependence, although half will regularly use alcohol as an anxiolytic. Measurement is a major problem, anxiety symptoms are very common and non-specific, symptoms alone do not make for a diagnosis, and misdiagnosis, particularly of alcohol withdrawal, is likely to occur if assessments are made during an episode of heavy drinking or immediately post-detoxification.

Allan (1995) recommended that patients presenting with anxiety and alcohol dependence should first be detoxified and reassessed after six weeks when an expected 10% will be found to have persistent symptoms amounting to an anxiety state. This can then be treated using conventional pharmacological or behavioural methods. She points out that patients may resist such an approach, preferring to deal with their psychological distress first. Clinicians can be more confident about reversing the order of treatment where it can be established that anxiety antedates alcohol misuse or is a specific trigger to drinking.

Depression

Davidson & Ritson (1993) found that many of the complex interactions existing in the relationship between alcohol use and anxiety also apply to alcohol use and depression. At low doses alcohol is generally reported to enhance mood, but at higher doses subjects report dysphoria and an aversion to continued drinking. Tolerance may necessitate an increasing level of alcohol intake in pursuit of a mood altering effect that is in reality no longer achievable. Similar problems to those described for anxiety apply when estimating the prevalence of depression. In hospitalised people with alcohol misuse 30–40% are found to be depressed, whereas in community samples less than 5% of people with alcohol misuse have both diagnoses.

People who are dependent on alcohol usually succumb to a number of financial, family, health and relationship problems and it is not surprising that many will complain of depression; equally it is not surprising that 80% or more will recover within a few weeks of abstinence without recourse to antidepressant treatment. While abstinence may enforce an acceptance of problems accumulated while drinking and this might be anticipated to increase depression, abstinence is also an opportunity to build self-efficacy and self-esteem, both of which are powerful psychological antidepressants. Pharmacological antidepressants should be avoided unless there is unequivocal evidence of a biological depression of mood.

In studies of completed suicides it is usual to find that 20–30% of cases misuse alcohol, however, the high rates of concurrence of depressive illness and alcohol misuse may exaggerate the influence of one or both factors. Murphy (1992) has identified seven risk factors for suicide in 'alcoholics':

(a) Depression.
(b) Suicidal thoughts.
(c) Poor social support.
(d) Physical illness.
(e) Unemployment.
(f) Living alone.
(g) Recent interpersonal loss.

The risks accumulate over a number of years suggesting that there is scope for preventive social and health care.

Personality disorder

Many patients who have a personality disorder also misuse alcohol and are often poly-drug users. Psychiatrists may be pessimistic about working with these patients, seeing custody as more appropriate, and yet most criminal justice system workers believe that therapy is better than custody. Patients with a dual diagnosis of personality disorder and substance misuse are frequently referred to addiction units. Walker (1992) has described the need to understand the psychopathology of personality disorder and

sees the inability of these patients to learn from the past or see into the future – a 'living for the moment' state of mind – as the central feature that informs the treatment plan. Accordingly, he does not suggest assigning people with a personality disorder diagnosis to a particular speciality, but rather to a psychiatrist with character traits to match the disorder. He sees these traits as being: self-confidence, truthfulness, neutral interaction, consistency, self-control and the ability to set limits. Such therapist variables may indeed be helpful in containing some personality problems but they fall short of a specific treatment or solution which should be resourced in a specialist service.

Summary

The key issue here is the ephemeral nature of comorbidity, notably so for anxiety and depression (Raimo & Schuckit, 1998), pointing to a need for restraint when prescribing for patients with a possible dual diagnosis. Obvious exceptions are Korsakoff's syndrome (Cook & Thompson, 1997) and other organic brain disorders which are normally the remit of rehabilitation teams, and alcoholic delirium which is typically treated within general medical or liaison psychiatry units. The clinician must, however, remain vigilant for psychiatric disorders, for example obsessional neurosis or manic depressive psychosis, which have been masked or partially treated by alcohol and may become more troublesome in the absence of alcohol.

A repertoire of treatment skills

The diagnosis and measurement of dependence tell the clinician what outcome goals are likely to be successful and how much treatment is needed; alongside this an understanding of motivation informs the kind of treatment needed. The Model of Change described by Prochaska & DiClemente (1984) is a motivational model widely used in the addiction field. The purpose of using the model is two-fold: first, to understand what is going on for a patient at a given time and second, to inform the choice of interventions (Box 1). People who are not motivated to change their drinking behaviour are said to be at the pre-contemplation stage, which is characterised by denial and rationalisation of drinking and its consequences. There are two strands to treatment strategy at this stage: one is to minimise the harm from drinking without expecting to change the drinking behaviour, for example by prescribing vitamin supplements or by providing shelter; the other is to introduce conflict about the drinking, for example by capitalising upon untoward alcohol-related life events. The temptation is to offer treatments aimed at changing drinking behaviour before the patient is ready to change. In such circumstances the treatment will always fail.

The experience of significant conflict about drinking, for example when drinking and driving is felt to be incompatible with a self-image of being a sensible and responsible person, or when the cost of drinking is causing family hardship, indicates movement into the contemplation stage. At this stage motivational interventions which may involve the use of simple clinical tools, for example the decision matrix, or may draw on more sophisticated skills, for example motivational interviewing (Tober, 1991), are indicated.

The action stage is reached when conflict is resolved and there is a commitment to change. A number of things will have happened at a psychological level: the person will believe that life will be better on stopping or controlling their drinking (positive outcome expectancy), will believe that they are able to change (self-efficacy), and will know how to change (skills learning). Elective detoxification is the most common medical intervention at the action stage and it is also one of the most frequently misused interventions in addiction. Not uncommonly patients who have yet to reach the action stage are offered detoxification, possibly because it gives the doctor a sense of helping and possibly because it colludes with a patient's wish to be seen to be having treatment. Not only is the intervention likely to fail if used in precontemplation, but failure is likely to reduce a patient's self-esteem or confirm their belief that they are 'a

---

> **Box 2.   Prescribing points**
>
> *Chlordiazepoxide*: drug of choice for de-toxification
>
> *Chlormethiazole*: in-patient detoxification if a history of seizures or delirium
>
> *Disulfiram*: adjunctive therapy in the main-tenance stage
>
> *Naltrexone or acamprosate*: adjunctive therapy in the maintenance stage
>
> *Antidepressants*: use with caution – assess indications post detox. where possible
>
> *Anxiolytics*: use with caution – assess indications post detox. where possible
>
> *Antipsychotics*: check for psychotomimetic drugs using toxicology screen

hopeless alcoholic'. On an out-patient basis, chlordiazepoxide 40–100 mg in divided doses is the drug of choice for detoxification on the grounds that it is effective, has a low addictive potential, low toxicity when mixed with alcohol, and a unique metabolite on urine screening (see Box 2). Chlormethiazole may be used on an in-patient basis when there is a history of seizures or delirium, but patients should not take this drug home because of its addictive potential and toxicity when mixed with alcohol.

The maintenance stage follows from behavioural change, the achievement of abstinence or controlled drinking. Maintenance of behaviour change may be assisted by an alcohol sensitising agent such as disulfiram 200 mg daily (Chick *et al*, 1992) or by reducing craving with naltrexone 50 mg daily (Volpicelli *et al*, 1995) or acamprosate (Sass *et al*, 1996). Pharmacological interventions are no more than an adjunct to the main task of achieving lifestyle change. Successful recovery requires that the patient has the confidence and skills to deal with drinking cues. The highest ambition would be to take on new activities, incompatible with drinking but at the same time exciting and enjoyable, for example, rock climbing may suit one person while the next will get a 'buzz' from doing voluntary work. The lowest ambition for lifestyle change would simply be to avoid drinking situations and friends. Attendance at Alcoholics Anonymous is very supportive of this limited goal, but has the disadvantage that group members are locked into the maintenance stage because of continuing self-definition as an 'alcoholic'.

> **Box 1.   Treatment strategy and stage of change**
>
> **Precontemplation**
>   Harm reduction measures
>   Introduce conflict about drinking
>
> **Contemplation**
>   Increase motivation to change
>
> **Action**
>   Preparation for behaviour change
>   Behaviour change
>
> **Maintenance**
>   Relapse prevention

Health of the Nation targets

Safer drinking limits

The *Health of the Nation* targets were cynically received, no doubt because of their political origins. Nonetheless, there is much to recommend pursuit of the targets relating to alcohol misuse. The scientific basis for proposing constraints on *per capita* consumption are detailed in *Alcohol Policy and the Public Good* (Edwards, 1994). Achievement of the *Health of the Nation* target to reduce the proportion of men drinking above low-risk limits to 18% and women to 7% by the year 2005 will require an effort by all doctors and many others. What will work and be acceptable to the public generally is everyone 'doing a bit' not a few 'doing a lot' (NHS Executive, 1998). Doctors are known to be effective communicators of brief health care messages (Heather, 1995). All psychiatrists should ensure that their clinics have suitable alcohol information leaflets available and should rehearse a 4–5 minute, brief intervention that includes an explanation of how alcohol misuse and dependence can impair mental health.

Suicide

General psychiatrists will be key players in achieving the target of reducing the overall suicide rates by 15% by the year 2000. Many of the factors associated with suicide in people with alcohol misuse problems are amenable to social care and vigorous pursuit of abstinence treatments. It is likely that a significant reduction in suicide can be achieved if social care resources are available and doctors redouble efforts to identify 'at risk drinkers'.

Referrals to specialists

There can be no hard and fast rules on referral: much will depend upon local agreement and available resources. Ideally a doctor with special knowledge of addiction should be available to general psychiatry colleagues to assess patients and advise on case management. However, few addiction teams are able to meet this demand, and as psychiatrists are dispersed into geographically separate community bases and trusts, even informal discussion becomes more difficult. Patients most likely to be referred on are those with uncomplicated but severe alcohol dependence and supplementary use of illicit drugs, especially if

this requires prescriptions for controlled drugs. It would be illogical to refer on patients requiring a brief intervention, or patients who are not amenable to treatment. Where there is a dual diagnosis the lead team should be agreed on the basis of what is thought to be the primary psychopathology. Ideally trusts should set up comorbidity services in accordance with correct models of care.

Conclusions

Many doctors are fearful of taking on people with substance misuse problems, perhaps thinking that as patients they will be disruptive. Doctors lacking in therapeutic confidence may find reasons to refer on rather than treat. Addiction teams can help by providing workshops on substance misuse for general psychiatry colleagues, as many have done for general practitioners. With a repertoire of skills the challenge of offering a more comprehensive care package for patients becomes less daunting and therapeutic success is certain to follow. With therapeutic success a more rounded approach to training and supervision of medical students and trainees is an inevitable bonus.

Acknowledgements

The 'Understanding dependence' section has drawn on the ideas of Gillian Tober and is taken from current work towards her PhD thesis. Thanks are due to Gail Crossley for expert secretarial support.

References

Allan, C. A. (1995) Alcohol problems and anxiety disorders – a critical review. *Alcohol and Alcoholism*, **30**, 145–151.

Ashton, C. H. & Kamali, F. (1995) Personality, lifestyles, alcohol and drug consumption in a sample of British medical students. *Medical Education*, **29**, 187–192.

Azrin, N. H., Sissons, R. W., Mayer, S. R., *et al* (1982) Alcoholism treatment by disulfiram and community reinforcement therapy. *Journal of Behaviour Therapy and Experimental Psychiatry*, **13**, 105–112.

Brooke, D. (1995) The addicted doctor. Caring professionals? *British Journal of Psychiatry*, **166**, 149–153.

Chappel, J. N. (1993) Training of residents and medical students in the diagnosis and treatment of dual diagnosis patients. *Journal of Psychoactive Drugs*, **25**, 293–300.

Chick, J., Gough, W., Falkowski, W., *et al* (1992) Disulfiram treatment of alcoholism. *British Journal of Psychiatry*, **161**, 84–89.

Cook, C. H. & Thompson, A. D. (1997) *British Journal of Hospital Medicine*, **57**, 161–165.

Davidson, K. M. & Ritson, E. B. (1993) The relationship between alcohol dependence and depression. *Alcohol and Alcoholism*, **28**, 147–155.

Edwards, G. (1994) *Alcohol Policy and the Public Good*. Oxford: Oxford University Press.

—— & Gross, M. M. (1976) Alcohol dependence: provisional description of a clinical syndrome. *British Medical Journal*, **1**, 1058–1061.

Heather, N. (1995) Interpreting the evidence on brief interventions for excessive drinkers: the need for caution. *Alcohol and Alcoholism*, **30**, 287–296.

Kosten, T. R., Rounsaville, J., Babor, T. F., *et al* (1987) Substance use disorder in DSM–III–R: Evidence for the dependence syndrome across different psychoactive substances. *British Journal of Psychiatry*, **151**, 834–843.

Murphy, G. E. (1992) *Suicide in Alcoholism*. New York: Oxford University Press.

NHS Executive (1998) *NHS Priorities and Planning Guidance 1997/98*. EL (96)45.Leeds: NHS Executive.

Office for National Statistics (1999) *General Household Survey*, pp. 180–181. London: The Stationery Office.

Orford, J. (1985) *Excessive Appetites*. Chichester: Wiley.

Penick, E. C., Powell, B. J., Liskow, B. I., *et al* (1988) The stability of coexisting psychiatric syndromes in alcoholic men after one year. *Journal of Studies on Alcohol*, **49**, 395–405.

Prochaska, J. O. & DiClemente, C. C. (1984) *The Transtheoretical Approach: Crossing Traditional Boundaries of Therapy*. Chicago, IL: Dow Jones-Irwin.

Raimo, E. B. & Schuckit, M. A. (1998) Alcohol dependence and mood disorders. *Addictive Behaviours*, **23**, 933–946.

Raistrick, D. S., Bradshaw, J., Tober, G., *et al* (1994) Development of the Leeds Dependence Questionnaire. *Addiction*, **89**, 563–572.

Ritson, E. B. (1990) Teaching medical students about alcohol. *British Medical Journal*, **30**, 134–135.

Robertson, I. (1986) A modest statistical phenomenon of little theoretical coherence. *British Journal of Addiction*, **81**, 190–193.

Room, R. (1989) Drugs, consciousness and self control: popular and medical conceptions. *International Review of Psychiatry*, **1**, 63–70.

Rounsaville, B. J., Dolinsky, Z. S., Babor, T. E., *et al* (1987) Psychopathology as a predictor of treatment outcome in alcoholics. *Archives of General Psychiatry*, **44**, 505–513.

Sass, H., Soyka, M., Mann, K., *et al* (1996) Relapse prevention by acamprosate. *Archives of General Psychiatry*, **53**, 673– 680.

Tober, G. (1991) Motivational interviewing with young people. In *Motivational Interviewing: Preparing People to Change* (eds W. Miller & S. Rollnick), pp. 248–259. New York: Guilford.

—— (1992) What is dependence and why is it important? *Clinical Psychology Forum*, **41**, 14–16.

Volpicelli, J. R., Watson, N. T., King, A. C., *et al* (1995) Effect of naltrexone on alcohol "high" in alcoholics. *American Journal of Psychiatry*, **153**, 613–615.

Walker, R. (1992) Substance abuse and b-cluster disorders. I. Understanding the dual diagnosis patient. *Journal of Psychoactive Drugs*, **24**, 223–232.

Young, R. M., Oei, T. P. S. & Knight, R. G. (1990) The tension reduction hypothesis revisited: an alcohol expectancy perspective. *British Journal of Addiction*, **85,** 31–40.

The management of anorexia nervosa

R. L. Palmer

The severity of anorexia nervosa can vary from mild to life threatening. It is sometimes transient but often chronic. Such variety in a disorder requires a variety of responses. The clinician must choose the right treatment to offer at the right time. The literature contains plenty of advice, but most of this is based upon experience and opinion rather than on systematic research and treatment trials. Anorexia nervosa is a disorder which is distinct from other psychiatric syndromes but is of uncertain cause. In the face of this uncertainty, treatment tends to be informed by the favoured formulation of the clinician, usually some sort of 'multi-factorial theory'. This chapter is no exception and will concentrate upon the management of anorexia nervosa in late adolescence and adulthood. The treatment of children requires a different approach (Lask & Bryant-Waugh, 1993). The emphasis here is upon what can go wrong as well as what may be the best interventions to offer. Often the things that go wrong have more to do with the context of treatment and the way in which it is offered rather than with the treatment intervention itself.

The nature of the problem

The core features of anorexia nervosa are well known and the criteria set out in ICD–10 (World Health Organization, 1992) and DSM–IV (American Psychiatric Association, 1994) are closely similar for practical purposes. Although atypical cases are not uncommon, making the diagnosis is not usually difficult. When there is real doubt the diagnostic puzzle can be tough and is worthy of a paper in its own right. What is not so easy is the development of a 'feel' for what eating disorders are about. In this respect it may be useful to think of anorexia nervosa as involving an entanglement of two sets of ideas and the consequences of that entanglement. One set of ideas concerns weight and eating control. The other concerns wider personal issues such as self-esteem, emotional control and self-image in the broadest sense. These issues are mixed up for many people in our society, especially for young women.

The idea that self-worth may be enhanced by slenderness is often, although not always, the initial motivation for the eating restraint which seems to be the necessary way into anorexia nervosa. Most slimmers give up restraint in the face of their bodies' regulatory responses. This is the arguably healthy 'what the hell; it's not worth it' response. For some reason those people with the potential to become anorexic persist and become caught up in what seems like a series of vicious circles. For whatever reason, the more the person tries to control his or her eating and weight, the more potentially out of control these issues feel and the more frightening seems the option of, in any sense, letting go. His or her ideas become more extreme. The person feels worse about him- or herself. He or she comes to feel like the driver of a car stuck with a foot flat down on both the accelerator and the brake. Too often it feels as though everyone else just wants to give him or her a push. Of course, the person needs to get moving – but simply pushing may make matters worse.

Assessment and engagement

The assessment involves more than just making the diagnosis. This chapter assumes that a diagnosis has been made and will discuss what management may appropriately follow. However, management begins within the context of the assessment interviews. It is important to remember that the patient is assessing the clinician every bit as much as the clinician is assessing the patient. Does the clinician seem knowledgeable, confident and trustworthy? Does he or she feel understood? Does he or she feel safer or more threatened as a result of the interview? How things proceed may depend on the patient's answers to these questions. The conclusions which he or she reaches are likely to be influenced by the way in which the assessment is conducted.

Anorexia nervosa is a disorder of fearful mixed feelings. Its management needs to take this into account from the beginning. Personally, I always start off the first assessment interview by asking the patient what he or she feels about coming along. This gives an opportunity for the expression of what are usually quite complicated feelings about the consultation. If the patient expresses only clear antipathy or resentment at having been pushed by others into coming along, I offer him or her the opportunity of opting out of the consultation. However, in several hundred such first interviews, only one sufferer has ever taken up my offer and she returned within a few weeks. Making the offer can change the nature of the interview and at least creates an early chance to explore any hostility and ambivalence.

Diagnostic issues

Apart from the diagnosis of the eating disorder itself, there is a need to consider both Axis I and II comorbidity. This does not involve much that is out of the ordinary. The important thing is to make the usual mental state examination even if the main diagnosis is evident and unequivocal. However, assessment of the more specific psychopathology and behaviours does require the clinician to ask

questions which would not be routinely explored in such detail. Likewise, the usual history should be supplemented with greater attention to issues of weight and eating even before the onset of frank disorder (see Box 1).

Assessment of special issues

Some issues require special attention in the assessment of someone with anorexia nervosa:

(a) Lifetime weight history, especially highest ever and premorbid stable weight. Premorbidly obese subjects may have difficulty sustaining an average weight without undue restraint. There may be no premorbid stable weight in an individual who has been eating-disordered (or has been slimming) since their teenage years. It is useful to ask what weight the person would prefer to be if they had a magic wand which erased problems of weight control.
(b) History of eating restraint.
(c) Use of abnormal weight control methods: vomiting, laxatives, diuretics, etc.
(d) Presence or absence of bingeing. Full bingeing involves eating larger quantities of food than would be expected in the particular circumstances and with a subjective sense of loss of control. Sometimes anorexia nervosa sufferers report any lapse from their habitual tight control as a binge.
(e) Ideas of loss of control of weight and eating.
(f) Disturbance of body image.
(g) Use of exercise as a method of attempted weight control.
(h) Beliefs about weight control and 'healthy eating'.

Various questions and standardised interviews are available for the assessment of these kinds of issues. However, they do not replace the clinical interview in practice. A brief review of such methods can be found in Garner (1995).

While listening to the history it is almost impossible not to entertain ideas as to why the patient has developed an eating disorder. How has weight and eating control come to be so tangled up with the person's sense of self-worth and self-control? What has undermined his or her self-esteem? Why has this person developed this illness at this time? What has it been like to be this person and to lead his or her life? And so on. It is important to think up possible answers to such questions. For instance, a history of childhood sexual abuse may be relevant. It is even more important to keep an open mind and not to be too convinced that one has the real answers. It is useful to generate hypotheses, or stories, as this

---

Box 1. Diagnostic issues

Assessment should include attention to the following:

Diagnosis of the eating disorder
Diagnosis of Axis I comorbidity
Diagnosis of Axis II comorbidity – especially obsessional traits or borderline personality disorder
Detection of physical complications
Description of the context of the illness
What 'story' can be told about the illness?

can aid understanding and empathy. But to elevate your favoured story to the status of 'the truth' about the matter is to risk being damagingly wrong.

It may often be useful to seek a collateral history from the patients' family or some other relevant informant. Some authorities frame the whole assessment within a family interview on the grounds that anorexia nervosa is best viewed as a product of a derailed adolescent development within the family (Crisp, 1980). While there is much to be said for this view, it is not always possible to work in this way. For instance, the patient may clearly want to present himself or herself alone. Issues of separation and individuation may be central and an important focus. However, these can be addressed in relation to the joint decision of the patient and the clinician as to whether to involve the family in the assessment and subsequent therapy.

Assessment needs to include the physical state of the patient. An obvious aspect of this is the act of weighing the patient. This may seem to be a simple matter. Often it is. Sometimes, however, the patient is reluctant to be weighed or even refuses. This faces the clinician with a dilemma. Is it better to push the matter and risk seeming to make weight 'too important', or worse, getting into a fight? Or is going along with not weighing the patient not only missing out on gaining important information, but also somehow unhelpfully endorsing the patients' fearful avoidance? A way forward is to use the situation as an opportunity to explore the patient's feelings and ideas about weight and the dilemmas which he or she is facing. Framed in this way the act of weighing can come to be a part of both assessment and engagement, perhaps even of therapy.

Physical assessment

Anorexia nervosa has a significant mortality from physical complications as well as from suicide. Initial assessment should include the physical state. Furthermore, there is a need for continued monitoring throughout treatment. There are many potential complications. The following are some pieces of general advice:

(a) Sufferers who are at a very low weight (BMI <15), feel weak or complain of physical symptoms should usually be examined and have an ECG as part of their initial assessment.

(b) Blood tests are indicated for almost all patients. Electrolyte disturbance, especially hypokalaemia, and dehydration are common in sufferers who vomit or misuse laxatives or diuretics. Potassium supplements may be

required as a first aid measure. Anaemia may occur. Moderate leucopenia is common and tends to remit with weight gain. Plasma proteins may be low.

(c) The results of the physical assessment should be discussed with the patient. Most of the physical complications are reversible consequences of the sufferer's behaviour. He or she needs an honest account of his or her current state and future prospects. Information helps the patient to define his or her dilemma. However, attempts to scare a person into changing are rarely successful. Osteoporosis may be less reversible although the optimal management to avoid or contain this problem is unclear.

(d) Oedema can be an alarming consequence of refeeding. This seems to occur especially in patients who misuse laxatives. The mechanism is unclear. Fluid retention may lead to weight gain of several kilogrammes over a few days, which can be extremely alarming to the sufferer. The condition is usually self-limiting but potassium-sparing diuretics may be required.

Useful reviews of the physical aspects of eating disorders, including the rarer complications, can be found in Sharp & Freeman (1993) and Treasure & Szmuckler (1995).

Brokerage of responsibility

Characteristically the anorexia nervosa sufferer has mixed feelings about his or her condition. He or she may feel in control but precariously so. He or she does not want to be as he or she is but at the same time he or she is wary at best (and terrified at worst) of the prospect of change. Any change seems to carry the risk of everything getting out of control, although this may be spoken of in terms of weight gain and fatness. He or she feels threatened not only by others' efforts to change him or her but also by his or her own urge to eat. The management of anorexia nervosa involves the management of such mixed feelings and the proper brokerage of responsibility. In my view, it is in this matter that things most commonly go wrong.

The transaction between doctor (or other clinician) and patient can become derailed easily. The person suffering from anorexia nervosa may provoke considerable anxiety in those around him or her. He or she may push one half of his or her mixed feelings onto someone who is sufficiently worried about him or her to fulfil that role. This may be the doctor, especially in severe cases. Then doctor and patient may come together to do battle. The patient is relieved of much of the internal struggle and can simply resist the change which is being thrust upon him or her. On the other hand, the doctor feels obliged to fight to overcome this resistance if the patient is to be saved. The most detached of clinicians may behave like a finger-wagging parent comforted by the feeling that the best is being done for a difficult patient. The whole business can come to have something of the character of a poker game. Each side 'ups the ante'. The patient refuses to eat at all and the doctor issues increasingly dire warnings and threats. It is possible that some of the disasters which occur in the management of anorexia nervosa can be understood as the tragic consequence of such interactions played out to the bitter end. It is better to avoid such battles (see Box 2).

Another trap involves the doctor and the patient slipping into a collusion around the idea that they need to get beyond the issue of weight and eating and tackle what are usually described as the underlying problems, using the metaphor of depth. Of course, this is in a sense true. However, to act as if weight and eating are not important (or only symbolically so) is to ignore something crucial. I prefer the metaphor of entanglement of weight and eating with personal issues because it avoids placing one side in a more basic position, which seems inevitable with language employing the idea of depth. Certainly, it is possible for therapist and patient to spend hours just talking around the wider issues without touching upon the tangles which entrap the sufferer. This too is better avoided.

Assessment usually culminates in the offer of a treatment plan. The tasks of recovery are the same, whatever help is offered (Box 3). There is a need for clinician and patient to find a common language in which to discuss them. Elsewhere, I have suggested one useful way of talking but there are clearly many

ways of doing this (Palmer, 1989). There may be room for compromise about some details but 'fudge' in response to the patient's ambivalence is not helpful. It is usually best if such ambivalence is explicit rather than acted out. The patient is faced with real choices. He or she can opt not to change or to change only a little. Except in rare circumstances his or her wish not to have active treatment should be respected. If someone does not want to change it is usually best not to press the matter too hard, but rather to remain in touch and keep the matter under review and the option of treatment open. People who are not chased rarely run away and often come to accept help when they feel less panicky about the prospect.

Treatment

The treatment of anorexia nervosa is rationally directed at all three tasks of recovery (see Box 3). A treatment package that omits attention to one or more task is unlikely to be optimal. This is an assertion based on principle and experience. It is unfortunately the case that there is only a limited base of relevant treatment trials. Furthermore much of the evidence that exists relates mainly to the promotion of weight gain (task one) and is short-term in a disorder which is usually chronic and notoriously subject to relapse. There is no evidence that drug treatments are helpful in changing weight or the core psychopathology of anorexia nervosa. They may have some role in the treatment of some symptoms (e.g. metoclopramide for bloating) and comorbidity.

Task one

If the anorexia nervosa sufferer is to eat more and gain weight he or she must overcome the feeling that everything will get out of control if he or she does so. Treatment needs to promote a situation in which he or she can feel safe enough to do this. For the majority of sufferers, out-patient contact suffices for this (Crisp *et al*, 1991). It is difficult to be sure which characteristics of this contact promote such a sense of safety. The research literature does not help much. I believe that the patient needs consistent and regular conversation with someone who seems to be confident and recognises the nature of his or her dilemma. Simply feeling understood may sometimes be enough to shift the balance in favour of change.

The sessions need to be predictable. Weekly meetings are usual to start with. Regular weighing by the therapist, diary keeping, encouraging a pattern to eating and advice about what to eat are

---

Box 2. Management of mixed feelings

Remember that the dilemma belongs to the patient

Give the patient information

Offer the patient ways forward and out of his or her disorder

Don't 'fudge' the issues

Allow the patient real choice about whether to try to change

Remain in touch even if help is initially rejected

> **Box 3. The tasks of recovery**
>
> However it is achieved, recovery from anorexia nervosa may be thought of as the accomplishment of three tasks:
>
> (a) Restoration of a weight that is normal, healthy and sustainable and a regular pattern of eating. This weight is usually an average one (BMI 18–25). People who have been obese may need to stabilise at a higher weight if they are to live without undue eating restraint
>
> (b) Disentanglement of ideas about weight and eating from wider personal issues such as self-esteem
>
> (c) Making progress with regard to such wider issues and problems. Problems of living and so on are seldom if ever fully 'sorted out' but once freed from the entanglement with weight and eating, life can move on again

further techniques. The last of these can come to be overemphasised. The patient may try to lead the conversation into prolonged negotiation about what to eat because of his or her anxieties. The therapist needs to give advice and structure but will often need also to edge the conversation toward more direct discussion of these anxieties and away from the details of diet. The skill lies in using the particular situation as a way of looking with the patient at the links with wider personal issues.

Detailed dietary advice, perhaps from a dietician, sometimes has a place. However, it is usually robust common sense about diet which is lacking in the patient's thinking. Most of the difficulties which arise are of a kind that require psychological rather than dietetic expertise. What is required is a mixed diet which is increased at a pace which is manageable for the patient. It is sensible to give vitamin supplements to chronically malnourished subjects.

Weight gain that is faster than a kilogramme, or at most two, per week is too fast once initial dehydration is rectified. It cannot be sustained and is likely be frightening. It raises the possibility that the patient is bingeing. Is he or she stuffing him- or herself in the hope of being let off some perceived hook? Families may need to be advised against constantly nagging the sufferer or tempting him or her to eat with favourite foods.

Weight gain that is slow or absent in the face of apparently adequate intake raises the question of the hidden use of vomiting, laxatives or diuretics. It is best to raise this suspicion and discuss the matter openly. It may be best to encourage the patient to eat only what he or she is willing to retain. Most patients can give up these behaviours when they resolve to do so. High doses of laxatives, for example, over 30 senna per day, are best tailed off in a stepwise fashion over a month or so. Repeated monitoring of urea and electrolytes is indicated in an unstable situation.

Some treatment plans seek to keep the supervision and promotion of weight gain separate from the exploration of wider personal issues. The patient might be provided with what amounts to two therapists, one who talks about eating and weight and one who talks about other matters in a more traditionally psychotherapeutic way. While I am sure that this can work if it is done with confidence, I see little advantage in it in the out-patient setting. It can promote splitting and furthermore may miss the little opportunities to explore the all important links between these two sets of issues which the one-therapist model allows.

In-patient treatment

In usual psychiatric practice, perhaps a third of sufferers will not make any progress with out-patient treatment alone. The patient feels stuck and too unsafe to allow change to occur. In these circumstances, it will be necessary to consider offering a more intensive treatment. This usually means hospital admission, although special day programmes are being developed and may be an alternative option (Freeman & Newton, 1992). The patient herself will be faced with the difficult choice of whether or not to accept admission. Only in exceptional circumstances should the adult patient be relieved of this decision. Indeed, the more the whole undertaking is discussed and the more the patient commits to the treatment plan before admission, the more likely things are to go smoothly after admission.

Indications for in-patient treatment

Admission to hospital should be considered under the following circumstances:

(a) If the physical status of the patient is such as to cause immediate danger to life.

(b) If suicide risk or comorbidity warrants admission.

(c) If no adequate out-patient treatment is available.

(d) If the patient has failed to progress with appropriate out-patient help.

Compulsory admission under a section of the Mental Health Act can be justified in either the first or second circumstance. However, detention for the treatment of anorexia nervosa alone is indicated only very rarely. It should usually be considered only in relation to admission to a specialist service and then in a small minority of cases.

Tasks two and three

The more specific aspects of psychotherapeutic treatment (see Box 4) aimed at helping with tasks two and three are usually best delivered in a one to one therapy session, on at least a weekly basis. When in-patient care is involved, it is ideal if the same therapist is able to see the patient before, during and after admission. However, in the context of admission there is a need to avoid undue splitting between the designated therapist and the rest of the team. The therapist needs to be seen to be a party to the in-patient enterprise and the ward staff need to be psychotherapeutically aware. Sometimes formal therapy is delayed until after in-patient weight restoration. Unfortunately, this is the pattern that has been employed in some research projects as a way of simplifying the design. They can therefore throw no light on whether this timing is optimal. My guess is that it is not.

As with any psychotherapy, sessions should be regular and predictable. The need to combine what might be called a degree of 'physicianly concern' (whatever the discipline of the therapist) with other more traditional psychotherapeutic skills means that the role demands flexibility and confidence. It also demands persistence since the whole process of recovery takes months and years even when it goes well. This can cause real problems when the patient lasts longer than the therapist, for example, if a junior doctor is assigned to that role. Non-medical therapists need the back-up of a doctor.

The style of therapy offered to anorexia nervosa patients varies. Unfortunately there is little in the literature which offers clear guidance. Provided the issue of weight and eating is not avoided, psychodynamically informed therapy and cognitive–behavioural therapy (CBT) seem equally appropriate. Neither can convincingly claim superiority (Garner & Garfinkel, 1997). The systematic evaluation of therapies which has made considerable progress in the field of bulimia nervosa has yet to occur to the same degree in the admittedly more difficult matter of the treatment of anorexia nervosa.

One clear finding from the first of an important series of psychotherapy research projects from the

> **Box 4. Most in-patient regimes should have the following characteristics**
>
> The patient should have real and informed choice about admission
>
> The regime and its aims should be worked out before admission
>
> These aims should include a target weight for the admission. The ultimate target should be restoration of a sustainable weight within the normal range
>
> There should be clear control of both the lower and the upper limit of what the patient is expected to eat. The patient needs to feel that it is safe to let go some of his or her own internal control because the regime will stop him or her from over-eating. All relevant staff need to understand this counterintuitive imperative and resist 'stuffing' the patient
>
> The whole regime should be predictable and 'safe' for the patient. The use of tight behavioural regimes in which weight gain is rewarded by increasing privileges after initial deprivation has been shown to have no advantages and can feel punitive
>
> 'Fights' should be avoided by allowing the patient to leave and think again about admission. The corollary of such a policy should be that the clinician remains willing to keep in touch with the patient and to continue to offer appropriate treatment opportunities including re-admission

Institute of Psychiatry (Dare & Eisler, 1995) relates to the superiority of family interventions for patients with an onset of disorder before age 18. This study compared the experimental therapies over the year after in-patient weight restoration (Russell et al, 1987). Family therapy was compared with individual supportive psychotherapy. In a further study of adolescent out-patients (Dare et al, 1990), family therapy was found to be comparable with 'family counselling' in which the patient and the family were seen separately. In both family interventions there was an emphasis upon helping the family take responsibility for feeding the patient; an approach which may be relevant only for young sufferers. There was also an avoidance of blaming the family; an unfortunate feature of some family therapies. In the first study, the differences in favour of family therapy were still evident after five years.

Psychiatric complications and comorbidity

People suffering from anorexia nervosa are often distressed and even suicidal. Sometimes they show all of the features of a major depression. Such depression may limit their capacity to appraise and change their situation. It may require treatment with antidepressant medication or occasionally with electroconvulsive therapy. The decision as to when to offer such treatments for comorbid depression is familiar territory for any psychiatrist. Of course, some degree of depression in the broadest sense is both understandable and appropriate. Indeed, anyone who is happy within his or her anorexia nervosa is unlikely to change.

Obsessional symptoms, alcohol or drug misuse, overdosing, self-cutting and other forms of self-harm often occur in people in treatment for anorexia nervosa. Such problems deserve assessment and intervention in their own terms and along lines which would be appropriate for other patients. The problem is to keep sight of all of the issues at once. It is rarely the case that treating a comorbid problem will lead the anorexia nervosa to remit. When present in its full form anorexia nervosa is usually the most persistent of a mixed Axis I psychopathology (Schork *et al*, 1994).

The most common mixture of other issues is of problems of personality and interpersonal relationships. Sometimes these amount to a diagnosable Axis II disorder. The important task is to seek to disentangle these issues from weight and eating control and not to allow the attempt to treat the disorder to emphasise still further such entanglement.

Chronicity

Anorexia nervosa is commonly a chronic disorder. Some people become firmly stuck within it. However, both clinical experience and research suggest that full recovery can occur even after many years (Herzog *et al*, 1992). No sufferer should be thought to have no chance to change. Nevertheless some people feel that the best they can manage is to live some sort of life within, and despite, the disorder. In such cases, the clinician needs to give support while keeping the door open for more ambitious treatment. Simply keeping in touch may be valuable (Yager, 1995).

Conclusions

The management of anorexia nervosa is never a straightforward matter of applying particular treatments. It involves the construction and use of an appropriate treatment alliance with the patient. Because of the fears and mixed feelings of the anorexia nervosa sufferer, building and maintaining this alliance can be a tricky business. The most commonly missing ingredient is probably clinician confidence rather than competence. There are real problems of generalisation from the limited research findings to ordinary clinical practice. Thus, it would be inappropriate to conclude that all younger anorexia nervosa sufferers are always best treated by any family therapy, or that because there are indications that a specialist day programme may be effective attending any general day hospital would achieve the same. The clinician must decide what is 'the best buy' locally rather than seeking to apply the headline messages of research in the manner of someone consulting a cookery book. This is not to disparage the available findings but rather to suggest that the small quantity of good research limits the confidence with which the results can be appropriately generalised.

It is a conundrum of service provision whether the interests of people with eating disorders are best promoted by the creation of specialist services or by making the treatment of anorexia the task of every psychiatric team. Almost certainly some kind of compromise is optimal in which improvement of general service combines with continuing specialist services for severe cases (Eating Disorders Association, 1995). The conundrum for the general psychiatrist considering the individual patient concerns when to seek more specialist help if things are not going well. At present, the provision of special services is patchy and haphazard.

References

American Psychiatric Association (1994) *Diagnostic and Statistical Manual of Mental Disorders* (DSM–IV)(4th edn). Washington, DC: APA.

Crisp, A. H. (1980) *Anorexia Nervosa: Let Me Be*. London: Academic Press.

——, Norton, K., Gowers, S., *et al* (1991) A controlled study of the effect of therapies aimed at adolescent and family psychopathology in anorexia nervosa. *British Journal of Psychiatry*, **159**, 325–333.

Dare, C., Eisler, I., Russell, G. F. M., *et al* (1990) The clinical and theoretical impact of a controlled trial family therapy in anorexia nervosa. *Journal of Marital and Family Therapy*, **16**, 39–57.

––– & ––– (1995) Family therapy. In *Handbook of Eating Disorders: Theory, Treatment and Research* (eds G. Szmuckler, C. Dare & J. Treasure), pp. 333–349. Wiley: New York.

Eating Disorders Association (1995) *Eating Disorders – A Guide for Purchasing and Providing Services.* Norwich: EDA.

Freeman, C. P. & Newton, J. R. (1992) Anorexia nervosa: what treatments are effective? In *Practical Problems in Clinical Psychiatry* (eds K. Hawton & P. Cowen), pp. 77–92. Oxford: Oxford University Press.

Garner, D. M. (1995) Measurement of eating disorder psychopathology. In *Eating Disorders and Obesity; A Comprehensive Handbook* (eds K. D. Brownell & C. G. Fairburn), pp. 117–121. New York: Guilford.

––– & Garfinkel, P. E. (1997) *Handbook of Treament for the Eating Disorders* (2nd edn). New York & London: Guilford.

Herzog, W., Deter, H-C. & Vandereycken, W. (1992) *The Long Term Course of Eating Disorders.* Berlin: Springer Verlag.

Lask, B. & Bryant-Waugh, R. (1993) *Childhood-Onset Anorexia Nervosa and Related Eating Disorders.* Hove: Erlbaum.

Palmer, R. L. (1989) The spring story: a way of talking about clinical eating disorder. *British Review of Anorexia Nervosa and Bulimia,* **3**, 13–16.

Russell, G. F. M., Szmuckler, G., Dare, C., *et al* (1987) An evaluation of family therapy in anorexia nervosa and bulimia nervosa. *Archives of General Psychiatry,* **44**, 1047–1056.

Schork, E. J., Eckert, E. D. & Halmi, K. A. (1994) The relationship between psychopathology, eating disorder diagnosis and clinical outcome at 10 year follow up in anorexia nervosa. *Comprehensive Psychiatry,* **35**, 113–123.

Sharp, C. W. & Freeman, C. P. L. (1993) The medical complications of anorexia nervosa. *British Journal of Psychiatry,* **162**, 452–462.

Treasure, J. & Szmuckler, G. (1995) Medical complications of chronic anorexia nervosa. In *Handbook of Eating Disorders; Theory, Treatment and Research* (eds G. Szmuckler, C. Dare & J. Treasure), pp. 197–220. Chichester: Wiley.

World Health Organization (1992) *The Tenth Revision of the International Classification of Diseases and Realated Health Problems.* (ICD–10). Geneva: WHO.

Yager, J. (1995) The management of patients with intractable eating disorders. In *Eating Disorders and Obesity; A Comprehensive Handbook* (eds K. D. Brownell & C. G. Fairburn), pp. 374–378. New York: Guilford.

The management of bulimia nervosa and other binge eating problems

Christopher G. Fairburn

This chapter is about the management of eating disorders in which binge eating is a prominent feature. These disorders include bulimia nervosa, the most common eating disorder, and 'binge eating disorder', a provisional new diagnosis included in DSM–IV (American Psychiatric Association, 1994). In addition, binge eating is seen in anorexia nervosa and in many atypical eating disorders.

Until recently, there was confusion over what constitutes a 'binge'. In general usage the term does not have a truly specific meaning; indeed, over the years dictionary definitions have changed. The *Oxford English Dictionary* traces the use of 'binge' back to the mid-19th century when it referred to "a heavy drinking bout, hence a spree", and this remains one of its meanings today. Only more recently has the word been applied to eating. Nowadays dictionaries refer to overeating, and the term 'indulgence' may be used. However, these definitions neglect a central characteristic of binge eating, as seen in people with eating disorders; namely, the accompanying sense of loss of control. It is this loss of control over eating that distinguishes binge eating from everyday over-eating and gluttony.

Technically, binges (or bulimic episodes) have two essential features: first, a large amount of food is eaten; and second, there is an associated sense of loss of control. Hence the DSM–IV definition:

"An episode of binge-eating is characterized by both of the following:

(1) eating, in a discrete period of time (e.g. within any two-hour period), an amount of food that is definitely larger than most people would eat during a similar period of time and under similar circumstances; and

(2) a sense of lack of control over eating during the episode (e.g. a feeling that one cannot stop eating or control what or how much one is eating)."

It is important to note that the evaluation of the amount eaten is contextual; that is, account is taken of what would be the usual quantity to eat under the circumstances. In clinical practice some patients are encountered whose binges involve the consumption of modest amounts of food, this being especially true of patients with anorexia nervosa. Such episodes do not fulfil the technical definition of a binge, although they may seem very similar. Sometimes they are referred to as 'subjective bulimic episodes' or 'subjective binges'. Table 1 shows the binge eating of a patient with bulimia nervosa.

Diagnostic characteristics

Figure 1 shows how binge eating problems are classified. The diagnostic criteria for the relevant eating disorders are described.

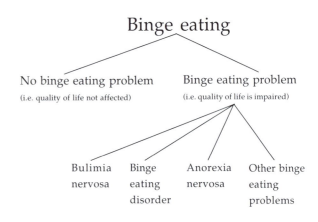

Fig. 1. The classification of binge eating. Adapted with permission from Fairburn, 1995.

Bulimia nervosa

Three features have to be present for someone to be said to have bulimia nervosa.

(a) The person must have frequent binges; that is, he or she must consume genuinely large amounts of food, taking into account the context in which the food is eaten, and the person must have a sense of loss of control at the time.

(b) The person must regularly use one of a variety of extreme measures for controlling shape or weight. These measures include self-induced vomiting, misusing laxatives or diuretics, overexercising and intense dieting or fasting.

(c) The person must be excessively concerned about his or her shape or weight or both. There should be an intense fear of fatness or weight gain, and self-worth should be judged largely or even exclusively in terms of shape or weight.

There is one other requirement; the person should not have anorexia nervosa. In effect, this means that the person should not be significantly underweight. In practice, the great majority of people with bulimia nervosa have a weight that is in the normal range.

Binge eating disorder

People with binge eating disorder have repeated binges in the absence of the extreme measures to control shape and weight that characterise bulimia nervosa (item 'b' above). In the past they have sometimes been called 'compulsive overeaters'. Among patient samples, many such people are overweight.

Anorexia nervosa

Three features must be present for someone to be said to have anorexia nervosa:

(a) The person should be significantly underweight, and this should be the result of his or her own efforts. A widely used weight threshold is being more than 15% below the expected weight for the person's age, gender and height.

(b) (Females only.) Should not be menstruating (unless she is taking an oral contraceptive).

(c) The person should be highly concerned about his or her shape or weight or both. However,

Table 1. Binge eating of a patient with bulimia nervosa: illustration of a food monitoring record that would be completed by the patient. B, binge; V, vomit; L, laxative. Adapted with permission from Fairburn, 1995

Time	Food and liquid consumption	Place	B	V/L	Comments
7.35	1 grapefruit	Kitchen			Feel really fat
	1 cup black coffee	Kitchen			
11.10	1 apple	Work			
3.15	2 Twix, 1 bread roll	High st.	*		
3.30	1 fruitcake, 2 chocolate eggs	Market	*		Everyone looked at me in the market. I'm out of control.
	2 bread rolls, ½ pint milk	Kitchen	*	V	I hate myself.
5.10	2 bowls cereal, 1 pita bread	Kitchen	*		I can't stop crying.
	with cottage cheese		*		
	1 glass water	Kitchen			
6.00	1 baked potato, 1 can Tab	Van outside	*	V	
9.00	1 cup slimline soup, ice cube	Kitchen			Weighed myself. 9st 7lb too heavy. Feel fat and ugly.
9.50	1 cup coffee	Kitchen			
10.00	1 coffee (black)	Sitting room			
11.20	1 coffee (black)	Kitchen	*		Why do I do this? I want to be thin.
	6 shortbread biscuits		*	V	
	4 pieces of chocolate		*	V	I can't help it.
	2 pieces of toast				
	2 glasses of water				Weighed 9st 7lb – fat.
				L	Took 24 Nylax.

rather than worrying about being under-weight, the person should be afraid of gaining weight. As in bulimia nervosa, self-worth should be judged largely or even exclusively in terms of shape or weight. People with anorexia nervosa are sometimes said to have a morbid fear of fatness and their dieting may be said to be driven by a relentless pursuit of thinness. These attitudes to shape and weight are similar to those found in bulimia nervosa.

The scale of the problem

Since 1980, there have been numerous studies of the prevalence of binge eating (for a review see Fairburn & Beglin, 1990). These studies have mainly focused on women aged between 14 and 40 years, as they are thought to be most at risk, and the majority have collected their data by asking subjects to complete simple pencil-and-paper questionnaires. They have found that many young women report "binge eating". Indeed, across the studies, over one-third do so and about 15% report that they binge at least weekly. For a number of reasons, these figures must be questioned. One is that most studies have not used the formal definition of a binge (described above). Instead, many have simply asked questions like "Do you binge?" and have then taken subjects' responses more or less at face value. As a result, the figures are more likely to reflect those for any form of perceived overeating, rather than true binge eating. Another problem is that over one-half of the studies have focused on female students and often those enrolled at prestigious American universities. Such subjects are unlikely to be representative of young women in general, who may have different rates of binge eating.

What is needed are studies in which representative general population samples are recruited and assessed by standardised interview, since such interviews are regarded as the best way of assessing binge eating (see Wilson, 1993). There has been one study of this type (based in Oxfordshire) and it found that among women aged between 16 and 35 years, 10% had at least monthly binges and 3% were binge eating at least weekly. These figures are much lower than those obtained using self-report questionnaires but they are likely to be more valid. There are no comparable data on the prevalence of binge eating among men or women outside the 16–35 year age range.

Of the 3% or so of young women who binged at least once a week, about one-half had bulimia

nervosa, a very small proportion had anorexia nervosa and most of the remainder fulfilled the criteria for the new diagnosis of binge eating disorder.

Management of bulimia nervosa

In the relatively short time since bulimia nervosa was first described, much has been learned about its treatment: indeed, over the past decade bulimia nervosa has been one of the most intensively studied psychiatric disorders.

In-patient treatment

Both clinical experience and research evidence indicate that the great majority of patients may be managed on an out-patient basis. The few indications for admission are: depression of such severity that out-patient treatment is not possible, poor physical health (for example, severe electrolyte disturbance), and the failure of appropriate out-patient treatment.

When hospitalisation is necessary, it should always be viewed as a preliminary to out-patient care. In most cases the goal of hospitalisation should be simply to correct the problem that is preventing out-patient treatment, be it the patient's physical state or their level of depression. Once this has been done arrangements may be made for treatment proper to start on an out-patient basis. Clinicians should not be misled by the improvements that usually occur on admission to hospital: they merely reflect the influence of the hospital environment and rarely do they persist following discharge.

There is no consensus regarding the best way to manage those patients who are hospitalised as a result of the failure of appropriate out-patient treatment. Lacey (1995) advocates a multi-faceted approach incorporating behavioural and psychodynamic elements, whereas Tuschen & Bents (1995) have described an intensive cognitive–behavioural approach.

Out-patient treatment

Antidepressant drugs

The only pharmacological treatment to have shown promise is the use of antidepressant drugs. Controlled trials indicate that over a matter of weeks these drugs produce, on average, a 50–60% reduction in the frequency of binge eating, together with a substantial decrease in the level of associated psychiatric symptoms (see Wilson & Fairburn, 1998). No single antidepressant drug seems to be superior to any of the others, nor do the patients have to be depressed to benefit. Unfortunately, the changes generally do not last. For example, Walsh *et al* (1991) found that of the 41% of their sample who had responded sufficiently well to justify continuing taking the antidepressant drug desipramine, almost one-third (29%) relapsed over the following three months. It is only a minority of these patients who obtain enduring benefit from antidepressant drugs. This is probably because the drugs fail to moderate the extreme and brittle dieting that is characteristic of bulimia nervosa and which is thought to maintain the binge eating.

Cognitive–behavioural therapy

The leading treatment for bulimia nervosa is a specific form of cognitive–behavioural therapy (CBT). This treatment is based on a cognitive view of the processes maintaining the disorder (Fairburn, 1997). According to this view (see Fig. 2) these patients' characteristically extreme concerns about shape and weight maintain the disorder through the influence of an extreme and rigid form of dieting. Various other vicious circles also operate, especially in those patients who attempt to compensate for their

binges by vomiting or misusing laxatives. CBT aims to disrupt these maintaining mechanisms through the use of a specific sequence of behavioural and cognitive procedures. A detailed description of the treatment has been published (Fairburn *et al*, 1993a) and Box 1 lists its main elements. Generally, the treatment involves about 20 sessions over four to five months. No single professional group is inherently best qualified to administer the treatment; for example, psychiatrists, clinical psychologists

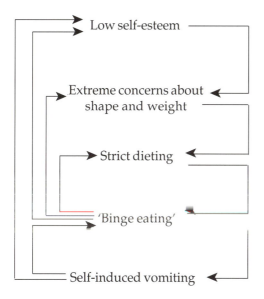

Fig. 2. The cognitive view of the maintenance of bulimia nervosa (adapted with permission from Fairburn *et al*, 1993a).

Box 1. The core elements of the cognitive–behavioural treatment for bulimia nervosa (adapted from Fairburn *et al*, 1993a).

Stage One
Presentation of the cognitive–behavioural view of the maintenance of bulimia nervosa
Establishing the self-monitoring of food and liquid intake and relevant cognitions
Education regarding body weight regulation, binge eating and the ineffectiveness of self-induced vomiting and laxative misuse as methods of weight control
Introduction of a pattern of regular eating
Use of alternative behaviour to help resist urges to binge

Stage Two
Cognitive restructuring applied to concerns about food, eating, shape and weight, and, where relevant, other general cognitive distortions (e.g. perfectionism, negative self-evaluation)
Use of procedures to erode the various forms of dieting, including the systematic introduction of avoided foods
Development of problem-solving skills to apply to difficulties which might otherwise trigger binges
Use of behavioural and cognitive procedures to tackle body-image misperception and body-image disparagement

Stage Three
Use of procedures to minimise the risk of relapse, including education to ensure that expectations are realistic and the formulation of a plan for use at times of difficulty

and nurse therapists are all equally appropriate. Nor is the therapist's gender necessarily relevant. Some patients might be better treated by a female therapist; others might be better treated by a male therapist. What is of far greater importance than gender is the therapist's overall level of competence at administering CBT.

CBT has been the focus of over 20 controlled treatment trials, the results of which have consistently supported its use. Three main findings have emerged from these studies (Wilson & Fairburn, 1998).

(a) CBT has a major beneficial effect on all aspects of the psychopathology of bulimia nervosa. There is a marked reduction (on average, about 80%) in the frequency of binge eating and associated vomiting and laxative misuse, a decrease in dietary restraint and lessening in the intensity of the patients' concerns about shape and weight. Associated with these changes is a decrease in the level of general psychiatric symptoms and an improvement in self-esteem and social functioning.

(b) The changes obtained with CBT appear to be well maintained. Although there is a definite need for further studies on the medium- to long-term outcome following CBT, the available data suggest that the changes are robust. Between one-half and two-thirds have an excellent outcome, which is well maintained over the following six months to one year. The one study of longer term outcome (mean (s.d.) length of follow-up 5.8 (2.0) years) found that two-thirds (63%) of the patients had no eating disorder and the great majority were functioning extremely well (Fairburn *et al*, 1995).

(c) CBT has been found to be superior to all but one of the treatments with which it has been compared. CBT has been compared with treatment with antidepressant drugs (and with antidepressant drugs and CBT combined), behavioural versions of CBT, exposure with response prevention, supportive expressive psychotherapy and interpersonal psychotherapy (IPT). It has been found to be superior to all these treatments, with the exception of IPT. Combining CBT and antidepressant drugs conveys no clear benefit.

Interpersonal psychotherapy

This is the one treatment that may be as effective as CBT. It is a short-term, focal psychotherapy developed by Klerman *et al* (1984) as a treatment for depression. The focus of the treatment is on helping patients identify and find solutions for current interpersonal problems. The one trial to have investigated IPT found that at the end of treatment it was less effective than CBT (Fairburn *et al*, 1991), but during follow-up the differences between the two treatments disappeared because of continuing improvement among the patients who received IPT (Fairburn *et al*, 1993*b*; 1995). Clinical experience suggests that IPT operates by improving interpersonal functioning, and thereby self-evaluation, which in turn results in a moderation of these patients' dependence upon shape and weight to evaluate their self-worth. As a result, weight control becomes of less importance to them, they diet less intensely and the eating disorder gradually erodes.

Before IPT can be recommended as an alternative to CBT it needs to be evaluated in further controlled trials. For the meantime, CBT must be regarded as the leading treatment for bulimia nervosa.

Simplified CBT

The main obstacle to the widespread use of CBT is the amount of therapist time that it takes. Training is less of an issue since CBT is not an unduly difficult treatment to master.

There is growing evidence that a subgroup of patients responds to simplified forms of CBT and that these treatments need not be administered by therapists with special training (for review see Carter & Fairburn, 1998). Of particular promise are the self-help books based on CBT. Two such books are available (Fairburn, 1995; Cooper, 1995), both of which are direct translations of the CBT for bulimia nervosa. Also, Schmidt & Treasure (1993) have published a more eclectic programme, which includes some elements of CBT. These books may be administered either on their own (pure self-help) or with guidance from a non-specialist therapist (guided self-help), the latter approach usually involving six to eight 20- to 30-minute sessions over three to four months. Clearly, pure self-help has the potential to be eminently disseminable but, not surprisingly, some patients have difficulty persevering with it. In contrast, adherence is generally good with guided self-help. However, it must be noted that the current enthusiasm for these simplified versions of CBT is outstripping the evidence supporting their effectiveness. The few studies to date have had important methodological shortcomings, the most significant being that there has been little attempt to study maintenance of change. This is an important limitation given the tendency of binge eating problems to run a chronic course.

Treatments for non-responders to CBT

CBT is far from being a panacea. In research trials (generally using secondary or tertiary referrals) between one-half and two-thirds of patients obtain a substantial and lasting benefit, but the remainder respond either partially or not at all. Accordingly, there is a need to develop other methods of treatment.

Wilson (1996) has reviewed the main alternatives to CBT. Antidepressant drugs and IPT are obvious options since both are established treatments in their own right. However, there is no *a priori* reason why they should benefit those who do not respond to CBT. Other alternatives include psychodynamic psychotherapy and family therapy. Once again, there is no reason to think that these treatments will succeed where CBT has failed. There has been just one controlled study of a psychodynamic treatment – supportive–expressive psychotherapy – and the results indicated that it was less effective than CBT (Garner *et al*, 1993). Similarly, a study of family therapy obtained disappointing results (Russell *et al*, 1987). In support of psychodynamic psychotherapy it is sometimes argued that it is particularly well suited to the treatment of patients with a coexisting personality disorder. Although it is certainly true that patients with severe personality disorders are over-represented among CBT non-responders, there is no evidence to suggest that psychodynamic psychotherapy is any more effective with this particular patient group.

Rather than replacing CBT with a different form of treatment, it is the author's view that there might be more to be gained by adapting CBT. Several possibilities suggest themselves. One would be to broaden the focus to address general issues such as self-esteem and interpersonal functioning. However, as Wilson (1996) points out, there is no evidence that 'broad' CBT is superior to a more focused approach, either with respect to this disorder or any other. Another possibility would be to incorporate features of Linehan's CBT for borderline personality disorder (Linehan, 1993). A third possibility would be to intensify the treatment in such a way as to ensure that adherence with key procedures is enhanced. It is common clinical experience that many people who do not respond to CBT have either failed to follow key assignments or have followed them to a limited extent. If their adherence were to be enhanced, the outcome might be improved. With this in mind, the cognitive–behavioural in-patient programme of Tuschen & Bents (1995) might have something to offer, especially since it could be adapted for use on a day patient or out-patient basis. Research on the best way to manage CBT non-responders is urgently needed.

Treatment of other binge eating disorders

Anorexia nervosa

In comparison with the large body of research on the treatment of bulimia nervosa, there has been little work on the treatment of the other disorders in which binge eating features. For example, comparatively little has been written on the management of those patients with anorexia nervosa who binge. (The management of anorexia nervosa is discussed in the previous chapter.) In my experience the best approach is to treat these patients in the same way as other people with anorexia, giving due priority to the need for weight gain. Once the patient's weight has been restored to a reasonable level, or earlier if need be, the binge eating may be addressed using procedures from CBT for bulimia nervosa.

Binge eating disorder

This disorder is attracting considerably more attention, particularly when it co-occurs with obesity. Not surprisingly, investigators are showing most interest in testing those treatments that have been shown to benefit patients with bulimia nervosa. Thus antidepressant drugs, CBT, IPT and cognitive–behavioural self-help have all been evaluated (Wilson & Fairburn, 1998). As in the treatment of bulimia nervosa, relapse appears to be a problem with the use of anti-depressant drugs. The outcome with CBT and IPT also seems disappointing, possibly because the studies have administered the treatment in a group rather than individual format. Much better results are being reported from a study from Pittsburgh in which CBT and a behavioural weight control programme were compared, both treatments being administered on a one to one basis. Substantial and sustained changes were obtained with both interventions and in the case of the behavioural weight control programme there was also significant weight loss. If this finding is confirmed, it would suggest that dietary/behavioural techniques alone may be sufficient to treat binge eating disorder, whereas their use is associated with relapse in bulimia nervosa. It is also of note that preliminary data from a trial evaluating cognitive–behavioural self-help suggest that a simple intervention of this type may also benefit some patients with binge eating disorder.

The notion of 'stepped care'

How can these research findings be implemented in routine clinical practice? It has been suggested that a 'stepped care' approach would be a logical way of managing many of these patients. In this approach, patients would be treated first with a simple treatment, and would move on to a more complex one only if they failed to respond. Two possibilities suggest themselves for the first step: either pure self-help or guided self-help. The research to date suggests that a worthwhile proportion would respond to one or other approach, although the stability of the response has not been established. Those who do not benefit from this initial intervention, or who make only temporary gains, would move on to the second step. In this case, full CBT would seem the most appropriate option. The choice of treatment for the third step is far from clear, given the uncertainty over how best to help CBT non-responders. At this point clinicians would need to rely on a trial-and-error approach.

References

American Psychiatric Association (1994) *Diagnostic and Statistical Manual of Mental Disorders* (4th edn) (DSM–IV). Washington, DC: APA.

Carter, J. C. & Fairburn, C. G. (1998) Cognitive–behavioural self-help for binge eating disorder: a controlled effectiveness study. *Journal of Consulting and Clinical Psychology*, **66**, 616–623.

Cooper, P. J. (1995) *Bulimia Nervosa and Binge-Eating: A Guide to Recovery*. London: Robinson.

Fairburn, C. G. (1995) *Overcoming Binge Eating*. New York: Guilford Press.

—— (1997) Eating disorders. In *Science and Practice of Cognitive Behaviour Therapy* (eds D. M. Clark & C. G. Fairburn), pp. 209–241. Oxford: Oxford University Press.

—— & Beglin, S. J. (1990) The studies of the epidemiology of bulimia nervosa. *American Journal of Psychiatry*, **147**, 401–408.

——, Jones, R., Peveler, R. C., *et al* (1991) Three psychological elements for bulimia nervosa: A comparative trial. *Archives of General Psychiatry*, **48**, 463–469.

——, Marcus, M. D. & Wilson, G. T. (1993*a*) Cognitive–behavioural therapy for binge eating and bulimia nervosa: A comprehensive treatment manual. In *Binge Eating: Nature, Assessment and Treatment* (eds C. G. Fairburn & G. T. Wilson), pp. 631–404. New York: Guilford Press.

——, Jones, R., Peveler, R. C., *et al* (1993*b*) Psychotherapy and bulimia nervosa: The long-term effects of interpersonal psychotherapy, behaviour therapy and cognitive behaviour therapy. *Archives of General Psychiatry*, **50**, 419–428.

——, Norman, P. A., Welch, S. L., *et al* (1995) A prospective study of outcome in bulimia nervosa and long-term effects of three psychological treatments. *Archives of General Psychiatry*, **52**, 304–312.

Garner, D. M., Rockert, W., Davis, R., *et al* (1993) Comparison of cognitive–behavioural and supportive–expressive therapy for bulimia nervosa. *American Journal of Psychiatry*, **150**, 37–46.

Klerman, G. L., Weissman, M. M., Rounsaville, B. J., *et al* (1984) *Interpersonal Psychotherapy of Depression*. New York: Basic Books.

Lacey, J. H. (1995) Inpatient treatment of multi-impulsive bulimia nervosa. In *Eating Disorders and Obesity: A Comprehensive Handbook* (eds K. D. Brownell & C. G. Fairburn), pp. 361–368. New York: Guilford Press.

Linehan, M. M. (1993) *Cognitive–Behavioural Treatment of Borderline Personality Disorder*. New York: Guilford Press.

Russell, G. F. M., Szmukler, G. I., Dare, F., *et al* (1987) An evaluation of family therapy in the treatment of anorexia nervosa and bulimia nervosa. *Archives of General Psychiatry*, **44**, 1047–1056.

Schmidt, U. & Treasure, J. (1993) *Getting Better Bit(e) by Bit(e)*. Hove: Lawrence Erlbaum.

Tuschen, B. & Bents, H. (1995) Intensive brief inpatient treatment of bulimia nervosa. In *Eating Disorders and Obesity: A Comprehensive Handbook* (eds K. D. Brownell & C. G. Fairburn), pp. 354–360. New York: Guilford Press.

Walsh, B. T., Hadigan, C. M., Devlin, M. J., *et al* (1991) Long-term outcome of antidepressant treatment for bulimia nervosa. *American Journal of Psychiatry*, **148**, 1206–1212.

Wilson, G. T. (1993) Assessment of binge-eating. In *Binge Eating: Nature, Assessment and Treatment* (eds C. G. Fairburn & G. T. Wilson), pp. 227–249. New York: Guilford Press.

—— (1996) Treatment of bulimia nervosa: When CBT fails. *Behaviour Research and Therapy*, **34**, 197–212.

—— & Fairburn, C. G. (1998) Eating disorder. In *A Guide to Treatments that Work* (eds P. E. Nathan & J. M. Gorman), pp. 501–530. New York: Oxford University Press.

Treatment of victims of trauma

Gwen Adshead

The psychiatric sequelae of trauma have been most often discussed in relation to disasters, both natural and man-made, and military conflict. This may sometimes lead psychiatrists to think of post-traumatic stress disorder (PTSD) and other post-traumatic mental illnesses as being somewhat exotic and unusual in general psychiatric practice. In this chapter, I propose that PTSD and related disorders are actually common psychiatric problems which require treatment.

The history of the concept will not be reviewed here; interested readers are referred to reviews by Trimble (1985) and Gersons & Carlier (1992). The problems of adult survivors of childhood trauma will not be discussed in detail here, but there are reasons for thinking that therapeutic approaches based on a PTSD model may sometimes be inappropriate. Concerning the specific problems of war veterans or children, readers are referred to the relevant chapters in textbooks such as Wilson & Raphael (1993).

Prevalence of post-traumatic disorders

The prevalence of PTSD and other disorders within a community will depend to some extent on the prevalence of traumatic events in the life of a community. Breslau et al (1991) found a prevalence of traumatic events of 39% in a heterogeneous community sample in the USA. Norris (1992) found a lifetime prevalence of traumatic events of 69%. Most common were bereavements by homicide, suicide or accident; least common was sexual assault.

Studies of prevalence of PTSD in the community have confirmed that PTSD is not a rare diagnosis. Two American studies suggest a lifetime prevalence rate of 1% for PTSD (Helzer et al, 1987; Breslau et al, 1991). The prevalence of chronic PTSD was 3.45% (Breslau et al, 1991). There are not yet any equivalent British studies; however,

the British Crime Survey of 1992 (Mayhew et al, 1993) found that over one million physical assaults were reported to the police. Between 500 and 600 people a year in England and Wales lose a relative by homicide, and 3000–4000 by fatal road traffic accidents in Britain. Although the level of criminal violence is lower here than in the USA, it is likely that the prevalence of PTSD within the British community may be similar to that of the USA. All psychiatric specialities may therefore expect to have to deal with PTSD and related disorders.

Normal responses to trauma

There is clearly nothing abnormal about feeling bad when bad things happen. It is equally clear that acute psychological stress reactions, however normal, are extremely distressing and uncomfortable. The best analogy is that of the fractured limb; the pain is entirely normal, but may be treated nonetheless. DSM–IV (American Psychiatric Association, 1994) and ICD–10 (World Health Organization, 1992) recognise acute stress reactions as diagnostic entities.

The features of acute stress reactions are described in Table 1. It is important to distinguish between normal stress reactions and PTSD. Both diagnoses have symptoms in common; for example, intrusive phenomena such as repetitive thoughts and nightmares. However, by 4–6 weeks, most acute stress reactions will be diminishing or much reduced. It appears that the majority of people surviving a traumatic event will make a spontaneous, if painful recovery. Only a minority will go on to develop PTSD and related disorders (about 25–40%; Green et al, 1990; Green, 1993). However, the subjective unpleasantness of acute stress reactions should not be underestimated, and clinicians may need to remind families of this. Recovery is the norm, but may be delayed where there is further stress.

Table 1.	Normal stress reactions after trauma
Time period	**Effects**
Anticipation phase (often not present)	Anticipatory anxiety/fear; denial
Immediate	Shock, numbness, disbelief Acute distress Dissociation and denial
Short-term (1–6 weeks)	High levels of arousal Intrusive phenomena of trauma: thoughts, flashbacks, nightmares Poor concentration Disturbed sleep, appetite, libido Irritability Persistent fear and anxiety, especially when reminded of trauma: leads to avoidance behaviour
Long-term (6 weeks to 6 months)	Features described above persist, but should decrease in intensity and frequency Increased avoidance behaviour Irritability is often most persistent Substance misuse is common as a way of managing arousal

DSM–IV criteria for acute stress disorder specify symptoms as not persisting for more than four weeks.

PTSD

Table 2 outlines the DSM–IV criteria for PTSD. The phrase "outside the range of usual human experience" has now been dropped from the definition. This is in part the result of research which suggests that the perception of fear and threat is crucial in the genesis of PTSD, so that PTSD is possible after events which are common but terrifying, such as road traffic accidents, or domestic violence (Walker, 1984; Mayou *et al*, 1993).

Risk factors for PTSD

Table 3 shows some of the risk factors for PTSD. Several studies have confirmed that the magnitude and degree of exposure to the stressor influence the

Table 2.	Criteria for post-traumatic stress disorder: DSM–IV (American Psychiatric Association, 1994)
Criterion	**Symptoms required to fulfil criterion**
A. The stressor criterion	Involves objective and subjective elements: 　(i) the person has been exposed to an event involving actual or threatened death, or serious injury, or threat to physical integrity of self or others 　(ii) the person's response involved intense fear, helplessness or horror
B. Intrusive phenomena	Persistent re-experiencing in at least one of five ways: intrusive recollections, dreams, flashbacks, psychological distress or physiological reaction when exposed to reminders of the trauma
C. Avoidance phenomena	At least three of seven ways of avoidance behaviour: e.g. avoidance of thoughts or feelings about trauma, amnesia, decreased interest, feelings of detachment
D. Hyperarousal phenomena	At least two of five possible symptoms: e.g. insomnia, irritability, poor concentration
E. Duration	At least one month
F. Impairment of social function	The symptoms must cause clinically significant distress or social dysfunction

Acute PTSD < 3 months duration; chronic PTSD > 3 months duration.

risk of developing PTSD. Previous personality traits, coping styles and experiences also influence the development of PTSD (McFarlane, 1988). There is evidence that those individuals with a pre-trauma psychiatric history are at increased risk of developing PTSD (Smith *et al*, 1990). Recent studies of soldiers suggest that those with histories of abuse in childhood are at increased risk of developing PTSD (Bremner *et al*, 1992). Although the adult sequelae of childhood trauma cannot be discussed here at any length, it is relevant to note that some workers have suggested that these problems may be conceptualised as chronic and 'complex' PTSD (Herman, 1992). In relation to crime, a previous history of victimisation increases the risk of developing PTSD. Once again, this suggests a complex interaction of constitutional responses to arousal, cognitive coping style and experience of new trauma.

The development of PTSD is therefore the complex result of the interaction of many factors. A clinical example I have seen makes the point. Five men were involved in a helicopter crash. Superficially, all were exposed to severe life-threatening trauma, involving grotesque imagery (a fellow passenger was decapitated and his mutilated remains spread over the crash site). On the basis of the nature of the trauma alone, one might expect all the survivors to develop PTSD. However, at 18 months post-trauma, only two of the five had failed to make a reasonable recovery after a normal stress response. Only one man developed PTSD. His subjective experience of the trauma was particularly unpleasant; there was also evidence that his pre-trauma personality put him at risk. The other man who failed to recover did not have PTSD, but instead was chronically anxious

in a way that severely affected his work performance. Each man's subjective account of the crash was different to the others, making the point that subjective experience interacts with objective severity to influence the development of psychopathology. It is therefore not possible to state that only extremes of trauma, or individual psychological vulnerability, lead to the development of PTSD. The relative contributions of both individual past and the traumatic experience need to be considered during assessment, and have implications for treatment choice.

Psychopathology and pathophysiology of PTSD

One of the principal debates about PTSD relates to whether PTSD is seen as an anxiety disorder or a mood disorder (Davidson & Foa, 1991). Other possible diagnostic categories are dissociative disorders, or a disorder of personality. The rationale for the various positions is detailed in Box 1.

Category definition has implications for treatment. Most treatment for PTSD is currently symptomatically based. The pathophysiology of PTSD remains relatively unclear, with research findings suggesting the involvement of the hypothalamic–pituitary axis (HPA), central monoamine regulation and endogenous opioids. In addition to the neurophysiological disturbances exhibited by patients with PTSD, there is also evidence of cognitive psychopathology, for

Table 3. Risk factors for PTSD	
Aspect of trauma	Risk factors
The stressor itself	Duration and magnitude of exposure to the stressor Stressors which: are sudden and/or occur with no warning; cause multiple loss of life; mutilate bodies or give rise to grotesque imagery; are caused by criminal violence, especially sexual
Experience during the trauma	When subject perceived life to be at real risk: "I thought I was going to die." Perceived uncontrollability of events, and helplessness Perception of grotesque imagery: especially of human remains, or of children Witnessing or carrying out atrocities, e.g. murder, torture
The individual subject	Previous psychiatric illness Previous neuroticism Previous exposure to trauma; especially childhood trauma Previous coping style Denial of trauma and/or avoidance
The post-traumatic environment	Denial of trauma by others or dismissal of experience: "not being believed"

Box 1. Models of psychopathology in PTSD

An anxiety disorder?
PTSD sufferers experience fear, anxiety and avoidance behaviour (like people with phobias)
Intrusive phenomena resemble obsessive–compulsive disorder phenomena
Introversion and neuroticism are common personality traits in both PTSD and anxious populations
Some patients improve with exposure therapy

A mood disorder?
Patients with PTSD experience sadness and grief, independent of bereavement
Comorbidity with depression is very common
Vegetative symptoms are very similar: loss of sleep, appetite, libido
Both groups experience avoidance, numbing and loss of interest

A dissociative disorder?
Flashbacks and amnesia are common in patients with dissociative disorder and PTSD

A personality disorder?
Considerable overlap of symptoms of PTSD with symptoms of borderline personality disorder
Some overlap of symptoms with those of antisocial personality disorder (e.g. antisocial behaviour, irritability)
Some evidence that trauma can induce personality change

A separate neurophysiological disorder?
Effects such as low monoamine oxidase activity, increased excretion of urinary beta-endorphin, therapeutic response to both serotonergic drugs, and drugs that affect the locus coeruleus, and HPA axis deregulation resulting in low cortisol levels

example, subjects with PTSD are more sensitive to percepts indicating threat, and respond more vigorously to such cues (Cassiday *et al*, 1992).

Other post-traumatic problems

It cannot be over-emphasised that PTSD is not the only problem that survivors of trauma face. 'Pure' PTSD after trauma is comparatively rare, and comorbidity is the norm. Depression is the most common co-diagnosis, and may be the most common post-traumatic disorder overall. Other post-traumatic psychiatric illnesses include anxiety disorders, such as panic disorder or phobic disorders. Full-blown PTSD is relatively uncommon, and partial PTSD may be more likely, particularly in a chronic form. Substance misuse may be the primary presenting problem, masking intrusive symptoms of PTSD. Marked changes in personality, in terms of personal interaction with others, may cause more problems than any of the other post-traumatic disorders, especially when this is accompanied by substance misuse or violent behaviour (Southwick *et al*, 1993).

As in general psychiatric practice, it is important to consider the influence of the patient's illness on other areas of his life, in relation to its effect on the process of recovery and the prognosis. The symptoms of many of the post-traumatic disorders may be troublesome for families and employers, particularly in the first 6–12 months after trauma. Patients may be chronically irritable and withdrawn for weeks on end, in a way which is alien to them and their families. Work performance deteriorates, but patients often find it impossible to discuss the reasons for this with their employers, who may not be sympathetic anyway. This is a particular problem when the trauma occurred at work (and compensation is being claimed), or where there is a work culture of denial of distress. Examples of this are the emergency or public services, and health care professionals. Even though the 'macho' culture is changing to some degree, especially within the emergency services, the process is slow, and patients may encounter hostility and rejection by their work-places.

Families, friends and employers are usually unfamiliar with the time-scale of normal recovery, let alone post-traumatic psychiatric illness. Most people do not realise that normal recovery may take six months, or longer if there are further stressors, and may become impatient with survivors who may be seen as being difficult or weak. Local social support often reduces as press reports of the trauma diminish, and it may seem, to health care professionals or family members, as though the trauma happened a long time ago. The pathology of PTSD, however, makes the trauma continually real to the survivor (Horowitz, 1973).

Many major personal disasters are never reported in the press at all. In peacetime, and between major disasters, the principal cause of traumatic stress responses is crime, of which the impact on the victim is rarely reported unless it is fatal (Kilpatrick *et al*, 1989). This applies to both men and women alike (Stanko & Hobdell, 1993). The best example of this is the plight of the families of murder victims. The killer is often a member of the family, and so relatives must cope with multiple losses. In one case known to me, a woman presented after her husband murdered their daughter. The killing took place to prevent the daughter from telling her mother about her father's 20-year affair with a family friend. This woman lost not only her daughter and her husband, she also lost her experience of her marriage and the support of a trusted friend. She was also without funds as the husband had been the principal earner, and she did not have access to the bank account. The trial did not take place for a year, and the funeral was delayed several times for post-mortem reports for both defence and prosecution. Other problems of families of murder victims are well described by other authors (Parkes, 1992; Black *et al*, 1993).

These social and legal aspects of post-traumatic dysfunction have a profound influence on the management and prognosis of PTSD, and can cause major setbacks in treatment. A man who becomes homeless because of domestic violence related to his post-traumatic irritability may be unable to cooperate, or tolerate a treatment programme which is quite taxing. In-patient treatment may be indicated for such patients. Patients with PTSD as a result of crime have particular problems. Not only may they be involved with reminders of the stressor, such as police identification parades or court appearances, they may be at continued risk of further trauma, such as threats from the defendant.

Assessment

The need for thorough assessment is particularly pressing for the post-traumatic disorders. It may not always be immediately apparent that the presenting complaint is post-traumatic in origin, and it is important to bear this possibility in mind. This is particularly so for victims of crime, especially sexual assault and domestic violence, who may find it difficult to tell others about their experiences, and who may not define their experience as a crime. There is some evidence that health care professionals do not ask enough about trauma, although there is evidence that patients do not resent this (Friedman *et al*, 1992). Patients suffering post-traumatic disorders may find it difficult to describe spontaneously their experiences, and appreciate a tactful enquiry. In addition, patients are frequently not referred to general practitioners (GPs) until some time after traumatic events, so that the importance of an event that may have taken place a year before may be overlooked.

Having enquired about trauma, the assessor must be prepared to hear the patient's account. This entails making enough time for the patient to do this comfortably. If a history of a trauma is already known at referral, then it may be helpful to suggest to patients that history-taking takes place in two stages: firstly, a general psychiatric history, and secondly, an account of the trauma and post-traumatic events. This gives the patients some warning, and allows them to prepare themselves, reducing anticipatory anxiety. If the trauma is disclosed *de novo*, and the patient wants to give an account of his experience, then it is important to allow this to take place. Patients with post-traumatic disorders are very sensitive to the understandable reluctance of others to hear their stories. It may be necessary to let the patient talk for a little time, then negotiate a time for the patient to return and for the assessment to continue.

What is not advisable is dismissing patients' disclosures of trauma. There is no evidence that patients benefit from being told to 'forget all about it' or 'put it out of your mind'. Intrusive phenomena which cannot be voluntarily excluded are characteristic of PTSD; patients are not actually capable of 'just forgetting'. Dismissal also gives a message to the patient that the health care professional does not want to hear, or does not believe what he is being told. Even in cases where the professional needs to maintain a true scepticism about the patient's account of events (such as in medico-legal work), this does not entail an unsympathetic manner, which in any case will impede the assessment.

Apart from tactfully and sensitively facilitating the patient's account of trauma, psychiatric assessment proceeds along usual lines. Interviews with family members may be invaluable for an impression of the pre-traumatic state of the patient, and may also give an insight into the course of the post-traumatic sequelae. Discussion with the GP and examination of the records may yield more valuable information about the patient's pre-traumatic state.

Box 2. Key questions in the assessment of post-traumatic disorders

When did the trauma occur?
How long has the person had symptoms?
How have they coped to date?
What resources do they have to support them?
Is there a previous history of trauma?
Is there a pre-traumatic history of psychiatric illness?
Was the trauma they suffered a 'risky' one? (e.g. criminal assaults of grotesque imagery)

Key questions in the assessment are outlined in Box 2. If the trauma happened only recently (say in the last 3–6 months), then some spontaneous progress may still be made, or augmented with support. Positive signs may be the diminishing frequency of nightmares, decreasing use of alcohol, and the return of appetite. Spontaneous progress may be retarded by degree of trauma, simultaneous losses and physical ill-health; patients may not begin the process of psychological recovery until their physical state allows. If they are making progress, then it may be that all they need is pharmacological support for the remaining symptoms, information about the natural course of stress reactions and advice from the GP. The support of community psychiatric nurses may be useful here.

GPs are obvious professionals to be involved in the management of stress reactions. If patients are referred to psychiatry while still in the acute phase of response, these possibilities may be considered:

(a) The patient's GP may lack information about PTSD, and may need information and consultation with the psychiatrist.
(b) The GP/practice counsellor/psychologist has particular concerns about the patient, because of the nature of his/her symptoms.
(c) The GP or practice team may not be able to provide the time needed for support.
(d) The nature of the trauma is particularly serious.

A case history may act as an example. Miss A was abducted on the street by strangers, and gang-raped in the back of a van for several hours before being released. She was reluctant to talk to her GP who was very concerned. Her family were distraught. She was referred to a general psychiatrist as an out-patient, for support and counselling.

It is important to enquire about any previous history of trauma. A previous psychiatric history may make the development of PTSD more likely. If the trauma is a criminal one, it is important to ascertain the state of any legal proceedings, since this will have an impact on treatment and progress.

Indications for treatment

Treatment approaches for the post-traumatic disorders need to be comprehensive, flexible and geared to what the patient can tolerate. The principal treatment modalities are:

(a) behavioural and cognitive strategies (Foa & Rothbaum, 1989);
(b) short- and long-term psychological therapies;
(c) medication (Davidson, 1992).

All three modalities may form part of different therapeutic strategies for the same patient over time, depending on the patient's needs (Southwick & Yehuda, 1993). Table 4 shows the range of treatments available, the optimal types of therapy for different disorders, and their timing.

The rationale for some behavioural and cognitive treatments is the breaking of the cycle of intrusion and avoidance described in Horowitz's model of PTSD. By exposing the patient to their feared memories, or their thoughts about the trauma, avoidance is reduced, and control over intrusion is introduced. Different types of exposure therapy include imaginal flooding, systematic desensitisation and exposure to the feared stimulus in both imagination (using tapes) and *in vivo*. Exposure therapy may be the first line of treatment, or may follow treatment for other post-traumatic disorders such as depression. Concurrent prescription of antidepressants in PTSD may be necessary to increase the patient's ability to tolerate the exposure programme. It is likely that exposure to feared memories is an important part of most post-traumatic therapies (Richards & Rose, 1991).

The other rationale for cognitive and behaviour therapies is based on PTSD as a failure of cognitive processing (Foa *et al*, 1989). Cognitive therapies have been shown to be effective for some types of trauma (Foa *et al*, 1991; Resick & Schnike, 1992). A more recent development in cognitive processing techniques using saccadic eye movement has been described by Shapiro (1989) and Page & Crino (1993). This technique remains controversial, and its relationship to other treatment modalities uncertain. Behavioural and cognitive strategies are probably indicated as first line treatments where there is good psychological health before the traumatic event, and where the event itself is discrete.

Brief and longer term psychodynamic psychotherapy, both group and individual, may be

Table 4. Indicated treatments for post-traumatic disorders	
Type of disorder	Indicated treatments
Acute stress responses	Debriefing Social supports Pharmacological supports, e.g. hypnotics Information and advice to families
Post-traumatic stress disorder (acute)	If intrusive phenomena prominent: exposure therapy may be the first line of treatment In addition/sequence: cognitive therapy; brief psychodynamic psychotherapy; antidepressants (especially where avoidance prominent)
Post-traumatic stress disorder (chronic)	Cognitive–behavioural approaches may still be effective: group or individual Long-term psychotherapy: group or individual Antidepressants/lithium Carbamazepine May be worth trying exposure therapy if trauma was never discussed before

indicated where there is prior history of trauma, psychological vulnerability, or where the trauma is the result of personal victimisation (Lindy *et al*, 1983). Group psychotherapy may be of particular use where the trauma occurs in a group context, such as occupational settings, or transport disasters. Therapeutic communities have been used principally in veteran populations (Silver, 1986). Brief group work is possible when the group focuses on a particular task, such as the Critical Incident Stress Debriefing model described by Mitchell (1983). Group work may be of particular use after sexual assaults, where by making the experience less individual, shame and guilt may be reduced (Roth *et al*, 1988).

Individual psychodynamic approaches may focus on restoring defences, and helping the patient to think about those events which appear to have no meaning (Garland, 1991). Short-term (12-week) packages of individual therapy have been described by Marmar (1991) and may be especially useful for a discrete event such as a traumatic bereavement. Such brief approaches are not indicated where there is extensive previous trauma or severe concurrent psychopathology. In such cases, where a traumatic experience resonates with prior losses or childhood trauma, long-term individual therapy may be indicated.

Medication has an important role in the treatment of post-traumatic disorders, both as symptomatic relief, but also as directly addressing pathology. A detailed account of the use of various types of medication is given in Davidson (1992). Antidepressants, especially the serotonergic agents, may be helpful, as may tricyclics because of their hypnotic effects. Medication alone is unlikely to be helpful, but may be necessary to enable patients to undertake other types of therapy later.

Once a diagnosis of PTSD has been made, treatment should be vigorous, because chronic PTSD is hard to treat. Even if the traumatic events took place some time before (>1 year), it may still be worth attempting exposure therapy, if the patient can tolerate it. Antidepressant treatment should also be instituted. However, the prognosis, after 1–2 years is not good. Although the natural history of the disorder is of very gradual improvement over time, the concurrent effects on family and work life continually retard this process. Once chronic PTSD is established, the therapeutic focus may need to be these concurrent problems (Hammarberg & Silver, 1994).

There are particular questions relevant to the selection of treatment.

What is the worst problem at the moment?

If intrusive phenomena are prominent, this may suggest exposure therapy as part of a cognitive–behavioural package. If depression and distress are worst, then regular supportive therapy sessions plus antidepressants may be most effective.

What supports does this person have?

Many forms of treatment for PTSD are quite stressful. It is therefore important to ensure that the patient will be well supported, and that the family supports are informed about the nature and process of therapy.

What solutions to stress is the patient adopting now?

If a patient is misusing alcohol or drugs as a means of managing his/her PTSD symptoms, then this problem needs to be addressed before any specific PTSD treatment can be implemented. Rarely, patients may present with acts of deliberate self-harm, such as overdoses, and these should not be dismissed as 'attention-seeking'.

Efficacy of treatment

There have been a number of studies pressing the efficacy of treatment for PTSD, although these have tended to focus mainly on psychological treatment. Two recent meta-analyses have been carried out (Sherman, 1998; Van Etten & Taylor, 1998). Studies using 'psychodynamic methods' were included in both analyses. Psychological therapies appear to be better than psychotropic medication, although both are better than controls. Sherman found significant effects for all psychological therapies, particularly for behavioural therapy, but found no support for one single rationale for therapy. A contrary view is put by Shalev *et al* (1996) who found less significant effects for psychological therapies. Methodological problems with PTSD treatment studies include the open-endedness of studies and short-term follow-up. Other difficulties include obtaining homogeneous samples and ethical concerns about the use of control subjects. Treatment for 'pure' PTSD can be successful, but this is an unusual presentation, and tends to be characteristic of research samples. In clinical settings there is often enormous variation in the symptom presentation and comorbidity, particularly with depression, and substance misuse is the norm.

In subjects with good pre-traumatic psychological health, and where there is a discrete traumatic event, cognitive–behavioural strategies can be highly effective. In more complex cases, especially where there are pervasive feelings of accompanying shame and guilt, individual or group therapy may be appropriate, combined with appropriate medication. Shame and guilt reactions are particularly likely after interpersonal traumatic violence, such as criminal assaults, domestic violence, or sexual assaults. Patients with symptoms of clinical depression are unlikely to be able to engage in exposure therapy until the depression has lifted. For those patients with long-standing post-traumatic problems, and where there is depressed or shameful affect, exposure therapy may make symptoms worse not better, particularly in the short-term, and therapy addressing the disturbed mood state is indicated as a first strategy.

There is currently a lack of information about the efficacy of treatment for victims of childhood trauma or chronic interpersonal violence, domestic violence or torture. In so far as complex past traumatic stress disorder reactions like this resemble borderline personality disorder (Roth *et al*, 1997) there may be some reason for thinking that cognitive approaches to affect and arousal regulation may be most helpful for these patients.

There has been considerable interest in the last 5–6 years in the efficacy of psychological interventions to prevent the development of PTSD which are given in the initial days or weeks after a trauma; so called 'psychological debriefing'. The briefing is offered in an initial post-traumatic stage (1–3 weeks) and is now standard procedure in some work places; legal actions have been mounted when such interventions have not been offered to workers. However, there is considerable uncertainty about the efficacy of briefing interventions. There appears to be little evidence that such interventions actually prevent the development of PTSD (Wessely *et al*, 1997; Avery & Orner, 1998; Bolwig, 1998). There is some reason to think that some vulnerable individuals may experience more symptoms as a result of debriefing interventions (Bisson *et al*, 1997). However, such data may also suggest that early interventions may be of value to some individuals who need to be appropriately identified. Given that most individuals who have experienced debriefing value it, it may be premature to abandon a debriefing before more research on different approaches is carried out (Mitchell & Everley, 1998).

Conclusions

Traumatic events are not uncommon in civilian life, especially as a result of crime. Survivors of traumata, both large and small scale, are likely to appear in general and specialist psychiatric clinics requiring treatment, and there is evidence to suggest that treatment for the post-traumatic disorders can be very effective. There is no evidence to suggest that the majority of patients who present with post-traumatic psychopathology are manufacturing those symptoms for the purposes of compensation. Although this view lingers rigidly on in the minds of some psychiatrists, 30 years of research suggest that there really are post-traumatic disorders which need and respond to treatment.

Helpful agencies

National Association of Victim Support Schemes	020 7735 9166
Compassionate Friends (help for families of murder victims)	01179 539639

Aftermath	01942 246017
(help for families of offenders)	
Cruse (help for the bereaved)	020 7431 7122
Medical Foundation for the Victims of Torture	020 7813 7777
Royal Free Clinic (for traumatised children)	020 7936 9000

References

American Psychiatric Association (1994) *Diagnostic and Statistical Manual of Mental Disorders* (4th edn) (DSM–IV). Washington, DC: American Psychiatric Press.

Avery, A. & Orner, R. (1998) First report of psychological debriefing abandoned – the end of an era? In *Traumatic Stress Points*, Volume 12, pp. 3–4. IL: ISTSS.

Bisson, J., Jenkins, P. L., Alexander, J., *et al* (1997) Randomised controlled trial of psychological debriefing for victims of acute burn trauma. *British Journal of Psychiatry*, **171**, 78–81.

Black, D., Harris-Hendriks, J. & Kaplan, A. (1993) *When Father Kills Mother*. London: Routledge.

Bolwig, T. (1998) Debriefing after psychological trauma. *Acta Psychiatrica Scandinavia*, **98**, 169–170.

Bremner, J., Southwick, S., Johnson, D., *et al* (1992) Child physical abuse and combat-related post-traumatic stress disorder. *American Journal of Psychiatry*, **150**, 235–239.

Breslau, N., Davis, G., Andreski, P., *et al* (1991) Traumatic events and PTSD in an urban population of young males. *Archives of General Psychiatry*, **48**, 216–222.

Cassiday, L., McNally, R. & Zeitlin, S. (1992) Cognitive processing of trauma cues in rape victims. *Cognitive Research and Therapy*, **16**, 283–295.

Davidson, J. (1992) Drug therapy of post-traumatic stress disorder. *British Journal of Psychiatry*, **160**, 309–314.

––– & Foa, E. (1991) Diagnostic issues in PTSD: Considerations for the DSM–IV. *Journal of Abnormal Psychology*, **100**, 346–355.

––– & ––– (1993) *PTSD: DSM–IV and Beyond*. Washington, DC: American Psychiatric Press.

Foa, E. & Rothbaum, B. (1989) Behavioural psychotherapy for PTSD. *International Review of Psychiatry*, **1**, 219–226.

–––, Steketee, G. & Rothbaum, B. (1989) Behavioural–cognitive conceptualisation of PTSD. *Behaviour Therapy*, **20**, 155–176.

Friedman, L. S., Samet, J. H., Roberts, M. S., *et al* (1992) Inquiry about victimisation experiences. *Archives of Internal Medicine*, **152**, 1186–1190.

Garland, C. (1991) External disasters and the internal world: an approach to the psychotherapeutic understanding of survivors. In *Textbook of Psychotherapy in Psychiatric Practice* (ed. J. Holmes). London: Churchill Livingstone.

Gersons, B. P. R. & Carlier, I. V. E. (1992) Post-traumatic stress disorder: the history of a recent concept. *British Journal of Psychiatry*, **161**, 742–749.

Green, B. (1993) Identifying survivors at risk. In *International Handbook of Traumatic Stress Syndromes* (eds J. Wilson & B. Raphael). Washington, DC: Plenum.

–––, Lindy, J., Grace, M., *et al* (1990) Buffalo Creek survivors in the second decade. *American Journal of Orthopsychiatry*, **60**, 43–54.

Hammarberg, M. & Silver, S. (1994) Outcome of treatment for PTSD in a primary care unit serving Vietnam veterans. *Journal of Traumatic Stress*, **7**, 195–216.

Helzer, J., Robins, L. & McEvoy, L. (1987) PTSD in the general population. *New England Journal of Medicine*, **317**, 1630–1634.

Herman, J. (1992) Complex PTSD: a syndrome in survivors of prolonged and repeated trauma. *Journal of Traumatic Stress*, **5**, 377–391.

Horowitz, M. (1973) Phase oriented treatment of stress response syndromes. *American Journal of Psychotherapy*, **27**, 506–515.

Kilpatrick, D., Saunders, B. E. & Amick McMullen, A. (1989) Victim and crime factors associated with the development of crime related PTSD. *Behaviour Therapy*, **20**, 199–214.

Lindy, J. D., Green, B., Grace, M., *et al* (1983) Psychotherapy with survivors of the Beverley Hills Supper Club. *American Journal of Psychotherapy*, **4**, 593–610.

McFarlane, A. (1988) The longitudinal course of PTSD: the range of outcomes and predictors. *Journal of Nervous and Mental Disease*, **176**, 30–39.

Marmar, C. (1991) Brief dynamic psychotherapy of PTSD. *Psychiatric Annals*, **21**, 405–414.

Mayhew, P., Maung, N. A. & Mirrlees-Black, C. (1993) *The 1992 British Crime Survey*. London: HMSO.

Mayou, R., Bryant, B. & Duthie, R. (1993) Psychiatric consequences of road traffic accidents. *British Medical Journal*, **307**, 647–651.

Mitchell, J. (1983) When disaster strikes … the critical incident stress debriefing process. *Journal of Emergency Medical Services*, **8**, 36–38.

––– & Everly, G. S. (1998) Critical incident stress management: a new era in crisis intervention. In *Traumatic Stress Point*, Volume 12, pp. 4–6. IL: ISTSS.

Norris, F. (1992) Epidemiology of trauma: frequency and impact of different potentially traumatic events on different demographic groups. *Journal of Consulting and Clinical Psychology*, **60**, 409–418.

Page, A. & Crino, R. (1993) Eye movement desensitisation: a simple treatment for PTSD? *Australia and New Zealand Journal of Psychiatry*, **27**, 288–293.

Parkes, C. M. (1992) Psychiatric problems following bereavement by murder or manslaughter. *British Journal of Psychiatry*, **162**, 49–54.

Resick, P. & Schnike, M. (1992) Cognitive processing therapy for sexual assault victims. *Journal of Consulting and Clinical Psychology*, **60**, 748–756.

Richards, D. & Rose, J. (1991) Exposure therapy for post-traumatic stress disorder. Four case studies. *British Journal of Psychiatry*, **158**, 836–840.

Roth, S., Dye, E. & Liebowitz, V. (1988) Group therapy for sexual assault victims. *Psychotherapy*, **25**, 82–93.

–––, Newman, E., Pelcovitz, D., *et al* (1997) Complex PTSD in victims exposed to sexual and physical abuse: results from the DSM–IV field trial for post-traumatic stress disorder. *Journal of Traumatic Stress*, **10**, 539–556.

Shalev, A., Bonn, E. O. & Eth, S. (1996) Treatment of post-traumatic stress disorder: A review. *Psychosomatic Medicine*, **58**, 165-182.

Shapiro, F. (1989) Efficacy of eye movement desensitisation procedure in the treatment of traumatic memories. *Journal of Traumatic Stress*, **2**, 199–223.

Sherman, J. J. (1998) Affects of psychotherapeutic treatments for PTSD: a meta-analysis of controlled trials. *Journal of Traumatic Stress*, **11**, 413–436.

Silver, S. M. (1986) An inpatient program for PTSD: context as treatment. In *Trauma and its Wake* (vol. 2) (ed. C. Figley). New York: Brunner-Mazel.

Southwick, S. & Yohuda, R. (1993) The interaction between pharmacotherapy and psychotherapy in the treatment of PTSD. *American Journal of Psychotherapy*, **47**, 404–410.

–––, –– & Giller, E. (1993) Personality disorders in treatment seeking combat veterans with PTSD. *American Journal of Psychiatry*, **150**, 1020–1023.

Smith, E., North, C., McCool, R., *et al* (1990) Acute post-disaster psychiatric disorders: identification of persons at risk. *American Journal of Psychiatry*, **147**, 202–206.

Stanko, E. & Hobdell, K. (1993) Assault on men. *British Journal of Criminology*, **33**, 400–415.

Trimble, M. (1985) Post-traumatic stress disorder: history of a concept. In *Trauma and its Wake* (vol. 1) (ed. C. Figley). New York: Brunner-Mazel.

Van Etten, M. L. & Taylor, S. (1998) Comparative efficacy of treatment for post-traumatic stress disorder: a meta-analysis. *Clinical Psychology in Psychotherapy*, **5**, 126–144.

Walker, L. (1984) *Battered Woman Syndrome*. New York: Springer.

Wessely, S., Rose, S. & Bisson, J. (1997) *A Systematic Review of Brief Psychological Interventions ('Debriefing') for the Treatment of Trauma Related Symptoms and the Prevention of Post-Traumatic Stress Disorder* (Cochrane Review). In The Cochrane Library, Oxford: Update Software.

Wilson, J. & Raphael, B. (eds) (1993) *International Handbook of Traumatic Stress Syndromes*. New York: Plenum.

World Health Organization (1992) *The ICD–10 Classification of Mental and Behavioural Disorders*. Geneva: WHO.

Index

Compiled by Caroline S. Sheard